# The Psychological Significance of the Blush

The blush is a ubiquitous yet little understood phenomenon which can be triggered by a number of self-conscious emotions such as shame, embarrassment, shyness, pride and guilt. The field of psychology has seen a recent surge in the research of such emotions, yet blushing remains a relatively neglected area. This unique volume brings together leading researchers from a variety of disciplines to review emerging research on the blush, discussing in depth issues that have arisen and stimulating new theorizing to indicate future directions for research. Topics covered include: the psychophysiology of the blush; developmental aspects; measurement issues; its evolutionary significance and the role of similar colour signals in the social life of other species; its relation to embarrassment, shame and social anxiety; and the rationale for, and clinical trials of, interventions to help people suffering from blushing phobia.

W. RAY CROZIER is Honorary Professor in the School of Social Sciences at Cardiff University.

PETER J. DE JONG is Professor of Experimental Psychopathology and Chair of Clinical Psychology at the University of Groningen, the Netherlands.

# The Psychological Significance of the Blush

*Edited by*

W. Ray Crozier and Peter J. de Jong

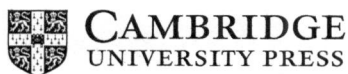
CAMBRIDGE
UNIVERSITY PRESS

CAMBRIDGE UNIVERSITY PRESS
Cambridge, New York, Melbourne, Madrid, Cape Town,
Singapore, São Paulo, Delhi, Mexico City

Cambridge University Press
The Edinburgh Building, Cambridge CB2 8RU, UK

Published in the United States of America by
Cambridge University Press, New York

www.cambridge.org
Information on this title: www.cambridge.org/9781107013933

© Cambridge University Press 2013

This publication is in copyright. Subject to statutory exception
and to the provisions of relevant collective licensing agreements,
no reproduction of any part may take place without
the written permission of Cambridge University Press.

First published 2013

Printed and bound in the United Kingdom by the MPG Books Group

*A catalogue record for this publication is available from the British Library*

*Library of Congress Cataloguing-in-Publication Data*
The psychological significance of the blush / edited by
W. Ray Crozier, Peter J. de Jong.
 p. cm.
 ISBN 978-1-107-01393-3 (Hardback)
 1. Blushing.  2. Psychophysiology.  I. Crozier, W. Ray, 1945–
II. Jong, P. J. de (Peter J.)
 QP401.P83 2012
 612.8–dc23
                                                                    2012025563

ISBN 978-1-107-01393-3 Hardback

Cambridge University Press has no responsibility for the persistence or
accuracy of URLs for external or third-party internet websites referred to
in this publication, and does not guarantee that any content on such
websites is, or will remain, accurate or appropriate.

# Contents

| | | |
|---|---|---|
| *List of figures* | | *page* vii |
| *List of tables* | | viii |
| *List of contributors* | | ix |
| *Foreword by Frans B. M. de Waal* | | xi |
| *Acknowledgments* | | xiii |
| 1 | The study of the blush: Darwin and after<br>W. RAY CROZIER AND PETER J. DE JONG | 1 |
| **Part I** | **The nature of the blush** | **13** |
| 2 | Psychophysiology of the blush<br>PETER D. DRUMMOND | 15 |
| 3 | Measurement of the blush<br>RUTH COOPER AND ALEXANDER L. GERLACH | 39 |
| **Part II** | **Theoretical perspectives on the blush** | **61** |
| 4 | Psychological theories of blushing<br>MARK R. LEARY AND KAITLIN TONER | 63 |
| 5 | Colours of the face: a comparative glance<br>JAN A. R. A. M. VAN HOOFF | 77 |
| 6 | Self-conscious emotional development<br>HEDY STEGGE | 100 |
| 7 | A biosocial perspective on embarrassment<br>RYAN S. DARBY AND CHRISTINE R. HARRIS | 120 |
| 8 | The affective neuroscience of human social anxiety<br>VLADIMIR MISKOVIC AND LOUIS A. SCHMIDT | 147 |

## Part III  The blush in social interaction — 183

9  The interactive origins and outcomes of embarrassment — 185
ROWLAND S. MILLER

10  Performing the blush: a dramaturgical perspective — 203
SUSIE SCOTT

11  Blushing and the private self — 222
W. RAY CROZIER

12  Signal value and interpersonal implications of the blush — 242
PETER J. DE JONG AND CORINE DIJK

## Part IV  Blushing problems: processes and interventions — 265

13  Red, hot and scared: mechanisms underlying fear of blushing — 267
CORINE DIJK AND PETER J. DE JONG

14  Psychological interventions for fear of blushing — 286
MICHELLE C. CAPOZZOLI, IMKE J. J. VONK,
SUSAN M. BÖGELS AND STEFAN G. HOFMANN

15  Psychophysiological aspects of rosacea — 308
PETER D. DRUMMOND AND DAPHNE SU

16  Conclusions, what we don't know and future directions for research — 327
W. RAY CROZIER AND PETER J. DE JONG

*Index* — 345

# Figures

| | | |
|---|---|---|
| 2.1 | Making a mistake evokes blushing | *page* 16 |
| 2.2 | Distribution of parasympathetic vasodilatation, sympathetic vasoconstriction and active sympathetic vasodilatation in the face | 17 |
| 2.3 | Effect of an injury to the sympathetic pathway to the face on facial flushing | 18 |
| 2.4 | Cognitive model of fear of blushing | 30 |
| 3.1 | Photoplethysmogram | 41 |
| 7.1 | Embarrassment and delay or avoidance of medical care | 135 |
| 8.1 | Midsagittal (a) and coronal (b) sections of the human brain | 150 |
| 15.1 | Hypothesized link between psychological factors and symptoms of rosacea | 318 |

# Tables

| | | |
|---|---|---|
| 8.1 | A selected summary of studies on the neural correlates of social anxiety | page 155 |
| 9.1 | The sources of embarrassment in social life | 187 |
| 9.2 | Actors' primary responses to their embarrassment | 196 |
| 11.1 | Categories in content analysis | 227 |
| 11.2 | Blushing episodes categorized as shame occasions | 228 |
| 11.3 | Distributions of numbers of categories coded within individual protocols (percentage data) | 228 |
| 14.1 | Summary of treatment studies for fear of blushing | 288 |

# Contributors

SUSAN M. BÖGELS Department of Developmental Psychopathology, University of Amsterdam, the Netherlands

MICHELLE C. CAPOZZOLI Department of Psychology, University of Nebraska-Lincoln, USA

RUTH COOPER Department of Clinical Psychology and Psychotherapy, University of Cologne, Germany

W. RAY CROZIER School of Social Sciences, Cardiff University, UK

RYAN S. DARBY Department of Psychology, University of California, San Diego, USA

PETER J. DE JONG Department of Psychology, University of Groningen, the Netherlands

FRANS B. M. DE WAAL Department of Psychology, Emory University, USA

CORINE DIJK Department of Clinical Psychology, University of Amsterdam, the Netherlands

PETER D. DRUMMOND School of Psychology, Murdoch University, Australia

ALEXANDER L. GERLACH Department of Clinical Psychology and Psychotherapy, University of Cologne, Germany

CHRISTINE R. HARRIS Department of Psychology, University of California, San Diego, USA

STEFAN G. HOFMANN Department of Psychology, Boston University, USA

MARK R. LEARY Department of Psychology and Neuroscience, Duke University, USA

ROWLAND S. MILLER Department of Psychology and Philosophy, Sam Houston State University, USA

VLADIMIR MISKOVIC McMaster Integrative Neuroscience and Discovery Graduate Program, Faculties of Science and Health Sciences, McMaster University, Canada

LOUIS A. SCHMIDT Child Emotion Laboratory, Department of Psychology, Neuroscience and Behaviour, McMaster University, Canada

SUSIE SCOTT Department of Sociology, University of Sussex, UK

HEDY STEGGE Division of Developmental Psychology, Free University of Amsterdam, the Netherlands

DAPHNE SU Clinical Psychologist, Department of Health, Western Australia

KAITLIN TONER Department of Psychology and Neuroscience, Duke University, USA

JAN A. R. A. M. VAN HOOFF Faculty of Biology, University of Utrecht, the Netherlands

IMKE J. J. VONK Department of Psychology, Boston University, USA

# Foreword

Blushing is remarkable for two reasons. First, it is the only expression for which there is no equivalent in any other animal. All of our facial expressions and many of our gestures can be found in our fellow primates. The way we frown, bare our teeth in a smile, or beg with open hand is all basic primate communication, yet the blush is not. I do not know of any instant face-reddening in monkeys or apes. Second, blushing is highly communicative yet involuntary. Even tears can be faked more easily than the blush. We are dealing with a signal, therefore, over which we lack control. We are unable to produce it on command, and unable to suppress it if we wish it to go away. In fact, the more aware we are that we are blushing the harder it is to make it disappear.

There was a time in which biologists held heated debates about whether communication is essentially cooperative (sharing of information) or manipulative (making others act to your advantage). Blushing never came up in this debate, however. It would have thoroughly upset those who advocated that all communication serves selfish ends. If this were true, would we not be far better off without blood uncontrollably rushing to our cheeks and neck, where the change in skin colour stands out like a lightning rod? Such a signal makes no sense for a born manipulator. Charles Darwin was so puzzled that he wrote letters to colonial administrators and missionaries all over the world to see if all members of our species blushed. He speculated about the effect of skin colour (with face-reddening standing out more against a lighter background), and the role of shame and moral standing. He did so long before blushing became the respected topic of study that it now is. His main conclusion was that shame was an innate, universal reaction in our species, and that blushing evolved to broadcast it to our surroundings.

Why would a species need a shame signal that other primates apparently do not need, and why did nature not grant us more control? The most likely framework to explain this trait is that we are a species that relies on cooperation and obedience to moral rules. Nothing is more telling than how we react to transgressions. We lower our face, avoid the gaze of others, slump our shoulders, bend our knees, and generally look diminished in stature. Our mouth droops and our eyebrows arch outward in a distinctly unthreatening expression. We feel ashamed, and hide our face behind our hands or 'want to sink into the ground'. This desire for invisibility is reminiscent of submissive displays in many animals. Chimpanzees crawl in the dust for their leader, lower their body so as to look up at him or turn their rump towards him to appear unthreatening. Dominant apes, in contrast, make themselves look larger and literally run or walk over a subordinate, who ducks into a fetal position. Daniel Fessler, an anthropologist who has studied shame in human cultures, compares its universal shrinking appearance with that of a subordinate facing an angry dominant. Shame reflects awareness that one has upset others, who need to be appeased. Whatever self-conscious feelings go with it, they are secondary to the much older hierarchical template.

But we add blushing to it, which is more than appeasement or subordination. It communicates to others that we are aware how our actions affect them. This fosters trust. We prefer people whose emotions we can read from their faces over those who never show the slightest hint of shame or guilt. We have another unique characteristic that fits this idea, which is the white sclera around the eyes. They make our eye movements stand out much more than those of, say, a chimpanzee, whose eyes are all dark, and recessed in the shade of a prominent eyebrow ridge. There is no way to tell where a chimp is looking from the eyes alone (even though I always feel that apes themselves are better at this than we humans), whereas humans have trouble obscuring their gaze direction or hiding a restless gaze. Also here, we have been self-handicapped in the domain of manipulation, which must mean that evolution has favoured honest communication. Probably, trustworthiness became such a premium during human evolution that we lost deceptive capacities in order to become more attractive as cooperation partners.

The present volume addresses a critically important topic, therefore, by delving more deeply into what at first sight looks like a very simple trait. It is one that has very complex ramifications if looked at from an evolutionary perspective, however. Blushing may be part of the same evolutionary package that gave us morality.

Frans B. M. de Waal

# Acknowledgments

We are grateful to the following colleagues for their help in planning and preparing this volume: Susan Bögels, Sandra Bonney, Hans Coveliers, Sandra Crozier, Robert Edelmann, Anja Eller, Agneta Fisher, Myra Hunter, Peter Marshall, Sandra Mulkens, Xueni Pan, Brian Parkinson, Gerrod Parrott, Louis Schmidt, Don Shearn, Lance Workman and Dan Zahavi.

We are grateful to all who read and commented upon draft chapters, including colleagues who preferred to remain anonymous. Thanks also to the School of Social Sciences, Cardiff University, the School of Social Work and Psychology, University of East Anglia, and the Department of Psychology, University of Groningen, for their support. Finally, we are grateful to Hetty Marx and her colleagues at Cambridge University Press for their advice and support.

# 1 The study of the blush: Darwin and after

*W. Ray Crozier and Peter J. de Jong*

**The blush as a puzzle**

The blush is ubiquitous yet scarcely understood. In the past it has attracted little scientific attention and it is only in recent years that it has begun to attract systematic investigation. We believe that the time is right for a volume that brings together the leading international researchers in this field to review and evaluate this emerging research, to discuss issues that have arisen, to stimulate new theorizing and to map future directions for research. The scientific neglect of blushing is surprising given that the facial expression of emotion has attracted so much research for many years and occupies a central place in the study of emotion. It is all the more surprising in the light of the surge of interest in recent years in the self-conscious emotions of shame, embarrassment, pride and guilt, all of which are associated with the circumstances of blushing.

Its neglect would be understandable if the blush was straightforward to understand or was of little psychological or social consequence. However, it presents many puzzles and, as we will show in this volume, has considerable psychological and cultural significance. Why does our reaction to a social predicament or to simply realizing that we are the object of others' attention take this form at this specific site on the body, particularly as it often results in drawing attention to ourselves just when we would least want it? Why should an expression of embarrassment, shame or shyness be highly visible when these emotions are associated with hiding, keeping in the background and covering oneself up? How does a blush differ from the facial reddening that is brought about by body temperature regulation mechanisms, that accompanies other emotions such as anger and indignation, that is a symptom of the skin condition rosacea or that is experienced by many women during the menopause? How does the blush of embarrassment and shyness relate to the pallor of fear? Why is a blush uniquely human? Are there comparable expressions in other species? When a sample of leading biologists was asked during the bicentenary celebrations of Darwin's birth to identify the largest gaps in his theory, Frans de Waal, one of the world's foremost authorities on primate behaviour, nominated the blush (de Waal, 2009). We have no convincing accounts of the evolutionary origins of the blush, its emergence in childhood, its significance in social life or how it has come to have significance. Textbooks on physiology, including specialist texts on the cardiovascular system, have little to say on its physiology. In the psychology of emotion the place of the blush in embarrassment, shyness, guilt and shame is contested or, more typically, tends to be passed over.

The blush represents a lacuna in our understanding of emotion. Indeed, knowing more about it would yield considerable insight into the nature of emotion and the autonomic neurophysiological processes involved, since, for example, a blush entails cognitive processes such as the appraisal of social contingencies, the involvement of the self in social encounters, and the contribution of the face and the body to social interactions, a contribution which has particular significance in that a blush is involuntary, uncontrollable and therefore cannot be feigned. The blush also draws attention to the moral dimension of emotion since it is associated with shame and guilt, compliance with personal and social moral standards, and our capacity to reflect upon our conduct and understand its implications for ourselves and others. Moreover, it would increase our understanding of the motivational and autonomic processes involved in people's responsiveness to interpersonal distress.

Research into the significance of the blush ought to extend beyond advancing knowledge in the psychology of emotion and interpersonal processes to embrace the problems that blushing causes many individuals. A blush is part of everyday life, a fleeting change in appearance that is typically accompanied by fluster and embarrassment and that can be psychologically uncomfortable for a time. For many of us this is a transient experience that we can readily cope with, even sometimes enjoy or find amusing or attractive. However, for many individuals their blushing is a source of great distress and they regard it as having a major and adverse impact on their life. Some are prepared to undergo irreversible surgery in order to prevent reddening from occurring. Fear of blushing (erythrophobia) has become recognized as a psychological problem and is now included as a symptom of the psychiatric condition of social anxiety disorder.

## Darwin on the blush

The *Oxford English Dictionary* defines the blush as a 'reddening of the face as a sign of shyness, embarrassment or shame'. It traces its origin to the Anglo-Saxon word *ablisian*, which is related to the Dutch word *blosen*. The *OED* provides examples of usage dating to the sixteenth century. In these sources the blush is regarded as a sign of shame although it is also mentioned in the context of modesty and sexual attraction. The word blush as a noun and verb, and its equivalent in other languages, has remained in common use, but it was only in the nineteenth century that the phenomenon it describes was submitted to systematic analysis. A London physician, Thomas Burgess, published *The Physiology or Mechanism of Blushing* in 1839. He made original observations on the blush, particularly on blushing in people of different 'races', and made a distinction between the 'true blush' as a sign of shame which served as a valuable social signal, and the 'false blush' as a symptom of over-sensitivity (Burgess 1839/2009). In doing so he anticipated much later work on individual differences in blushing propensity. However, scientific investigation began with the seminal chapter in Darwin's *The Expression of the Emotions in Man and Animals*, published in 1872. For many years the chapter provided the definitive account of the phenomenon in the scientific literature, and it remains common for it to be cited in articles on blushing (including the chapters within this volume).

Darwin's approach to the blush exemplifies the systematic collection of evidence that characterized all his scientific endeavours. He dispatched questionnaires to correspondents around the world requesting information on cross-cultural similarities in expressions. He reports on correspondence with Dr Crichton Browne, a doctor in a mental institution, and with colleagues overseas, aiming to establish whether people who are blind and those of low intelligence blush, whether young children do, and whether people of all skin tones do so. Darwin raised questions that we have only recently started to address through the collection of systematic empirical evidence and the development of theoretical accounts.

Darwin proffered an explanation of blushing, its relation to emotional experience, its causes and psychophysiological mechanisms. He regarded the blush as an expression of shame, modesty and shyness. He argued that it is caused by attention directed towards the self: '... originally self-attention directed to personal appearance, in relation to the opinion of others, was the exciting cause; the same effect being subsequently produced, through the force of association, by self-attention in relation to moral conduct' (Darwin, 1872/1999, p. 324). It is found only among humans not because only they have a developed moral sense but because they alone have a sufficiently sophisticated capacity for cognitive self-representation. He speculated on the mechanism by means of which self-attention to one's appearance could produce a blush, proposing that attention paid to a particular area of the body triggers vasodilatation of blood vessels in that area, resulting in increased blood flow (p. 336). Darwin played down adaptive or communicative functions of the blush, arguing, for example, that 'those who believe in design, will find it difficult to account for shyness being the most frequent and efficient of all the causes of blushing, as it makes the blusher to suffer and the beholder uncomfortable, without being the least service to either of them' (p. 335). As Dixon (2003, p. 168) remarked, commenting on the lack of emphasis on the utility of emotional expression and indeed on natural selection or sexual selection in Darwin's account, a more appropriate title for the book might have been '*The Inheritance of Useless Habits in Man and Animals*'. Dixon argued that Darwin's neglect of the utility of expressions and his emphasis on the inheritance of acquired habits rather than on adaptation reflected his opposition to the theological explanation of the blush proposed by Burgess, and his reluctance to yield any ground to this position in his defence of an evolutionary thesis. Has Darwin's theory stood the test of time? This introductory chapter considers the issues that Darwin raised and indicates how these have been addressed in subsequent chapters.

### The nature of the blush

Since the publication of Darwin's chapter much progress has been made in understanding mechanisms involved in the regulation of blood circulation. This includes factors involved in vasodilatation and vasoconstriction of the various types of arterial and venous vessels as these have received considerable attention in scientific research: for example, in the context of thermoregulation and physical exertion. We now have a much more comprehensive understanding of both the anatomy of the circulatory system and factors involved in controlling the circulation through vasodilatation and vasoconstriction. Research shows that blushing is the product of a much more complex process than that envisaged by Darwin.

The role of vasodilatation and vasoconstriction of blood vessels – for example, in thermoregulation – has received considerable attention in basic and more applied research: for example, in the physiology of physical activity (Astrand *et al.*, 2003). Vasodilatation of blood vessels has been shown to be controlled by several factors: action of the sympathetic nervous system, catecholamines circulating in the blood stream, and local factors that originate either in the blood vessels themselves – endothelial or myogenic factors – or in metabolic and other activities in tissue surrounding the vessels. The network of blood vessels in the 'blush region' has a distinctive structure that facilitates the movement of a large volume of arterial blood close to the surface of the skin as well as the capacity to create a 'reservoir' in the facial veins ('blood pooling'), which may both result in visible facial reddening. Yet we do not yet understand which specific processes are involved in blushing as opposed to other forms of circulation-induced reddening of people's skin. It is generally assumed that sympathetic nervous system activity is somehow involved: for example, seminal findings reported by Mellander, Andersson, Afzelius and Hellstrand (1982) showed that electrical stimulation of beta-adrenoceptors in a section of human facial vein removed from the cheek region produced rapid vasodilatation; furthermore, this effect was eliminated when a beta blocker drug was administered. Also, surgical techniques that prevent the sympathetic branch from connecting with the facial veins seem effective in reducing people's ability to blush (see Chapter 2). Peter Drummond has undertaken a substantial body of research into the psychophysiology of the blush, combining psychophysiological measurement techniques and experimental methods in order to identify the mechanisms involved in the blush. In Chapter 2 of this volume he provides an overview of this research, demonstrating the complexity of this phenomenon and how much remains to be learned.

Perhaps the major problem facing researchers in the past was that they had no means of recording or measuring the blush for analysis. For example, Darwin used photography to illustrate facial expressions, but it was impossible to capture a blush with the technology that was available to him at the time. Photography – and subsequently moving film, videotape and computer technology – has become profoundly influential in the development of the psychology of emotion, not only in providing empirical evidence for testing hypotheses about the universality of certain facial expressions but also in shaping the classification of basic emotions. The involuntary, transient reddening of the face escaped capture and this may be one reason why it has never occupied a prominent place in theorizing the emotions.

The lack of suitable psychophysiological techniques may also have contributed to the neglect of the blush. In the 1990s Don Shearn and his colleagues (Shearn et al., 1992; Shearn et al., 1999) were the first to tailor the available techniques in the context of blushing. Currently available instruments rely on techniques that measure changes in facial skin temperature such as thermistors and infrared cameras and techniques that measure changes in blood flow such as laser Doppler flowmetry and photoplethysmography. In Chapter 3 of this volume Ruth Cooper and Alexander Gerlach provide a systematic, critical overview of the strengths and limitations of the methods available to researchers.

They also compare these physiological measures with participants' and observers' reports on embarrassment and blushing during the experiments. As is evident in other chapters in this volume these measures have been used to address significant questions about the blush, including its communicative function, and the relation between subjective reports of blushing and physiological measures in both non-clinical and clinical samples.

## Theoretical perspectives on the blush

Even if we understood the physiological mechanisms involved in blushing we would still not have provided an explanation of the blush. This question is addressed throughout this volume and is central in chapters that comprise Part II.

Darwin's explanation in terms of the direction of attention has been highly influential in psychological theories of blushing. Mark Leary and Kaitlin Toner (Chapter 4) compare three such theories: undesired social attention, communicative and remedial, and exposure theories. They review the available evidence for each of these theories and discuss their limitations. The theory of undesired social attention clearly follows from Darwin's account and was developed in a seminal paper by Leary, Britt, Cutlip and Templeton (1992), where they argued that undesired attention can be positive, negative and neutral. This theory aims to accommodate findings that a blush can be triggered by public praise or by being wished a happy birthday, and simply by realizing that you are the object of attention: for example, appearing on a public platform without necessarily having to perform. This approach links blushing to the self-conscious emotions, where research emphasizes the ability to take another perspective on the self and see oneself through the eyes of others. The blush entails inter-subjectivity, a capacity that seems absent in other species.

While Darwin seems correct in his often cited observation that the blush is uniquely human, bodily signs of dominance and submission relations are nevertheless common among nonhuman primates as are colour changes that may (just like the blush) also serve as a signalling device. The evolution and functions of animal displays have been extensively studied in ethology. In Chapter 5 Jan van Hooff surveys the role of displays across species, relating the evolution of colour vision to the functions that colour displays serve: for example, the associations among colour, social success, circulating levels of hormones and sex, where redness increases as social status (particularly among males) rises and levels of testosterone increase. He discusses the hypothesis that trichromatic vision may have evolved in primates for discriminating changes in skin colour that are associated with sexual and emotional states: for example, the red face of rage.

Darwin argued that infants and young children do not blush because they lack self-consciousness in the early years. Research within the 'theory of mind' paradigm suggests that this capacity can be detected in children from the third year. However, there has been scarcely any research into blushing in childhood, and there is insufficient evidence to conclude whether cognitive self-representations are necessary or sufficient for blushing or even at what age the blush emerges in childhood. The paucity of this research is in marked contrast to a large body of theory and empirical research into childhood self-awareness, self-consciousness, shyness and social anxiety. Hedy Stegge (Chapter 6) discusses this research in the domain of developmental psychology in an attempt to provide a foundation for the future study of childhood blushing.

The remaining two chapters in this section build further on the link proposed by Darwin between blushing and particular emotional experiences. More specifically, these chapters take the psychophysiology of embarrassment and social anxiety as their starting point and consider how this might inform us about the mechanism involved in the blush. One strand of psychological theorizing initiated by Buss (1980) and Schlenker and Leary (1982) construes embarrassment as a form of social anxiety with the implication that the blush is a bodily expression of anxiety. Thus, embarrassment is a response to threat, of loss of reputation or of social rejection, and a blush is triggered by stimulus cues for threat. This immediately raises questions about the nature of the psychological and psychophysiological mechanisms involved in reactions to social threats: how does embarrassment differ from fear?

Ryan Darby and Christine Harris (Chapter 7) consider the, possibly unique, 'signature pattern of cardiovascular reactivity' in embarrassment where, for example, instead of the correlation between increased heart rate and blood pressure typically found in fear, there is a decoupling of heart rate and blood pressure. They argue that embarrassment is not linked to one specific area of the brain, but is associated with regions of the brain that seem to be important to theory of mind, self-awareness and the regulation of social behaviour, specifically the medial prefrontal cortex, temporo-parietal region, the basal temporal cortex and the orbitofrontal cortex. Vladimir Miskovic and Louis Schmidt (Chapter 8) review research into social anxiety, including social anxiety disorder – the fear and avoidance of interpersonal interactions, especially those with potential for scrutiny and evaluation. They review research into the neural substrates that may underlie social anxiety, drawing upon functional neuroimaging and experimental studies. Their account emphasizes the key roles played by the various divisions of the amygdala and the prefrontal cortex in identifying and responding to sources of threat. Both chapters indicate the role of the sympathetic nervous system and raise the question whether separate mechanisms are involved in embarrassment and fear, with different pathways between a threat stimulus and an emotional response. Under what circumstances would, say, the prospect of speaking up in front of others trigger a blush as opposed to the pattern of anxious reactions associated with stage fright?

## The blush in social interaction

Darwin's chapter makes no explicit reference to embarrassment, even though the usage of the word was current at that time. In apparent contrast with Darwin's view, it is now widely assumed that the blush is a sign of embarrassment – according to Buss (1980), even the hallmark of embarrassment – and a component of its characteristic display. Rowland Miller (Chapter 9) focuses upon the role of embarrassment in social interactions, presenting a catalogue of the kinds of circumstances that give rise to embarrassment and discussing its consequences for social encounters. He compares a social evaluation model of the causes of embarrassment with a dramaturgic self-presentation model and sets out arguments and supporting evidence for preferring the former model. He argues that the consequences of embarrassment are seldom as bad as people anticipate, in that there are social pressures to overcome the awkwardness that can ensue and help the individual out of his or her predicament. The negative view that people have of embarrassment is shared in many psychological accounts, which tend to regard it as an aversive state. Blushing also tends to be regarded in a negative light. In this chapter Miller argues that embarrassment and blushing do in fact serve valuable social functions and can enhance the pleasantness of interpersonal encounters.

Clearly, Miller's chapter questions Darwin's view that the blush 'makes the blusher only to suffer and the beholder uncomfortable, without being the least service to either of them'. The contribution of Susie Scott (Chapter 10) continues on this theme and provides more detailed insight into the potential impact of the blush on the blusher's beliefs and behaviours. She discusses the blush from a dramaturgic perspective within the theoretical tradition of symbolic interactionism, which she describes as the analysis of 'how social actors collaboratively work to negotiate shared "definitions of the situation" by interpreting the meaning of each other's symbolic gestures'. She draws upon protocols from a set of interviews to analyse the circumstances that evoke a blush and the blusher's understanding of the consequences of the blush in terms of what it reveals. She distinguishes between the incompetent self that the shy person fears he or she will reveal – 'the discredit*able* stigma, one that could potentially be hidden but which threatens to reveal itself at any moment – and the blush as discredit*ing* stigma, which is already socially visible and cannot be concealed'.

Although Darwin emphasized the importance of undesirable social attention, Ray Crozier (Chapter 11) argues that not all episodes of blushing are responses to undesired attention. On the basis of analysis of circumstances where respondents to a questionnaire recall occasions when they blushed and novelists describe scenes where a character blushes, his contribution sets out 'exposure theory'. This theory aims to explain why blushing may sometimes occur in the complete absence of direct social attention, and where the blush in itself may even be the trigger for getting undesired social attention. It is explored whether perhaps the blush may be triggered by the blusher's sudden awareness of how they might be seen in a particular situation, especially in situations where something may be revealed that the blusher prefers to keep hidden. Consistent with Darwin's view, this account implies that adopting an other-perspective on the self is essential for a blush to occur.

In spite of Darwin's sceptical attitude regarding the functional value of the blush, the question of the blush as communication has attracted a substantial body of research, which is reviewed and evaluated by Peter de Jong and Corine Dijk in Chapter 12. De Jong and his co-researchers have undertaken a series of investigations into the interpretations that people make when they see someone blush. In short, their research has established that actors who have committed some misdemeanour are perceived less negatively and their actions are judged to be less serious if they are portrayed as blushing than if they are portrayed as shamefaced or as showing no reaction. Yet a blush does not always have a positive effect; what a blush conveys depends on its context. De Jong and Dijk provide a thorough analysis of the factors that influence the communicative significance of a blush. Whether or not the blush evolved to function as a signal, this chapter argues that at the very least Darwin was premature in deciding that it does not serve as one.

### Blushing problems: processes and interventions

Whether or not blushing is an anxious response it is evident that many people are anxious about their blushing, and epidemiological research shows that fear of blushing is comorbid with social anxiety disorder. Dijk and de Jong (Chapter 13) discuss the psychological processes involved in sustaining fear of blushing. Many individuals regard their blushing as the source of their anxieties, not just as a symptom of them, and the question arises whether they do blush more frequently or intensely than others do or whether their anxieties owe more to their beliefs about their blushing, including their belief that a blush creates a poor impression on others, who will think badly of them because of their reddening. Dijk and de Jong address this issue in Chapter 13, where they assess evidence on the roles that beliefs about blushing and about its social costs, as well as tendencies towards self-focused attention, play in influencing fear of blushing; they outline a cognitive model that shows how these elements come together to produce fear of blushing.

In light of the profound consequences of blushing phobia, it seems important to design interventions to help people to overcome their fear of blushing. Michelle Capozzoli, Imke Vonk, Susan Bögels and Stefan Hofmann (Chapter 14) provide a review of studies that evaluate the effectiveness of the currently available psychological interventions. There have been few randomized controlled clinical trials of psychological interventions, but the authors show that current cognitive behavioural therapeutic approaches have proved moderately successful. On the basis of this review the authors sketch options for how to improve further the available interventions to overcome fear of blushing.

In the final chapter of Part IV, Peter Drummond and Daphne Su (Chapter 15) discuss the links between blushing and rosacea. Rosacea is a disorder of the facial skin characterized by extremely sensitive skin, burning and stinging sensations, and persistent flushing of the cheeks, nose, chin or forehead accompanied by acne-like facial pustules. The disorder is widespread: the National Rosacea Society estimates that it affects some 16 million Americans (National Rosacea Society, 2011). For many sufferers it reduces the quality of their life, lowering their self-esteem and self-confidence and leading to avoidance of social situations. Drummond and Su assess the prevalence of anxiety and depression in patients with the condition. They consider the relation between blushing and rosacea and whether the former plays a causative role in the latter. Finally, they review the role of psychological interventions in helping sufferers cope with their anxiety, and discuss how this may also provide fresh clues for the treatment of blushing phobia as described in Chapter 14.

## Conclusion

The volume aims to review theory and empirical research into blushing from a number of perspectives, to address the issues raised in this introductory chapter, and to suggest future directions in research. In the closing chapter (16) we highlight some of the important progress that has been made but also identify significant gaps that still call for an answer through further investigation. Blushing has been a neglected area of research yet we hope that we will manage to convey that it is a rich topic and that its study has the potential to illuminate many areas of life.

REFERENCES

Astrand, P.-O., Rodahl, K., Dahl, H. A., & Stromme, S. B. (2003). *Textbook of work physiology*, 4th edn. Champaign, IL: Human Kinetics Publishers.

Burgess, T. H. (1839/2009). *The physiology or mechanism of blushing.* Charleston, SC: BiblioLife, 2009.

Buss, A. H. (1980). *Self-consciousness and social anxiety.* San Francisco: Freeman.

Darwin, C. (1872/1999). *The expression of the emotions in man and animals.* Corrected 3rd edn with an introduction, afterword, and commentaries by Paul Ekman. London: HarperCollins.

De Waal, F. (2009). Evolution: the next 200 years. *New Scientist*, **2693**, 28 January.

Dixon, T. (2003). *From passions to emotions: the creation of a secular psychological category.* Cambridge University Press.

Leary, M. R., Britt, T. W., Cutlip, W. D., & Templeton, J. L. (1992). Social blushing. *Psychological Bulletin*, **107**, 446–60.

Mellander, S., Andersson, P. O., Afzelius, L. E., & Hellstrand, P. (1982). Neural beta adrenergic dilatation of the facial vein in man: possible mechanism in emotional blushing. *Acta Physiologica Scandinavica*, **114**, 393–9.

National Rosacea Society (2011). *What is rosacea?* Available at www.rosacea.org/index.php. Accessed 15 November 2011.

Schlenker, B. R., & Leary, M. R. (1982). Social anxiety and self-presentation: a conceptualization and model. *Psychological Bulletin*, **92**, 641–9.

Shearn, D., Bergman, E., Hill, K., Abel, A., & Hinds, L. (1992). Blushing as a function of audience size. *Psychophysiology*, **29**, 431–6.

Shearn, D., Spellman, L., Meirick, J., & Stryker, K. (1999). Empathic blushing in friends and strangers. *Motivation and Emotion*, **23**, 307–16.

*Part I*

# The nature of the blush

# 2  Psychophysiology of the blush

*Peter D. Drummond*

In Darwin's view, blushing was 'the most peculiar and most human of all expressions' (1872/1965, p. 309). However, over the past twenty-five years an accumulating body of programmatic research has begun to shed light on the psychophysiological mechanisms and emotional correlates of blushing. This research is reviewed below.

## Physiological mechanisms that may contribute to blushing

Blushing refers to reddening of the face in emotionally charged situations, typically in association with feelings of embarrassment, guilt or shame. The reddening is due to an accumulation of red blood cells in the superficial venous plexus in the facial skin. This appears to involve an active dilatation of the arterial supply because vascular pulsations increase markedly during blushing (Figure 2.1). In addition, as facial veins are supplied with β-adrenoceptors (Mellander *et al.*, 1982), a β-adrenergic mechanism that contributes to the dilatation of veins may increase their capacity to hold blood.

The neural regulation of blood flow is more complex for the face than for most other regions of the body, because facial blood vessels supply the sensitive membranes of the eyes, nose and mouth in addition to the skin. Thus, broadly distributed sympathetic vasoconstrictor and dilator reflexes, locally distributed parasympathetic reflexes and vasodilator reflexes mediated by sensory nerves all influence facial blood flow. In addition, substances that arrive in the bloodstream (e.g., hormones, vasoactive peptides, dietary products and drugs), or that are produced locally by the vascular endothelium, add an extra level of control over facial blood flow. Potentially, each of these influences could contribute to blushing, although some of these influences clearly are more important than others.

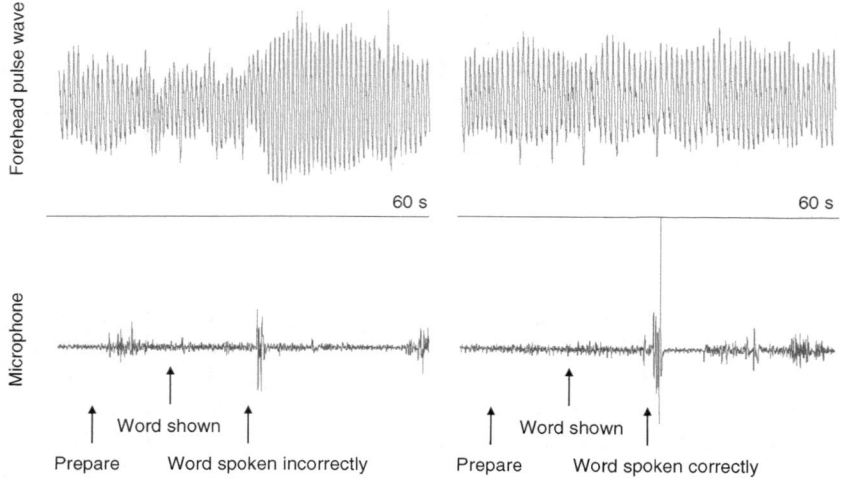

Figure 2.1 Making a mistake evokes blushing (Drummond, 2012). Pulse amplitude was recorded from the forehead via a Grass Instruments photoplethysmograph that was attached a few centimetres above the eyebrows with an adhesive washer, and protected from ambient light with a black headband. Pulse amplitude increased when the participant was corrected for mispronouncing an unfamiliar word (e.g., 'demesne') but did not change after a familiar word (e.g., 'ache') was pronounced correctly.

## Sympathetic vasoconstrictor influences on facial blood flow

Heat is distributed around the body in the bloodstream. In cold environments, repetitive discharge of sympathetic vasoconstrictor nerves decreases the calibre of cutaneous blood vessels, thereby limiting blood flow through the skin and heat loss from exposed parts of the body. Sympathetic vasoconstrictor discharge also prevents blood from pooling in the lower parts of the body when the body is upright; it also prepares the body for action by shunting blood away from the skin to skeletal muscles in threatening situations and before and during the early stages of exercise. In the face, vasoconstrictor tone is greatest in the ears, nose and lips, as these parts are most likely to be exposed to cold (Blair et al., 1961; Fox et al., 1962) (Figure 2.2). Release of this vasoconstrictor influence results in minor increases in blood flow in most parts of the face in warm environments, during the early stages of exercise and in response to limb pain (Drummond & Finch, 1989; Drummond, 1997a; Drummond & Granston, 2003; Drummond, 2006). However, release of sympathetic vasoconstrictor tone probably plays only a minor role in

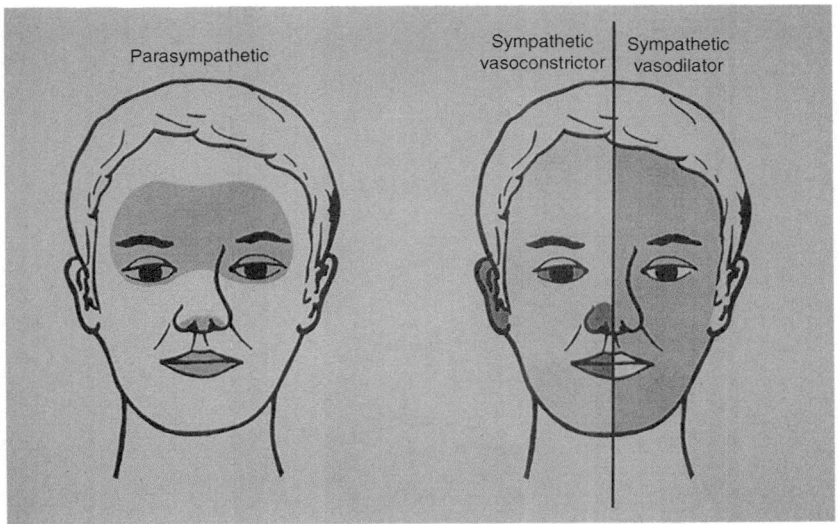

Figure 2.2 Distribution of parasympathetic vasodilatation, sympathetic vasoconstriction and active sympathetic vasodilatation in the face. Parasympathetic vasodilatation spills over from the facial glands to blood vessels in the lips, nostrils and forehead. Vasoconstrictor innervation is greatest in the lips, ears, eyes and nose, whereas active sympathetic vasodilatation predominates in other parts of the face. Reproduced from Drummond (1999b) with permission from Oxford University Press.

blushing because resting tone is relatively weak in most parts of the face (Blair *et al.*, 1961; Fox *et al.*, 1962).

*Active sympathetic vasodilatation*

Active sympathetic vasodilatation predominates when body temperature rises (Figure 2.2) (Drummond & Finch, 1989). This produces dramatic results in patients with an injury to the sympathetic supply on one side of the face, as these vessels can no longer dilate to assist the release of heat from the body (Figure 2.3). Microelectrode studies have demonstrated that bursts of sympathetic activity in the supraorbital nerve precede vasodilator responses and sweating in the forehead during psychological stress as well as body heating (Nordin, 1990), indicating that psychological stimuli can trigger active sympathetic vasodilatation. Thus, this mechanism is likely to be important for blushing.

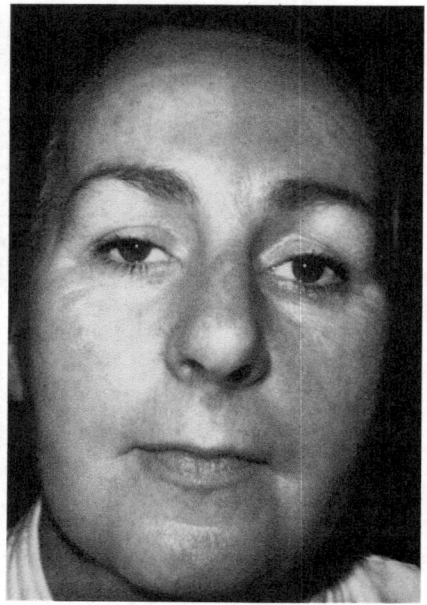

Figure 2.3 Effect of an injury to the sympathetic pathway to the face on facial flushing. Despite release of sympathetic vasoconstrictor tone, the right side of the face remained relatively pale during body heating compared with the uninjured left side. Reproduced from Drummond and Lance (1987) with permission from Oxford University Press.

### Parasympathetic influences on facial blood flow

Parasympathetic vasodilator fibres supply the secretory glands of the nose, eyes and mouth to enable the rapid production of secretory products when their sensitive membranes are irritated. These secretions help to dilute and wash away potentially harmful substances. The parasympathetic vasodilator supply overflows to the cutaneous circulation of the lips and forehead (Drummond, 1992, 1995; Izumi, 1999) (Figure 2.2), so that blood flow increases in these regions when the secretory glands are active. For example, eating food spiced with chili peppers produces facial flushing in association with salivation and lacrimation (Drummond 1995). Similarly, a drop of soapy water in the eye not only stimulates tear secretion to remove the source of irritation but also evokes parasympathetic vasodilatation in nearby parts of the forehead (Drummond, 1992). However, parasympathetic vasodilatation is unlikely to contribute much to blushing due to the limited distribution of parasympathetic vasodilator nerve fibres in the face.

## Local autoregulatory mechanisms

The major sensory nerve of the face, the trigeminal nerve, supplies all of the tissues of the face including deep and superficial blood vessels. Injury or painful stimulation of the facial skin initiates local vasodilatation via an axon-reflex mechanism that discharges neuropeptides such as substance P and calcitonin-gene-related peptide from the cutaneous terminals of sensory nerves into the skin. Among other functions, neuropeptides increase the calibre and permeability of blood vessels, thereby allowing large proteins and white blood cells to move from the bloodstream to the source of injury to combat infection and to begin repair. Axon reflexes may also protect the skin by dispersing heat and other potentially harmful substances (Magerl & Treede, 1996). The vascular endothelium produces vasoactive substances in response to changes in the local environment (e.g., in blood flow or oxygenation, neurotransmitters, hormones or inflammatory products). These endothelial substances not only regulate local blood flow but also contribute to inflammatory responses by attracting and activating white blood cells (Lindsey et al., 2000). Discharge of inflammatory mediators from cutaneous mast cells and keratinocytes may amplify the inflammatory response at sites of injury (Drummond, 2004). Pro- and anti-inflammatory substances then act on sensory nerves to fine-tune the inflammatory response by adjusting the gain of axon reflexes. Because of their limited distribution, these local autoregulatory mechanisms are unlikely to be the primary mediators of blushing. However, they might delay the resolution of blushing if they are activated by surges of blood flow or by neurotransmitters or hormones released during the acute stage of blushing.

## Pyschophysiology of blushing

Emotions provoke a spectrum of colour change, ranging from the pallid face of fear through to the blush of embarrassment and the flush of rage. Indeed, primate colour vision may have evolved to detect these colour changes because they provide useful information about the mood and possible intentions of other members of the same species (Changizi et al., 2006). Blushing is most visible in the cheeks but also extends to the forehead (Drummond & Lance, 1987; Voncken & Bögels, 2009) and sometimes to the neck and upper chest (Leary et al., 1992). Blushing forms part of a broad increase in sympathetic activity characterized by increases in heart rate, sweating in the hands and vasoconstriction in the fingers (Gerlach et al., 2001; Shearn et al., 1990; Vassend & Knardahl,

2005; Voncken & Bögels, 2009). Increases in forehead blood flow during embarrassment coincide with increases in forehead sweating and cheek blood flow (Drummond, 1989), suggesting that vasodilatation in the cheeks and forehead is associated with heightened sympathetic activity.

Cutaneous vasodilatation may be most prominent in the face because of the high density and close proximity of blood vessels to the skin surface (Wilkin, 1988). During emotional reactions such as rage, the hormonal and neural vasodilator responses that mediate flushing appear to form part of the classic 'fight or flight' response, as blood is directed towards the face during 'confrontational defence' responses in animals (Carrive & Bandler, 1991). This vasodilator response is coupled with activity in the jaw and facial muscles involved in snarling and biting. Conversely, blood is directed away from the facial skin to the muscles of the hind limbs during fear (Carrive & Bandler, 1991), possibly accounting for facial pallor.

The acute stage of blushing appears to be regulated primarily by sympathetic vasodilator nerves that directly supply the blood vessels of the face, as injury to these nerves disrupts blushing (Drummond & Lance, 1987). An additional minor component of blushing may involve hormonal release of catecholamines into the bloodstream, because β-adrenoceptor blockade partly inhibits dilatation of facial blood vessels during psychological stress and embarrassment (Drummond, 1997a).

Whether the parasympathetic nervous system also contributes to blushing has never been directly evaluated. Gerlach, Wilhelm and Roth (2003) reported that social anxiety and embarrassment were associated with physiological signs of sympathetic arousal (increased heart rate and skin conductance) whereas an index of cardiac parasympathetic control (respiratory sinus arrhythmia) showed no evidence of heightened activity. In contrast, Laederach-Hofmann and colleagues (2002) reported that heart rate and mid- and high-frequency heart rate spectra (indices of cardiac parasympathetic control) were greater in patients with a fear of blushing than in controls during mental stress. Nonetheless, as noted above, it seems unlikely that parasympathetic vasodilatation contributes directly to blushing because of the limited distribution of parasympathetic vasodilator nerve fibres in the face.

## Surgical treatment of blushing

As blushing is mediated primarily by cervical sympathetic outflow, some surgeons now advocate the use of endoscopic thoracic sympathectomy (ETS) to eliminate blushing, thereby helping to alleviate acute social anxiety (e.g., Pohjavaara *et al.*, 2003). Preganglionic sympathetic nerve and core body temperature of up to 1.2°C during exercise (Nielsen, 1988) due, in part, to diversion of cool venous blood from the face and nasal cavity to intracranial venous channels (Nagasaka et al., 1998). More generally, heat loss from the face and nasal cavity may contribute to selective brain cooling in hyperthermic conditions (Irmak et al., 2004).

Cooling of venous blood during blushing may also help to reduce brain temperature. Brain warming is unpleasant whereas selective brain cooling is associated with pleasurable sensations (Zajonc et al., 1989). Thus, blushing may help to re-establish emotional equilibrium by replacing unpleasant emotions with more pleasant sensations.

## Psychophysiological studies of blushing

Changes in facial blood flow that reflect blushing are generally monitored with laser Doppler fluxmetry or photoplethysmography. One limitation of these methods is that the signal cannot be calibrated in units of blood flow, because of substantial variability in the microvasculature and skin characteristics between recording sites. Preferably, then, values should be expressed relative to a baseline measurement taken at the same site. Changes in skin temperature provide an additional index of changes in blood flow. This index is non-linearly related to blood flow as skin temperature cannot increase beyond core temperature (around 37°C in resting humans) despite further increases in flow. In addition, changes in skin temperature lag far behind abrupt changes in blood flow.

One of the first psychophysiological studies of blushing was carried out by Shearn, Bergman, Hill, Abel and Hinds (1990). They measured changes in cheek and ear blood flow with photoplethysmographs (specifically the DC component expressed in arbitrary units, reflecting changes in facial coloration), cheek temperature and finger skin conductance responses while undergraduate students watched a videotape of themselves singing and another videotape of a frightening movie segment. Increases in facial coloration were greater during embarrassment than during fear, as were increases in cheek temperature and skin conductance. In addition, increases in cheek temperature were greater during embarrassment in women than in men, and women were judged to be blushing more often than men at the peak of the plethysmographic response when the videotape was viewed by raters afterwards. We recently observed similar sex differences in blushing when participants sang a children's song (Drummond & Su, 2012). As increases in cheek temperature lagged well behind the peak plethysmographic response, Shearn and colleagues (1990) speculated that blushing might be noticed by others before it was detected by the blusher. In a follow-up study, Shearn, Bergman, Hill, Abel and Hinds (1992) reported that responses in each physiological modality were greater with an audience of four than with an audience of one during embarrassment than during fear.

Whether blushing might reflect empathy was investigated by Shearn, Spellman, Straley, Meirick and Stryker (1999). In an initial experiment, the performer, a friend of the performer and a stranger watched a videotape of the performer singing. Increases in facial coloration of the cheek (expressed in arbitrary units) were greater in the friend than in the stranger, consistent with empathic blushing. In a second experiment, responses were recorded while participants watched a videotape of themselves singing; while participants who had previously sung watched a videotape of someone else singing (the empathic condition); while participants who had previously sorted cards watched a videotape of someone else singing; and while participants who had previously sung watched a videotape about making a violin. Responses were greater in the empathic than in the card-sorting condition. Thus, prior singing may have evoked empathic blushing when participants watched someone else singing. Alternatively, the participant may have been reminded of his or her previous embarrassment when they had sung.

Much evidence has been gathered to support the view that blushing transmits nonverbal signals of social discomfort that evoke affiliative responses (e.g., de Jong, 1999; Dijk, de Jong *et al.*, 2009). However, this probably applies more to people with fair than with dark skin because blushing is difficult to detect in dark-skinned people. Indeed, we found evidence that the subjective experience of blushing differs between people with dark and fair skin during embarrassing social encounters, implying that blushing may have different social connotations for fair- and dark-skinned races (Drummond & Lim, 2000). In contrast, increases in forehead pulse amplitude (expressed as the percentage change from baseline) and cheek temperature were similar in both groups.

Although traditionally blushing is associated with emotions such as embarrassment and shame, similar psychophysiological responses are associated with emotions such as joy and anger. For example, in a study in our laboratory, cheek pulse amplitude (expressed as the percentage change from baseline) increased when participants received an unexpected reward, and forehead pulsations increased in line with ratings of pleasure (Drummond, 1994b). In a subsequent study, anger ratings and forehead pulsations (expressed as the percentage change from baseline) also increased over the course of a difficult task (assembling a three-dimensional jigsaw puzzle using just one hand), and increased further when participants were criticized (Drummond, 1999a). In contrast, finger pulsations decreased. Whether the response to provocation was elicited by anger or embarrassment is uncertain, because forehead pulsations also increased following more supportive comments. In a related study, the effect of anger expression on facial blood flow was investigated by comparing responses when angry incidents were described loudly and rapidly versus quietly and slowly (Drummond & Quah, 2001). Forehead pulsations (expressed as the percentage change from baseline) increased during anger expression, regardless of the anger expression style, whereas finger pulsations decreased. Curiously, forehead pulsations also decreased when participants read aloud, despite slight increases in embarrassment. Together, these findings suggest that a range of emotions influence facial blood flow, some evoking vasoconstriction and others vasodilatation. Whether vasodilatation predominates may depend not only on the type of emotion but also on its intensity.

In Darwin's view, the primary stimulus for blushing was concern about personal appearance while being scrutinized closely by others (Darwin, 1872/1965). To test this idea, we viewed the participant's facial profile from a distance of 40 cm while the participant sang a children's song (Drummond & Mirco, 2004). Surprisingly, increases in cheek temperature were greater on the observed than on the unobserved side when participants sang. To confirm that scrutiny evoked this asymmetrical response, changes in forehead blood flow were monitored using laser Doppler fluxmetry, again while participants sang a children's song. This time, the experimenter observed the participant's profile through a glass window. Once more, increases in blood flow (expressed as the percentage change from baseline) were greater on the observed than on the unobserved side. This asymmetrical blushing is reminiscent of the local effect of hypnotic suggestions on skin blood flow (Zachariae et al., 1994) and of biofeedback-assisted temperature asymmetry in the hands (Roberts et al., 1975). Thus, there may be some support for Darwin's assertion that 'attention closely directed to any part of the body tends to interfere with the ordinary and tonic contraction of the small arteries of that part' (1872/1965, p. 337).

Somewhat counterintuitively, blushing does not seem to be related in any direct way to personality traits such as neuroticism or extroversion. This issue was explored by Vassend and Knardahl (2005) in a study of fifty-eight women while they read aloud, delivered a speech about themselves and tracked the movement of a target on a computer screen. Facial blood flow (expressed in arbitrary units and as the percentage change from baseline) was recorded from the masseter region via a laser Doppler flow probe. Significant increases in flow while reading and during the speech were unrelated to measures of neuroticism or extroversion or to ratings of negative or positive affect. Similarly, in a study in our laboratory, increases in forehead and cheek pulse amplitude during mental arithmetic were unrelated to neuroticism or extroversion scores (Drummond, 1994b).

## Relationship between blushing and subjective estimates of blushing propensity

Leary and Meadows (1991) introduced the concept of blushing propensity as 'a measure of individual differences in the tendency to blush' (p. 256). They developed the Blushing Propensity Scale which requires respondents to rate how often they feel themselves blushing in a range of situations (e.g., when called on by a teacher in class; when talking to someone about a personal topic; or when embarrassed). High scores on this scale are associated with self-focused attention and social anxiety (Bögels et al., 1996; Edelmann & Skov, 1993; Leary & Meadows, 1991; Neto, 1996). Surprisingly, however, blushing propensity scores appear to be, at best, only loosely related to the intensity of blushing during embarrassment. For example, Mulkens and colleagues (1997) compared physiological responses in people with high or low blushing propensity scores while participants watched a videotape of themselves singing, a frightening movie scene and a neutral test pattern. Increases in cheek temperature and coloration (expressed in arbitrary units) were similar in both groups when they watched themselves singing, despite greater increases in ratings of blushing and anxiety about blushing in the group with high blushing propensity scores. Within the group with low blushing propensity scores, judgments about blushing intensity corresponded closely with raters' judgments. However, these two measures were unrelated in participants with high blushing propensity scores. Together, these findings suggest that people with high blushing propensity scores overestimate the intensity of blushing in embarrassing situations. In a follow-up study, similar results were obtained in participants selected to be high or low in fear of blushing (Mulkens et al., 1999).

In a study carried out in our laboratory, changes in forehead blood flow were assessed using laser Doppler flowmetry in twenty-one participants with high blushing propensity scores and another twenty-one with low blushing propensity scores during mental arithmetic and when they sang a children's song (Drummond, 1997a). By and large, ratings of embarrassment, self-consciousness and negative affect were greater in the high than in the low blushing propensity group during these tasks. However, increases in blood flow were similar in both groups during singing, averaging around 35 per cent greater than baseline. To investigate the adrenergic component of blushing, the α-adrenergic blocker phentolamine and the β-adrenergic blocker propranolol were administered by iontophoresis into small patches of skin in the forehead. Phentolamine had no effect on forehead blood flow during either task. Importantly, however, β-adrenergic blockade inhibited increases in blood flow in people with low blushing propensity scores during mental arithmetic and partly blocked increases in both groups during singing. Thus, a β-adrenergic mechanism appears to contribute to blushing, perhaps more so in people with low than with high blushing propensity scores.

Effects of feedback about blushing on subjective and physiological responses during embarrassing laboratory tasks have been explored in several studies. In the first such study, effects of true and false feedback were compared in groups with high or low blushing propensity scores during singing and reading (Drummond, 2001). Like in previous studies, people with high blushing propensity scores reported more embarrassment and blushing during the experiment than people with low scores. However, feedback had some influence both on subjective ratings and on physiological signs of blushing.

In the first part of the study, singing was repeated three times – once without feedback, once with true feedback, and once with 'false-negative' feedback that indicated no change in blushing irrespective of true changes. Forehead pulse amplitude (expressed as the percentage change from baseline) increased more in people with high than with low blushing propensity scores during the first round of singing, due to differences between groups when participants received 'false-negative' feedback. Expecting to blush apparently helped to provoke blushing, because forehead pulsations increased only in the group with high blushing propensity scores. If this also applies during social encounters, expecting to blush may become a self-fulfilling prophesy that heightens expectations about blushing during subsequent encounters. The 'false-feedback' effect on facial blood flow disappeared during the second and third rounds of singing, possibly because the task quickly lost its novelty. Nevertheless, ratings of blushing were greater during all three rounds in people with high than with low blushing propensity scores.

In the second part of the study, participants read a script aloud either with no feedback or while receiving 'false-positive' feedback that indicated that blushing was increasing. Vascular responses were similar in both groups during both trials when participants read aloud. Curiously, however, forehead pulsations *decreased* more during 'false-positive' feedback than in the no-feedback condition when participants read aloud, even though participants reported mild embarrassment. As forehead and finger pulsations decreased in parallel, these responses presumably were mediated by increased sympathetic vasoconstrictor tone. Vasodilator influences might overshadow the vasoconstrictor component in facial blood vessels during more intense emotions.

In a follow-up study, participants sang a children's song, read aloud and listened to an audiotape of themselves singing and reading (Drummond et al., 2003). After each task, half of the participants were told that they had blushed during the preceding task (the blushing condition) whereas the others were told that they hadn't blushed (the non-blushing condition). When expressed as the percentage change from baseline, forehead pulse amplitude increased progressively across the course of the experiment in the blushing condition in participants with high blushing propensity scores. In contrast, forehead pulsations returned to baseline after each task in the non-blushing condition. Before any feedback had been given, people with high blushing propensity scores were more embarrassed and gave higher ratings of blushing after they sang than people with low blushing propensity scores. However, feedback about blushing influenced embarrassment and blushing ratings – boosting ratings in the blushing condition in people with low blushing propensity, and suppressing ratings in the non-blushing condition in people with high blushing propensity scores. Effects of blushing propensity and feedback were weaker for the other tasks, possibly because they were inherently less embarrassing.

## Relationship between blushing and social anxiety

Social anxiety disorder (social phobia) is characterized by a marked and persistent fear of interpersonal evaluation in situations that may lead to embarrassment or humiliation (American Psychiatric Association, 1994). Many people who suffer from social anxiety disorder are concerned about autonomic and somatic cues of anxiety that might reflect social ineptitude, such as blushing, sweating and trembling (Amies et al., 1983; Cuthbert, 2002; Rapee & Heimberg, 1997). In particular, some people with social anxiety disorder are especially frightened of blushing (Voncken & Bögels, 2009).

Whether blushing is greater than normal in people with social anxiety disorder was investigated by Gerlach and colleagues (2001). In this study, participants watched a videotape of themselves singing, held a conversation with a stranger of the opposite sex, and prepared and delivered a talk. Blushing ratings were greater in people with social anxiety disorder than in controls during each of these tasks. Facial coloration (expressed in arbitrary units) was greater in people with social anxiety disorder than in controls when they first watched the pre-recorded videotape, but did not differ between groups during the other tasks. Within the group with social anxiety disorder, facial coloration in people who were primarily concerned about blushing was similar to coloration in others without this complaint. Gerlach and colleagues suggested that people with social anxiety disorder focus more intently than controls on internal sensations during social interactions, and thus might overestimate autonomic responses such as blushing. These conclusions were echoed by Edelmann and Baker (2002), who could find no differences in cheek temperature or other measures of physiological activity between people with social anxiety disorder, people with other anxiety disorders and healthy controls during a variety of tasks (riding an exercise bicycle, mental arithmetic, imagining an anxiety-provoking situation and having a conversation). Despite this, ratings of the intensity of somatic symptoms generally were greater in patients than in controls during socially engaging tasks.

In a similar vein, Voncken and Bögels (2009) compared patients with social anxiety disorder, with or without a fear of blushing, with normal controls during a conversation and a prepared speech. Responses to the tasks were combined in the statistical analysis. Observers reported that blushing was greater in patients with a fear of blushing than in the other participants. In terms of facial coloration, the most striking difference between groups appeared to be a smaller increase in coloration (expressed in arbitrary units) during the tasks and a reduced rate of recovery after the tasks in patients without a fear of blushing, perhaps due to the inhibitory effects of sympathetic vasoconstriction on facial blood flow. Importantly, increases in facial coloration in patients with a fear of blushing were similar to responses in controls. Increases in cheek temperature were similar in all three groups during the social tasks. Nonetheless, the cheeks of patients with a fear of blushing were warmer throughout the study than those of other participants. The heightened cheek temperature (and hence blood flow) might have increased the visibility of blushing in patients who were afraid of this response.

The effect of an introductory conversation, delivering a speech and listening to the speech afterwards was investigated in our laboratory in sixteen people who answered an advertisement that offered treatment for fear of blushing (Drummond et al., 2007). They were matched with sixteen controls of similar age and sex distribution. The blush of embarrassment typically develops and resolves rapidly (Figure 2.1). Although this was the case for controls, forehead pulsations (expressed as the percentage change from baseline) increased progressively over the course of the experiment in participants with a fear of blushing. These findings are consistent with the concept of a 'creeping blush' that sometimes is seen in speakers delivering prepared presentations to an audience (Leary et al., 1992) – over a period of several minutes a rash that resembles hives spreads from the upper chest to the neck and face. Alternatively, blushing might have provoked residual flushing in people with a fear of blushing. Further clarification of this is important, as the residual response might augment sensory cues of blushing and add to emotional distress.

The effect of false feedback of blushing on cheek temperature, facial coloration, judgments about how much they blushed and the costs of blushing were compared recently in people with a high or low fear of blushing (Dijk, Voncken et al., 2009). The participants initiated and maintained a 5-minute conversation with two strangers while receiving 'feedback' from a vibrating device attached to the finger. Approximately half of the participants were told that vibrations varied in proportion to the intensity of their own blushing, whereas the others were told that the vibrations varied in proportion to the intensity of blushing in another participant. The vibrations actually increased to a fairly intense level in all participants after the first 30 seconds of the conversation. In the 'yoked control' condition, participants with a fear of blushing gave higher blushing ratings than participants without a fear of blushing. However, in the false-feedback condition, ratings were similar in both groups. Irrespective of fear of blushing, participants in the false-feedback condition both anticipated and received a more negative evaluation of their conversational performance than participants in the control condition. Thus, the conviction that one is blushing may hinder performance in social encounters. Increases in facial coloration (expressed in arbitrary units) were greater in the control condition in people with high than with low fear of blushing but did not differ between groups in the false-feedback condition. In addition, for participants in the low-fear group, the facial coloration response was greater in the false-feedback than in the control condition but was similar in both conditions for participants in the high-fear group. Together, these findings suggest that false feedback raised awareness of blushing in people without a fear of blushing. This not only increased the perception of blushing but also increased blushing itself. False feedback appeared to have less effect in the high-fear group, presumably because their expectations about blushing already were high.

We recently investigated the relationship between blushing propensity, social anxiety and facial blood flow during embarrassment in eighty-six normal participants when they sang a children's song

Drummond & Su, 2012). Increases in facial blood flow were greatest in participants with elevated blushing propensity and social interaction anxiety scores. However, this was due primarily to social anxiety because the link with blushing propensity disappeared when social interaction anxiety scores were controlled. In sum, anxiety associated with heightened expectations of blushing may augment blushing, thus fulfilling those expectations and reinforcing anxiety. However, as people are generally unaware of how intensely they are blushing, contextual or emotional cues rather than physiological cues of blushing may reinforce blushing in people who are frightened of this response (Figure 2.4).

There is some overlap between concepts of social anxiety disorder and shyness, perhaps with more emphasis being placed on clinical diagnostic criteria for social anxiety disorder than for shyness (generally considered to be a personality trait or behavioural predisposition rather than a

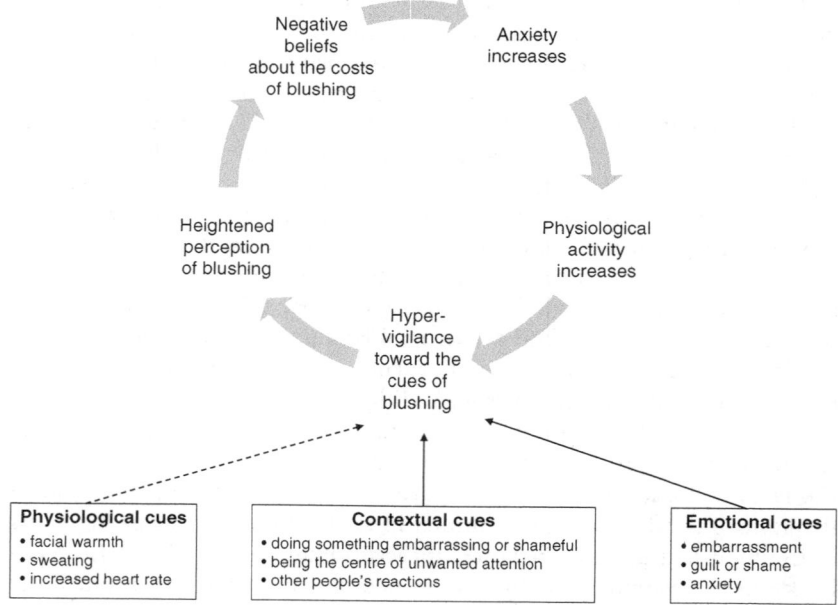

Figure 2.4 Cognitive model of fear of blushing (adapted from Dijk et al., 2009b). In this model, contextual, emotional and possibly physiological cues (represented by the dotted line) raise concerns that blushing might have begun. Apprehension about the negative consequences of blushing heightens stress responses and focuses attention on the cues of blushing, thereby increasing fear.

disorder). Hofmann, Moscovitch and Kim (2006) investigated whether shy people blush more than other people during an impromptu speech, singing and watching these performances on videotape. In general, increases in facial coloration (expressed as the percentage change from baseline) were greater during these tasks in shy than in non-shy participants. Surprisingly, however, ratings of embarrassment were similar in both groups throughout the experiment, as were scores on the Blushing Propensity Scale (Leary & Meadows, 1991) and the Embarrassability Scale (Modigliani, 1968). These findings reinforce the view that blushing often is out of step with emotional experiences.

Fear of scrutiny and interpersonal evaluation typically provoke avoidance behaviours such as gaze aversion (Baker & Edelmann, 2002; Horley et al., 2003), suggesting that eye contact raises anxiety in evaluative situations. Whether eye contact also evokes blushing in socially anxious people was investigated recently in our laboratory (Chen & Drummond, 2008). Physiological activity was recorded while participants sang, during 3 minutes of scrutiny (half with and half without prolonged eye contact), and while participants listened to an audiotape of themselves singing. Sweating and blushing (measured as the percentage change in forehead pulsations) increased during eye contact, and prior eye contact augmented blushing when participants listened to the audiotape. Prior eye contact also augmented somatic symptoms in people with high scores on the Fear of Negative Evaluation (FNE) Questionnaire (a key feature of social anxiety; Watson & Friend, 1969). In addition, ratings of anxiety, embarrassment and trembling were elevated in people with high FNE scores throughout the experiment, and sensations of facial warmth increased more in people with high FNE scores when they sang. Nevertheless, physiological activity did not differ between people with high or low FNE scores during any of the social-evaluative tasks. Together, these findings indicate that eye contact in evaluative situations is unpleasant, particularly for people with a fear of negative evaluation. However, misattribution of the cues of emotional arousal seems to be more important than aberrant physiological activity for generating symptoms of social anxiety.

To investigate the physiological basis of flushing in patients with social anxiety disorder, Bouwer and Stein (1998) administered 100 mg niacin (which mediates vasodilatation by formation of prostanoids) to six male patients who attended an anxiety disorders clinic for treatment of generalized social phobia, and to six healthy male controls. Flushing was greater in patients than in controls, but whether this was due to a specific effect of niacin or to anxiety is uncertain because placebo effects were not controlled. To explore this further, we recently administered 100 mg niacin or placebo double-blind to a non-clinical sample of young adults, and investigated flushing in relation to fear of negative evaluation while the participants rested quietly (Drummond & Lazaroo, 2012). In the niacin condition, increases in facial blood flow were greater in people with high rather than low fear of negative evaluation whereas, in the placebo condition, increases were minimal in both groups. Ratings of anxiety and embarrassment were similar in both groups before drug administration, and did not change over the 20-minute interval of monitoring. Thus, a physiological predisposition may augment blushing in people with social anxiety.

## Future directions

As noted above, we now have some insight into the neural regulation and triggers of blushing, the psychophysiological pattern of this response, and individual differences that influence awareness of and beliefs about blushing. However, there are still many unanswered questions.

From a psychophysiological perspective, we need to clarify the factors that determine whether emotional arousal evokes blushing or facial pallor. A start was made on this in a vignette study that required respondents to rate their expected facial coloration in various hypothetical situations that involved the expression or suppression of anger (Drummond, 1997b). Most respondents thought that their face would flush rather than blanch in anger-provoking situations, particularly when anger was expressed. Conversely, facial pallor was associated with fear and, in one situation, with embarrassment (silently receiving a speeding fine). Respondents with high scores on the Blushing Propensity Scale (Leary & Meadows, 1991) and the 'angry reaction' subscale of the Anger Expression Inventory (Spielberger, 1991) reported the highest flushing ratings. These leads need to be explored in psychophysiological studies.

Whether physiological factors might also increase the predisposition to blush deserves further investigation. For instance, an elevated density of $\beta$-adrenoceptors in facial blood vessels could increase the likelihood of blushing and flushing across a range of situations (Mellander et al., 1982). In addition, an increased sensitivity to prostanoids might augment or prolong blushing in people with social anxiety (Bouwer & Stein, 1998; Drummond & Lazaroo, 2012). Speculatively, a deficiency of $\alpha$-adrenoceptors in facial blood vessels might also augment blushing fibres that supply vasodilator neurons in the superior cervical ganglia exit from the spinal cord predominantly through the second to fourth thoracic roots. Postganglionic sympathetic vasodilator neurons then project from the superior cervical ganglia along cranial blood vessels and cranial nerves to the facial skin (Drummond, 1994a). The best outcome after ETS appears to be achieved by cutting or clipping the sympathetic chain at the level of the third or fourth thoracic roots, as procedures above this level are associated with an increased incidence of side-effects (Sugimura et al., 2009). Although blushing generally is abolished after ETS, troublesome side-effects such as compensatory sweating below the level of the lesion, ultimately may result in dissatisfaction (Drummond, 2000; Malmivaara et al., 2007). In addition, the post-surgical development of aberrant gustatory sweating and flushing in sympathetically denervated skin (Drummond & Lance, 1992) sometimes is as distressing as uncontrolled blushing.

The side-effects and overall satisfaction rates of ETS for facial blushing and/or excessive sweating were investigated recently in a survey of 3,015 patients who had undergone ETS 13–22 years previously (Smidfelt & Drott, 2011). Compensatory sweating was reported by 80 per cent of the 1,700 patients who responded to the survey (a response rate of 56 per cent). The proportion of patients who regretted having had ETS had risen over time from 7.8 per cent in a previous survey to 13.5 per cent in the current survey. Within the group who had undergone the procedure for facial blushing, 26.5 per cent ultimately were dissatisfied with the outcome or regretted having had ETS. Part of this dissatisfaction may have been due to the persistence of slowly emerging or blotchy blushing, which might not be mediated by cervical sympathetic outflow.

Some surgeons place clips on the sympathetic chain, to crush rather than sever nerve fibres, so that the procedure can more easily be reversed. Preferably, however, the clips should be removed before sympathetic nerves degenerate (i.e., within several weeks or months); thus, the reversal is not always effective (Chou et al., 2006; Sugimura et al., 2009).

## Selective brain cooling during blushing?

From a basic physiological perspective, parallels between the mechanisms of blushing and thermoregulatory facial flushing suggest that there may also be functional parallels. Dilatation of facial blood vessels brings warm blood to the surface, thereby facilitating transfer of body heat to the environment. Heat loss from the human face may result in differences between tympanic temperature (which reflects brain temperature) by decreasing the intensity of vasoconstrictor responses that could otherwise mask blushing during emotional arousal.

Irrespective of any physiological predisposition, the situational context clearly has a major influence on blushing. Perhaps the clearest illustration of this to emerge in our own research was the inhibitory effect of 'false-negative' feedback on blushing during singing in people with low blushing propensity scores (Drummond, 2001). That 'false-negative' feedback had no effect on blushing in people with high blushing propensity scores suggests that anxiety about blushing may alter the situational context in such a way that blushing becomes a self-fulfilling prophecy. If so, this vicious circle could lie at the heart of a fear of blushing (Figure 2.4).

The type of emotional response elicited by situational cues may also determine whether emotional arousal is associated with blushing. For instance, a tendency to amplify threats to social standing or self-esteem might evoke blushing and flushing, whereas a sense of danger may induce pallor (Drummond, 1997b). Separate motor programmes for each of these response patterns have been identified in the midbrain periaqueductal grey (Carrive & Bandler, 1991). Whether active sympathetic vasodilatation overshadows simultaneous sympathetically mediated vasoconstriction needs to be investigated not only during embarrassment (Drummond, 1997a) but also in other emotions (e.g., shame, guilt, anger and fear).

Many other issues remain unresolved. For instance, does blushing depend on age and, if so, why? What cues do socially anxious people use to decide whether or how intensely they are blushing? In particular, are interoceptive sensations such as engorgement or throbbing in the face, or increases in facial warmth or sweating, as important as appraisal of situational or interpersonal factors, or emotions such as embarrassment, fear or shame? Identifying these cues could be crucial for correcting faulty assumptions about blushing in people who are frightened of this response.

And finally, what are the psychophysiological consequences of recurrent blushing? Heightened blood flow increases the frequency of collisions between red blood cells and the vascular endothelium, resulting in the release of endothelium-derived vasodilating factors such as nitric oxide (Fleming, 2010). Local vasodilatation might reduce the rate of recovery after recurrent blushing episodes (Drummond *et al.*, 2007), particularly if physiological cues such as facial warmth or throbbing evoke further anxiety and blushing. Answers to these questions could help to make blushing less peculiar but still the 'most human of all expressions' (Darwin, 1872/1965, p. 309).

## REFERENCES

American Psychiatric Association (1994). *Diagnostic and statistical manual of mental disorders*, 4th edn. Washington, DC: American Psychiatric Association.
Amies, P. L., Gelder, M. G., & Shaw, P. M. (1983). Social phobia: a comparative clinical study. *British Journal of Psychiatry*, **142**, 174–9.
Baker, S. R., & Edelmann, R. J. (2002). Is social phobia related to lack of social skills? Duration of skill-related behaviours and ratings of behavioural adequacy. *British Journal of Clinical Psychology*, **41**(3), 243–57.
Blair, D., Glover, W., & Roddie, I. (1961). Cutaneous vasomotor nerves to the head and trunk. *Journal of Applied Physiology*, **16**, 119–22.
Bögels, S. M., Alberts, M., & de Jong, P. J. (1996). Self-consciousness, self-focused attention, blushing propensity and fear of blushing. *Personality and Individual Differences*, **21**(4), 573–81.
Bouwer, C., & Stein, D. J. (1998). Hyperresponsivity to nicotinic acid challenge in generalized social phobia: a pilot study. *European Neuropsychopharmacology*, **8**(4), 311–13.
Carrive, P., & Bandler, R. (1991). Control of extracranial and hindlimb blood flow by the midbrain periaqueductal grey of the cat. *Experimental Brain Research*, **84**(3), 599–606.
Changizi, M. A., Zhang, Q., & Shimojo, S. (2006). Bare skin, blood and the evolution of primate colour vision. *Biology Letters*, **2**(2), 217–21.
Chen, V., & Drummond, P. D. (2008). Fear of negative evaluation augments negative affect and somatic symptoms in social-evaluative situations. *Cognition and Emotion*, **22**(1), 21–43.
Chou, S. H., Kao, E. L., Lin, C. C., Chang, Y. T., & Huang, M. F. (2006). The importance of classification in sympathetic surgery and a proposed mechanism for compensatory hyperhidrosis: experience with 464 cases. *Surgical Endoscopy*, **20**(11), 1749–53.
Cuthbert, B. N. (2002). Social anxiety disorder: trends and translational research. *Biological Psychiatry*, **51**(1), 4–10.
Darwin, C. (1872/1965). *The expression of the emotions in man and animals.* University of Chicago Press.
de Jong, P. J. (1999). Communicative and remedial effects of social blushing. *Journal of Nonverbal Behavior*, **23**(3), 197–217.
Dijk, C., de Jong, P. J., & Peters, M. L. (2009). The remedial value of blushing in the context of transgressions and mishaps. *Emotion*, **9**(2), 287–91.
Dijk, C., Voncken, M. J., & de Jong, P. J. (2009). I blush, therefore I will be judged negatively: influence of false blush feedback on anticipated others' judgments and facial coloration in high and low blushing-fearfuls. *Behaviour Research and Therapy*, **47**(7), 541–7.
Drummond, P. D. (1989). Mechanism of emotional blushing. In N. W. Bond & D. A. T. Siddle (Eds.), *Psychobiology: issues and applications*. Amsterdam: Elsevier, 363–70.
  (1992). The mechanism of facial sweating and cutaneous vascular responses to painful stimulation of the eye. *Brain*, **115**(5), 1417–28.

(1994a). Sweating and vascular responses in the face: normal regulation and dysfunction in migraine, cluster headache and harlequin syndrome. *Clinical Autonomic Research*, **4**(5), 273–85.

(1994b). The effect of anger and pleasure on facial blood flow. *Australian Journal of Psychology*, **46**(2), 95–9.

(1995). Mechanisms of physiological gustatory sweating and flushing in the face. *Journal of the Autonomic Nervous System*, **52**(2–3), 117–24.

(1997a). The effect of adrenergic blockade on blushing and facial flushing. *Psychophysiology*, **34**(2), 163–8.

(1997b). Correlates of facial flushing and pallor in anger-provoking situations. *Personality and Individual Differences*, **23**(4), 575–82.

(1999a). Facial flushing during provocation in women. *Psychophysiology*, **36**(3), 325–32.

(1999b). Autonomic disorders affecting cutaneous blood flow. In C. J. Mathias & R. Bannister (Eds.), *Autonomic failure*, 4th edn. New York: Oxford University Press, 487–93.

(2000). A caution about surgical treatment for facial blushing. *British Journal of Dermatology*, **142**(1), 194–5.

(2001). The effect of true and false feedback on blushing in women. *Personality and Individual Differences*, **30**(8), 1329–43.

(2004). The effect of cutaneous mast cell degranulation on sensitivity to heat. *Inflammation Research*, **53**(7), 309–15.

(2006). Immersion of the hand in ice water releases adrenergic vasoconstrictor tone in the ipsilateral temple. *Autonomic Neuroscience*, **128**(1–2), 70–5.

(2012). [Making a mistake evokes blushing]. Unpublished raw data.

Drummond, P. D., Back, K., Harrison, J., Helgadottir, F. D., Lange, B., Lee, C., Leavy, K., Novatscou, C., Orner, A., Pham, H., Prance, J., Radford, D., & Wheatley, L. (2007). Blushing during social interactions in people with a fear of blushing. *Behaviour Research and Therapy*, **45**(7), 1601–8.

Drummond, P. D., Camacho, L., Formentin, N., Heffernan, T. D., Williams, F., & Zekas, T. E. (2003). The impact of verbal feedback about blushing on social discomfort and facial blood flow during embarrassing tasks. *Behaviour Research and Therapy*, **41**(4), 413–25.

Drummond, P. D., & Finch, P. M. (1989). Reflex control of facial flushing during body heating in man. *Brain*, **112**(5), 1351–8.

Drummond, P. D., & Granston, A. (2003). Facilitation of extracranial vasodilatation to limb pain in migraine sufferers. *Neurology*, **61**(1), 60–3.

Drummond, P. D., & Lance, J. W. (1987). Facial flushing and sweating mediated by the sympathetic nervous system. *Brain*, **110**(3), 793–803.

Drummond, P. D., & Lance, J. W. (1992). Pathological sweating and flushing accompanying the & Lance, J. W. trigeminal lacrimal reflex in patients with cluster headache and in patients with a confirmed site of cervical sympathetic deficit: evidence for parasympathetic cross-innervation. *Brain*, **115**(Pt 5), 1429–45.

Drummond, P. D., & Lazaroo, D. (2012). The effect of niacin on facial blood flow in people with an elevated fear of negative evaluation. *European Neuropsychopharmacology*, **22**(3), 200–4.

Drummond, P. D., & Lim, H. K. (2000). The significance of blushing for fair- and dark-skinned people. *Personality and Individual Differences*, **29**(6), 1123–32.

Drummond, P. D., & Mirco, N. (2004). Staring at one side of the face increases blood flow on that side of the face. *Psychophysiology*, **41**(2), 281–7.

Drummond, P. D., & Quah, S. H. (2001). The effect of expressing anger on cardiovascular reactivity and facial blood flow in Chinese and Caucasians. *Psychophysiology*, **38**(2), 190–6.

Drummond, P. D., & Su, D. (2012). The relationship between blushing propensity, social anxiety and facial blood flow during embarrassment. *Cognition and Emotion*, **26**(3), 561–7.

Edelmann, R. J., & Baker, S. R. (2002). Self-reported and actual physiological responses in social phobia. *British Journal of Clinical Psychology*, **41**(1), 1–14.

Edelmann, R. J., & Skov, V. (1993). Blushing propensity, social anxiety, anxiety sensitivity and awareness of bodily sensations. *Personality and Individual Differences*, **14**(3), 495–8.

Fleming, I. (2010). Molecular mechanisms underlying the activation of eNOS. *Pflugers Archiv: European Journal of Physiology*, **459**(6), 793–806.

Fox, R. H., Goldsmith, R., & Kidd, D. J. (1962). Cutaneous vasomotor control in the human head, neck and upper chest. *Journal of Physiology (London)*, **161**, 298–312.

Gerlach, A. L., Wilhelm, F. H., Gruber, K., & Roth, W. T. (2001). Blushing and physiological arousability in social phobia. *Journal of Abnormal Psychology*, **110**(2), 247–58.

Gerlach, A. L., Wilhelm, F. H., & Roth, W. T. (2003). Embarrassment and social phobia: the role of parasympathetic activation. *Journal of Anxiety Disorders*, **17**(2), 197–210.

Hofmann, S. G., Moscovitch, D. A., & Kim, H. J. (2006). Autonomic correlates of social anxiety and embarrassment in shy and non-shy individuals. *International Journal of Psychophysiology*, **61**(2), 134–42.

Horley, K., Williams, L. M., Gonsalvez, C., & Gordon, E. (2003). Social phobics do not see eye to eye: a visual scanpath study of emotional expression processing. *Journal of Anxiety Disorders*, **17**(1), 33–44.

Irmak, M. K., Korkmaz, A., & Erogul, O. (2004). Selective brain cooling seems to be a mechanism leading to human craniofacial diversity observed in different geographical regions. *Medical Hypotheses*, **63**(6), 974–9.

Izumi, H. (1999). Nervous control of blood flow in the orofacial region. *Pharmacology and Therapeutics*, **81**(2), 141–61.

Laederach-Hofmann, K., Mussgay, L., Buchel, B., Widler, P., & Ruddel, H. (2002). Patients with erythrophobia (fear of blushing) show abnormal autonomic regulation in mental stress conditions. *Psychosomatic Medicine*, **64**(2), 358–65.

Leary, M. R., Britt, T. W., Cutlip, W. D. II, & Templeton, J. L. (1992). Social blushing. *Psychological Bulletin*, **112**(3), 446–60.

Leary, M. R., & Meadows, S. (1991). Predictors, elicitors, and concomitants of social blushing. *Journal of Personality and Social Psychology*, **60**(2), 254–62.

Lindsey, K. Q., Caughman, S. W., Olerud, J. E., Bunnett, N. W., Armstrong, C. A., & Ansel, J. C. (2000). Neural regulation of endothelial cell-mediated inflammation. *Journal of Investigative Dermatology Symposium Proceedings*, **5**(1), 74–8.
Magerl, W., & Treede, R. D. (1996). Heat-evoked vasodilatation in human hairy skin: axon reflexes due to low-level activity of nociceptive afferents. *Journal of Physiology (London)*, **497**(3), 837–48.
Malmivaara, A., Kuukasjarvi, P., Autti-Ramo, I., Kovanen, N., & Makela, M. (2007). Effectiveness and safety of endoscopic thoracic sympathectomy for excessive sweating and facial blushing: a systematic review. *International Journal of Technology Assessment in Health Care*, **23**(1), 54–62.
Mellander, S., Andersson, P. O., Afzelius, L. E., & Hellstrand, P. (1982). Neural beta-adrenergic dilatation of the facial vein in man: possible mechanism in emotional blushing. *Acta Physiologica Scandinavica*, **114**(3), 393–9.
Modigliani, A. (1968). Embarrassment and embarrassability. *Sociometry*, **31**(3), 313–26.
Mulkens, S., de Jong, P. J., & Bögels, S. M. (1997). High blushing propensity: fearful preoccupation or facial coloration? *Personality and Individual Differences*, **22**(6), 817–24.
Mulkens, S., de Jong, P. J., Dobbelaar, A., & Bögels, S. M. (1999). Fear of blushing: fearful preoccupation irrespective of facial coloration. *Behaviour Research and Therapy*, **37**(11), 1119–28.
Nagasaka, T., Brinnel, H., Hales, J. R., & Ogawa, T. (1998). Selective brain cooling in hyperthermia: the mechanisms and medical implications. *Medical Hypotheses*, **50**(3), 203–11.
Neto, F. (1996). Correlates of social blushing. *Personality and Individual Differences*, **20**(3), 365–73.
Nielsen, B. (1988). Natural cooling of the brain during outdoor bicycling? *Pflugers Archiv: European Journal of Physiology*, **411**(4), 456–61.
Nordin, M. (1990). Sympathetic discharges in the human supraorbital nerve and their relation to sudo- and vasomotor responses. *Journal of Physiology (London)*, **423**, 241–55.
Pohjavaara, P., Telaranta, T., & Vaisanen, E. (2003). The role of the sympathetic nervous system in anxiety: is it possible to relieve anxiety with endoscopic sympathetic block? *Nordic Journal of Psychiatry*, **57**(1), 55–60.
Rapee, R. M., & Heimberg, R. G. (1997). A cognitive-behavioral model of anxiety in social phobia. *Behaviour Research and Therapy*, **35**(8), 741–56.
Roberts, A. H., Schuler, J., Bacon, J. G., Zimmermann, R. L., & Patterson, R. (1975). Individual differences and autonomic control: absorption, hypnotic susceptibility, and the unilateral control of skin temperature. *Journal of Abnormal Psychology*, **84**(3), 272–9.
Shearn, D., Bergman, E., Hill, K., Abel, A., & Hinds, L. (1990). Facial coloration and temperature responses in blushing. *Psychophysiology*, **27**(6), 687–93.
(1992). Blushing as a function of audience size. *Psychophysiology*, **29**(4), 431–6.
Shearn, D., Spellman, L., Straley, B., Meirick, J., & Stryker, K. (1999). Empathic blushing in friends and strangers. *Motivation and Emotion*, **23**(4), 307–16.

Smidfelt, K., & Drott, C. (2011). Late results of endoscopic thoracic sympathectomy for hyperhidrosis and facial blushing. *British Journal of Surgery*, **98**(12), 1719–24.

Spielberger, C. D. (1991). *State-trait anger expression inventory professional manual*, rev. research edn. Odessa, FL: Psychological Assessment Resources.

Sugimura, H., Spratt, E. H., Compeau, C. G., Kattail, D., & Shargall, Y. (2009). Thoracoscopic sympathetic clipping for hyperhidrosis: long-term results and reversibility. *Journal of Thoracic and Cardiovascular Surgery*, **137**(6), 1370–6; discussion 1376–7.

Vassend, O., & Knardahl, S. (2005). Personality, affective response, and facial blood flow during brief cognitive tasks. *International Journal of Psychophysiology*, **55**(3), 265–78.

Voncken, M. J., & Bögels, S. M. (2009). Physiological blushing in social anxiety disorder patients with and without blushing complaints: two subtypes? *Biological Psychology*, **81**(2), 86–94.

Watson, D., & Friend, R. (1969). Measurement of social-evaluative anxiety. *Journal of Consulting and Clinical Psychology*, **33**(4), 448–57.

Wilkin, J. K. (1988). Why is flushing limited to a mostly facial cutaneous distribution? *Journal of the American Academy of Dermatology*, **19**(2) (Pt 1), 309–13.

Zachariae, R., Oster, H., & Bjerring, P. (1994). Effects of hypnotic suggestions on ultraviolet B radiation-induced erythema and skin blood flow. *Photodermatology, Photoimmunology and Photomedicine*, **10**(4), 154–60.

Zajonc, R. B., Murphy, S. T., & Inglehart, M. (1989). Feeling and facial efference: implications of the vascular theory of emotion. *Psychological Review*, **96**(3), 395–416.

# 3 Measurement of the blush

*Ruth Cooper and Alexander L. Gerlach*

On first sight, one might think that measuring blushing is simple. After all, do we not see people blush all the time? Should it not be simple to derive a measure that captures this obvious physical symptom? However, although the naïve observer may claim to be easily able to assess reliably whether a person blushed, in fact this is not the case. At least, when observational measures of blushing are related to physiological measures such as an increase in blood flow at the blushing region, naïve observers do not perform above chance level (Gerlach, 1998). As early as 1968, Lang (cf. Lang, 1993) established the view that the assessment of emotion and related phenomena should include three response systems: overt behaviour, self-report and physiology. Lang's system has both been criticized and praised (Hugdahl, 1981; Lang *et al.*, 1983). Generally, the need for multiple measures from all three response systems is acknowledged. However, since concordance of individual measures even within these three systems is often absent, it remains questionable whether the grouping into response systems can substantially contribute to the understanding of psychopathological behaviour (Hugdahl, 1981). Nonetheless, collecting a large amount of data of different types will help to ensure that assessment of psychopathological reactions addresses the complexity of these basic human responses to the environment. In consequence, the blushing reaction has been captured in different ways, often leading to different results regarding its occurrence. Its physiological correlates – that is, the facial blood flow or the temperature changes – can be measured by a variety of methods. Self-reported blushing may be assessed using questionnaires, and the visibility of the blushing reaction can be rated by an observer on different dimensions.

In this chapter, we aim to give an overview about the specific principles and problems that arise within each of the measurement approaches.

### The physiological measurement of the blushing response

The first study that tried to capture the underlying physiological changes during a blushing response by experimentally inducing a blush was conducted by Schandry and Poth (1983). Assuming that vasodilatory processes at the facial surface are caused by thermoregulatory mechanisms, the authors expected a close correlation between visible facial blood flow and surface temperature. To investigate physiological concomitants of the blush, the authors elicited a blushing response by asking embarrassing questions (e.g., 'Do you think you look good?'). Indeed, the authors found a slight temperature increase during the first 30 seconds after the blush's onset, which was determined visually by the experimenter.

As of today, various mechanisms of measuring, parameterizing and operationalizing the physiological blushing response have emerged, which we will explain in more detail in the next sections.

*Blood flow measures*

The most commonly used methods to measure facial blushing are based on the direct recording of the facial blood flow in a given situation. Although these data do not directly indicate the extent of the visibility of the blushing reaction, facial blood flow is the closest physiological concomitant to the visible blushing response (Shearn et al., 1990). In the next sections, we will give an overview of the measurement principles, parameterization, and caveats concerning the measurement of the intensity of the facial blood flow.

**Measurement principles.** First used by Hertzman in 1938, the most common technique to measure the blushing response is to detect the magnitude of the facial blood flow photoplethysmographically (Hertzman, 1938). The recording instrument, a photoplethysmograph, consists of a light-emitting diode and a photoelectric detector which are located right next to each other. The measurement principle is the following: light is emitted from the diode into the skin and is partially absorbed by the skin tissue and surrounding blood vessels. Other parts are reflected by the same structures and recorded by the detector. If the wavelength of the emitting light is in the near-infrared spectrum (e.g., the often used UFI model 1020 photoplethysmograph emits and recodes light at 950 nM), the attenuation by skin tissue is small and constant (Weinman, 1967). Variations in recorded reflections can therefore give a measure of the ongoing blood flow. Although multiple processes are involved in the light attenuation of blood, including absorption, multiple scattering and reflection, it can generally be determined that the more blood is present in the skin, the greater is the attenuation of light, and the less is reflected to and consequently recorded by the detector (Challoner & Ramsay, 1974). Other factors influencing the magnitude of light

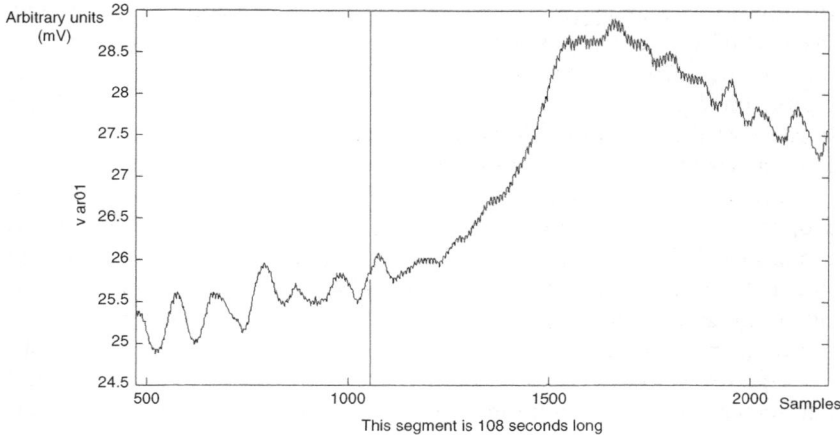

Figure 3.1 Photoplethysmogram
*Note:* A photoplethysmogram of a blushing reaction measured on the forehead. The vertical line indicates the onset of the blushing induction.

detection are the opacity of other tissue components (e.g., skin, muscles, bones); however, the small variations in light-detection intensity (about 1–2 per cent of the total light reflection) are a result of changes in the amount of blood: for example, as a result of arterial pulsations (Nijboer, Dorlas & Mahieu, 1981). The detected intensity of the reflected light is then usually converted to a DC voltage, electronically amplified and recorded as a plethysmogram (see Figure 3.1). The advantages of using DC instead of AC coupling, as usually done for photoplethysmographic recordings (i.e., pulse oximetry), lie at hand: although AC coupling renders a signal from which pulse waves can be obtained quite well, information regarding the overall blood volume in the respective vessels is lost due to AC's inherent high-pass filtering processes. However, this information is crucial for the blushing measurement since a visible blushing response, in addition to heightened pulse amplitudes (e.g., Drummond et al., 2007), is reflected by a comparably slow increase in the overall blood volume. Disadvantages are related to the sensitivity to overall levels: orthostatic changes (such as slight head movements) have a large effect on the signal intensity; in addition, the DC signal is more prone to artefacts induced by extraneous light. Nonetheless, since the time course of the blushing reaction is regularly in the focus of studies, DC coupling normally is the method of choice. Concerning filtering processes, it is useful to implement a lowpass filter at 30 Hz to protect the signal from measurement artefacts due to fluorescent lights which usually operate at a wavelength around 50–60 Hz and are commonly used in office rooms. Since the blushing reaction is much slower than 30 Hz, the lowpass filter does not affect the signal detection. On the other hand, implementing an additional highpass filter is not recommended: because of the long time course of a blushing response, filtering out low frequencies may actually result in filtering out the blushing signal itself.

Similar to the detection method of photoplethysmography, laser Doppler flowmetry is also based on the reflection of previously emitted red or near-infrared light by the red blood cells. The main difference is that flowmetry additionally investigates the *velocity*, and not only the photoplethysmographically detected amount of facial blood flow, by recording the frequency change (also called Doppler shift) that moving blood cells undergo respective to the point of measurement. The most often reported parameter, 'flux' (Drummond, 1997; Drummond & Mirco, 2004; Katzman et al., 2003), is an arbitrary unit that represents the product of the number of moving red cells approximately 1–2 mm beneath the skin and their mean velocity. Aside from recording the fluctuations of frequency, the measurement principles regarding the signal detection and recording are similar to the explained photoplethysmographic methods.

**Parameterization.** The first published investigation that photoplethysmographically recorded a previously elicited blushing response was conducted by Shearn and colleagues in 1990. To elicit the blushing response, healthy volunteers were asked to watch along with confederates a previously recorded video of themselves singing, which is a common procedure to heighten embarrassment and induce emotional blushing (e.g., Gerlach et al., 2001; Hofmann et al., 2006). Shearn and co-authors (1990) recorded cheek and ear blood flow, cheek temperature and skin conductance. For all four measures, the authors calculated a simple difference score between a baseline value and the maximum score recorded during the experimental induction of embarrassment. Similar methods and parameterizations for the induction and analysis of the blushing response were used by Mulkens and colleagues (1997, 1999) who calculated a difference score between a mean baseline score and a single maximum value during the blushing induction. Although this procedure seems very practical and reasonable at first glance, the single-value approach has one big caveat: the lack of reliability, which is especially problematic when considering the plethysmogram's susceptibility to measurement artefacts (see section 'Caveats' below). Later investigations addressed this problem: to ensure a certain degree of reliability, Gerlach and co-authors (2001) calculated the difference between the means of the 30-s periods before and after the onset of the experimental manipulation, which also consisted of watching along with an audience a previously made singing recording. Mean difference scores were also used by Dijk and colleagues (2009), who induced blushing by accusing the subject of blushing. Similarly, Bögels and colleagues (2002) operationalized the blushing response as mean values over measurement periods of interest; however, instead of implementing baseline difference scores, the authors analysed the respective values as repeated measures in a mixed model ANOVA.

A different parameterization is used by Peter Drummond, who particularly analyses the relative change in pulse *amplitude* (Chen & Drummond, 2008; Drummond, 1999, 2001; Drummond et al., 2007; Drummond et al., 2003; Drummond & Lim, 2000). The blushing reaction is operationalized in such a way that the bigger the pulse amplitude appears, the higher is the arterial inflow as compared to the venous outflow, which is the necessary physiological prerequisite for a blushing reaction. The mean amplitude from the photoplethysmographically measured trough-to-peak height of arterial pulsations is calculated for both the baseline and experimental periods. The parameter of interest is expressed as percentage increase of amplitude in the experimental as compared to the baseline condition.

Concerning the parameters obtained by Doppler flowmetry, blood flow can be parameterized in a similar manner: Drummond (1997; Drummond & Mirco, 2004) operationalizes blushing intensity as percentage increase of 'flow' (i.e., the product of the amount of red blood cells and their velocity) in the experimental condition as compared to the baseline. A more elaborated procedure to parameterize blood flow was conducted in a study by Katzman and colleagues (2003). The authors analysed 'flux' data that were recorded during a pharmacologically elicited blushing reaction by means of nonlinear curve fitting. This procedure yielded parameters of flux baseline, maximal level of change, maximal slope, and delay of reaction, which were all entered in a statistical analysis.

As of today, the most common approach to record and parameterize the blushing response is by calculating the photoplethysmographically recorded blood flow data as mean scores over a defined period of interest, which is then subtracted from or otherwise controlled for inter-individual baseline differences.

**Caveats.** A problem particularly related to the methods of recording the facial blood flow is their very principle of measurement: the sensitivity to light. The photoelectric sensor does not only record the reflected light specifically emitted from the diode but also light resulting from stray radiation from other light sources that are partially absorbed and reflected by the skin. Although most instruments work in the near-infrared spectrum and consequently do not record reflections of most artificial light sources, some parts of normal daylight are located within the infrared spectrum. Therefore, to ensure the signal quality of the recording, it is crucial that the measurement is conducted in the absence of normal daylight. Also, the investigator should check the device carefully for its recording frequencies and make sure that no light sources used during the investigation operate in the same spectrum. Additionally, the investigator can ask the subject to wear an opaque headband over the sensor, which will also prevent the recording of stray radiation from other light sources.

Another issue to be careful about is that the sensor is extremely vulnerable to movement due to a variety of reasons. First, even only slight detachments or dislocations of the sensor will lead to the recording of unwanted stray light radiation. Again, wearing a tight headband can be of help to prevent the sensor from detachment. Second, facial movement (such as speaking, frowning, etc.) will lead to a physiologically based increase in blood flow which, on the signal level, cannot be differentiated from the emotional blushing response. To address this problem, it is useful to conduct the measurement of the blush on the forehead instead of on the cheek, as was originally done by Shearn and colleagues (1990): the emotional blushing reaction can also be reliably detected on the forehead right above the root of the nose (Drummond, 1997; Drummond & Lance, 1987), where comparably little muscle activation takes place. Voncken and Bögels (2009) correlated forehead and cheek measures during a blushing reaction: albeit the correlation was found to be moderate in size ($r = .25$), it reached significance; additionally, both measures yielded very similar results in subsequent analyses. According to Drummond (2001), both cheek and forehead measures indeed capture the same blushing mechanism. Reasons for the comparably low correlation may stem from skin differences between forehead and cheek (i.e., opacity, density of blood vessels), slight differences in the temporal course of the blushing reaction in the respective areas, and different angles of sensor attachment and resulting skin reflection. Therefore, to minimize artefact contamination due to muscle innervation, the measurement on the forehead is recommended. Nonetheless, it is still important to keep the subject as passive as possible since even movement of the sensor's cable (especially if fibre-optic cables are used; Vongsavan & Matthews, 1993) can lead to artefacts in the recorded signal. As a result, possible experimental procedures to elicit a blushing response are restricted to passively embarrass the participant in a given situation, which sometimes questions the ecological validity of respective investigations.

Next to problems related to the photoplethysmographic measurement, some issues have to be addressed considering the signal parameterization: we already mentioned the reliability issues concerning the analysis of single values that arise when extracting one maximal value out of a measurement segment. However, even when using mean values, it is crucial to carefully inspect the raw data of the photoplethysmograph's output due to its proneness to artefacts. Since these are not always easily detectable, it may be useful to keep in mind how quickly a signal change can be expected to happen: as arterial blood flow is detected, increases and decreases in signal strength following the pulse frequency of the subject are often visible. Consequently, fast changes in signal intensity which clearly exceed the expected or measured pulse frequency will most likely be artefacts. Additionally to the pulse, the respiration circles are often visible as more or less defined waves at a frequency spectrum of 10–15 Hz. The comparably slow blushing reaction can be seen as the linear trend in the photoplethysmogram that usually reaches its maximum within 10 seconds after the onset of the blush (see Figure 3.1).

Finally, another caveat considering the yielded parameter of the measured blood flow relates to its ipsative nature. It is not possible to analyse meaningful absolute values of facial blood flow due to inter-individual differences in the density and depth of cutaneous vessels and the opacity of the skin, which directly influence photoplethysmographic and flowmetric recordings (Cook, 1974; Drummond & Lance, 1981; Stern, Ray & Davis, 1980). Therefore, it is crucial to control the blood flow parameter for a baseline or otherwise-obtained reference point. These reference points are quite different on an inter-individual level. Nonetheless, the reference points are in most cases simply differentiated from the experimental parameters although it is not yet investigated whether the same *recorded* increase when based on different reference points is indeed equivalent to the same *actual* increase in facial blood flow. In other words, the independence of the signal's slope from its baseline has still to be demonstrated. In addition, not too much is known regarding ceiling and floor effects of facial blood flow although it is quite obvious that a subject with an already red face in the baseline period will most likely not be able to blush as much as someone whose facial blood flow is on a comparably low level during the baseline assessment. However, our own experiences with the pharmacologically induced blushing reaction (also called 'flushing'), which may serve as an indicator of the physiological blushing capabilities of the facial blood vessels using niacin, demonstrated that the intensity of this pharmacologically induced reaction much exceeds the intensity of facial reddening elicited by emotional and/or social stimuli. Nonetheless, to prevent any preexisting emotional blushing effects from contaminating the results, the baseline period should be chosen with great care. Especially when working with patients suffering from fear of blushing and/or social anxiety disorder, the experimenter should carefully consider if the baseline period does indeed serve as a true baseline for all participants and does not entail any characteristics (the presence of other people, anticipatory anxiety, etc.) that might potentially evoke a blushing response in the anxious group.

### Temperature measures

Another attempt to physiologically measure the blushing response is by recording the facial temperature. On first glance, this approach seems very evident since the subjective experience of a blushing reaction consists in noticing an increase in facial or cheek temperature (Bögels & Reith, 1999; Poth & Schandry, 1983). As compared to blood flow measures, temperature recordings are less prone to movement and other artefacts, therefore resulting in a much more stable signal. However, temperature recordings as the only measures of facial blushing are only rarely used (Edelmann & Baker, 2002). More often, facial temperature recordings are incorporated additionally to blood flow measures (Drummond & Lim, 2000; Drummond & Mirco, 2004; Mulkens et al., 1997; Mulkens et al., 1999; Voncken & Bögels, 2009). The most common method to detect physiological temperature changes is the utilization of so-called 'thermistors', which change their resistance according to a given temperature. More specifically, the sensor consists of an electric circuit with an implemented resistor. When the sensor is attached to the skin, the temperature of the resistor will converge on the skin's temperature after a given period and allow for a correlated amount of electricity to pass. Consequently, the intensity of the recorded electric signal varies with the detected temperature and can therefore be used as a direct indicator of skin temperature.

When considering the measurement principle, one important caveat of the temperature measurement for indicating a blushing response is immediately obvious: as compared to blood flow measures, the temperature recording is working with a substantial delay from the actual blushing reaction to the consequent temperature recording (Shearn et al., 1990). For a blushing reaction to be recorded on a temperature-based method, the increase in blood flow has to affect the temperature of the surrounding tissue, which subsequently heightens the temperature of the sensor's resistor. Shearn and colleagues (1990) report roughly five times longer response latencies for the temperature recordings as compared to photoplethysmographic blood flow measures. In absolute terms, the peak temperature was detected 92.2 seconds after the onset of the blushing-eliciting situation whereas the peak blood flow appeared after 18.7 seconds. Additionally, observer judgments of the blushing reaction coincided with peak blood flow but not with peak temperature, indicating again the latency of the temperature recording. This issue is also reflected in the often reported non-significant correlations between blood flow and temperature measures during a blushing reaction (Drummond & Lim, 2000; Shearn et al., 1990, 1992), indicating again the different time course of temperature and blood flow recordings. However, Shearn and colleagues' (1990) notion that others are able to observe a blushing response before the blusher himself or herself can feel the actual temperature change may be an overestimation of the temperature effect latency. Due to the described latencies within the measurement setup and considering that thermoreceptors indicating warmth lie in deeper skin structures beneath the epidermis (i.e., within the upper and middle layer of the corium; Birbaumer & Schmidt, 2010), it is more likely that the rise in facial temperature will be experienced at a time when the epidermis' and thermistor's temperature still has to increase in order to indicate a temperature change on the signal level.

Another surprising issue related to temperature recordings was demonstrated by Schandry and Poth (1983). The authors elicited a blushing response by asking subjects embarrassing questions and recorded the cheek temperature throughout the experiment. For all cases in which a visible blush reaction was detected by the experimenter, the authors calculated mean pre- and post-blushing-eliciting temperature scores. Interestingly, the authors found that subjects with a comparably high pre-blush temperature (34–36°C) were more likely to show a *decrease* in facial temperature after the embarrassing questions, whereas for participants with a low pre-blush temperature (32–34°C), an *increase* in facial temperature occurred more often. A reason for this irritating finding might be that increased facial sweating occurred in the high temperature group, which may have led to evaporation and consequently cooling of the skin's surface. The further implications concerning this problem are clear: on the signal level, the skin's inherent temperature regulation processes are indistinguishable from the effects of a facial blushing response and can consequently lead to contaminated results. Therefore, it is important to choose an experimental procedure in which the temperature can be controlled thoroughly. Additionally, the baseline period should be long enough to allow for proper adjustment of the participant to the given room temperature.

On the other hand, next to the comparably low proneness to artefacts, the advantage of temperature recordings consists in the utilization of absolute values. As long as the sensor is calibrated accurately, absolute temperature units can be reported.

### Other physiological measures of the blushing reaction

**Infrared thermography.** Another approach to measure facial blushing was implemented by Mariauzouls (1996) by using an infrared camera to capture facial temperature differences. In addition to using Doppler flowmetry during a blushing inducing condition, the temperature of the left side of participants' faces was captured and averaged every 10 seconds into a condensed heat image. For the further analyses of the thermal data, difference pictures were generated for each participant in which each pixel of a baseline heat picture was differentiated from a corresponding pixel of a heat picture after the induction of a blushing response. Based on these difference pictures, individual nose and cheek areas were defined for each participant in whom temperature differences were especially pronounced. Subsequently, all pixels within these areas were averaged for each point of measurement, yielding one cheek and one nose temperature value every 10 seconds, which were then used in the statistical analyses. Thermography has one potential advantage over all other measurements: it is able to capture blushing within a large area, not just one specific measuring point. This is clearly a quite relevant advantage since some individuals blush not evenly but rather show a blotchy blushing pattern. However, when compared to direct blood flow data, limitations of thermographical measures lie at hand as well. First, the same disadvantages apply for thermography as they do for any other temperature-based method of measuring facial blushing (i.e., response latency, contamination by thermoregulatory mechanisms). Second, a detailed heat picture which is recorded at an appropriate sample rate needs much more memory capacity as compared to any of the so-far reviewed recording methods. Consequently, it can be difficult or even impossible to obtain both high time resolutions and high picture resolutions for the thermographic data (Mariauzouls, 1996), so that data have to be reduced at the recording level already. Finally, it is unclear whether the distribution of heat follows the pattern of visible redness on the skin.

**Colour analysis of visual recordings.** An intriguing question concerning the blushing response, especially when reviewing its possible communicative functions, consists in the measurement of its visibility.

Some promising approaches in how to capture the skin's colour come from the area of computer graphics (i.e., Vezhnevets *et al.*, 2003; Weyrich *et al.*, 2006), in which researchers try to quantize the colour of the facial skin by parameterizing picture and video material. Weyrich and co-authors (2006) have developed a parameter-based skin reflectance model in order to create graphic faces indistinguishable from real ones. For this reason, they measured real faces' parameters: participants were asked to sit quietly in a 'face-scanning dome' that implemented 16 digital cameras, 150 LED light sources and a 3D face-scanning system in order to capture facial images that were later used for parameter estimation. Although facial colour and other parameters could be obtained with high resolution, this approach is clearly not useful when it comes to the measurement of a blushing reaction: putting aside the unfeasible setup, the measuring process is too slow to reliably measure *changes* in facial colourization, which is a crucial feature when dealing with the facial blush. However, another investigation (Yamada & Watanabe, 2007), albeit methodologically questionable, addressed the issue of measuring facial colour change due to emotion induction. While subjects participated in a neutral and an anger-inducing conversation, their faces were recorded by a digital video camera. From these video recordings, different facial areas were analysed off-line by using the hue saturation value (HSV) colour space expression method. Facial colour change due to the emotion induction was found to especially impact the hue parameter on the cheek and forehead. Although no specific blushing reaction was induced and measured, this investigation is intriguing: given that visibility is a key feature for blushing, the idea of measuring the colour profile of respective skin areas is intuitively appealing (see also Pan *et al.*, 2011). Nonetheless, many questions have to be answered in order to validly measure the colour profile: how big is the impact of movement and resulting differences in light angles and skin reflection on the measurements? Which facial areas should be chosen for the investigation? Can colour parameters, such as hue, saturation and value, actually be treated as interval scaled variables; in other words: are colour measures indeed comparable between participants? Also, a number of technical difficulties have to be considered: most modern video cameras automatically adjust lens and white balance, which may affect the recording of the blush. It would clearly be advantageous for the research on social effects of the blushing response to look into the measurement of its visibility in more depth.

**Facial sweating.** Heinrichs and co-authors (Sansen *et al.*, 2010) misguidedly suggested that facial skin conductance can be used as a valid indicator for a blushing response. Although sweating and blushing rely on mainly sympathetic innervation (Gerlach et al., 2003), facial sweating has not been reported as a commonly co-occurring symptom of blushing (Poth & Schandry, 1983). In addition, the specific mechanism of blushing involves beta-adrenergic vasodilatation (Mellander et al., 1982), indicating that alpha-adrenergic release of sympathetic vasoconstrictor tone, the common pathway to thermoregulation of the skin, does not substantially influence blushing (Drummond, 1997). Note that a recent study demonstrated that localized beta-adrenergic receptor blockade does not affect the sweating response (Buono et al., 2011). In addition, although facial sweating does indeed occur as a reaction to anxiety-provoking situations in some participants (Allen et al., 1973), it has not been investigated yet whether facial sweating is also an inherent part of the physiological response to embarrassment. Furthermore, it may be difficult to disentangle the source of the facial sweating response from thermoregulatory mechanisms (which can also occur after an emotional blushing response; see above) and emotional processes. Taken together, blood flow or temperature measures are much more valid indicators of a facial blushing response.

## Self-report measures of the blushing response

Having reviewed the most important methods regarding the measurement of the facial blush, we will now proceed to describe the two most commonly used questionnaires regarding self-reported blushing: the Blushing Propensity Scale (BPS; Leary & Meadows, 1991) and the Blushing, Trembling and Sweating Questionnaire (BTS-Q; Bögels & Reith, 1999).

### Blushing Propensity Scale

The first instrument that was specifically designed to assess self-reported blushing in various situations is the BPS (Leary & Meadows, 1991). The fourteen-item questionnaire asks for the subjective blushing propensity in various common situations: for example, being introduced to someone unknown. The frequency with which the blush is experienced in the given situation is rated on a 5-point Likert scale (1 = 'I never feel myself blush in this situation'; 5 = 'I always feel myself blush in this situation'). The internal consistency of the instrument was satisfactory (Cronbach's $\alpha = .86$). Also, test-retest reliability after four weeks was high ($r = .81$), indicating the stability of self-reported blushing propensity. A German translation of the questionnaire has similar psychometric properties and is available from the authors (cf. Domschke et al., 2009). The aim of the questionnaire development was to examine differences between self-reported frequent and infrequent blushers. In order to support the communicative theory of blushing (i.e., blushing as a sign of remediation; Castelfranchi & Poggi, 1990), the authors additionally administered several personality and anxiety scales. Given that a blushing response is thought to be closely related to concerns about others' evaluations and also its function as an involuntary display of remediation when one's position in a social group is in jeopardy, the authors hypothesized frequent blushers to be more fearful regarding negative evaluation and also to report higher levels of embarrassability and social anxiousness. Furthermore, blushing propensity should be associated with the importance placed on social relationships. However, while Leary and Meadows could confirm their hypotheses, the question remains whether self-reported blushing propensity can indeed be equated to the physiological blushing propensity.

A questionnaire study conducted by Bögels, Alberts and de Jong (1996) investigated the relationship between blushing propensity, blushing frequency, fear of blushing, attentional focus and self-consciousness. Interestingly, the authors found that the highest correlations with the BPS were with the Social Phobia and Anxiety Inventory (Turner et al., 1989; $r = .63$), with the 'social anxiety' subscale of the Self-Consciousness Scale (Fenigstein et al., 1975; $r = .58$) and with an instrument assessing fear of blushing ($r = .56$). The latter measure had been specifically developed for the aims of the study. To measure the frequency of blushing, participants were asked with one single question how often they had blushed during the past week. The relationship of the blushing frequency and the BPS reached significance ($r = .25$). However, it is small in comparison to the referred correlations of the BPS and social anxiety measures. These results again suggest self-reported blushing propensity to be most closely related to the concept of social anxiety, a finding that other authors have confirmed (e.g., Stevens et al., 2008).

*Blushing, Trembling and Sweating Questionnaire*

To directly examine the relationship between fear of bodily symptoms and social anxiety, Bögels and Reith (1999) developed the BTS-Q, which assesses a wide range of frequently reported physiological symptoms of social anxiety. To validate the newly developed questionnaire, the authors investigated a clinical sample of ninety-two outpatients meeting DSM-IV criteria (American Psychiatric Association, 2000) for social anxiety disorder and sixty-five healthy control participants. A fear of somatic reactions was the main complaint in forty of the ninety-two socially phobic individuals, whereas the remaining fifty-two patients did not fear blushing, trembling and/or sweating predominantly. The BTS-Q consists of six subscales with altogether 115 items, which are all scored by means of visual analogue scales (0–100). The subscales measure (1) the fear of blushing, trembling and sweating; (2) the experience of physical symptoms of blushing, trembling and sweating; (3) avoidance behaviour concerning these symptoms; (4) behavioural problems resulting from these symptoms; (5) beliefs concerning these symptoms; and (6) the frequency with which those symptoms are experienced. The BTS-Q had an overall satisfactory reliability in this sample, ranging from Cronbach's $\alpha = .67$ to $\alpha = .98$. Scores on each of the BTS-Q subscales discriminated patients from control participants. In addition, the 'fear' subscale and, to a smaller extent, the 'avoidance' subscale successfully discriminated social anxiety disorder patients with predominant complaints of bodily symptoms from social anxiety disorder patients without these complaints, whereas responses to the remaining subscales did not differ between these two subgroups. In consequence, the authors proposed that the central maintaining factor of a predominant fear of somatic reactions is primarily avoidance behaviour, whereas cognitive factors, such as negative expectations and beliefs concerning the consequences of displaying bodily symptoms, maintain the psychopathology to a lesser extent.

Due to economic reasons, most studies assessing self-reported fear of blushing apply the six-item BTS-Q 'fear of blushing' subscale only (de Jong & Peters, 2005; Dijk & de Jong, 2009; Drummond et al., 2007; Heinrichs et al., 2006; Mulkens & Bögels, 1999; Mulkens et al., 2001; Mulkens et al., 1999; Zou et al., 2007). Individuals with a mean score of 50 and higher are usually interviewed for a clinical fear of blushing (Heinrichs et al., 2006). Mulkens and colleagues (2001) reported pre-treatment mean scores of a socially phobic patient sample with a fear of blushing as the predominant complaint to be 65.7 for women and 77.0 for men.

## Observational measures of blushing

Observer judgments of a participant's blushing reaction are conducted to establish an indicator of the often feared *visibility* of the blush. As already noted, physiological measures such as blood flow or temperature data provide only an indirect implication of visibility due to inter-individual differences in skin characteristics. Similarly, self-report measures such as the BPS do not allow for direct inferences to the actual visibility of the experienced blushing reaction. However, observational measures of blushing are incorporated only rarely. Reasons for this include the necessary involvement of specifically trained and costly personnel, the current lack of standardized instruments or procedures, and the low reliability and validity of the methodology used so far. The next sections give a brief overview of the observational measures of blushing.

### Naïve observer

Perhaps the least laborious method for incorporating an observational measure of blushing is to ask observers and/or confederates a single question about how much the participant blushed, as was done, for example, by Bögels and Lamers (2002). After an experimental conversation task, the participant, two confederates and four video observers rated the intensity of the participant's blushing on a single visual analogue scale. For the subsequent analyses, difference scores between the participant's self-rating and the combined judges' ratings were used. However, the reliability of the observer-rated blushing scores was low: confederates had an average correlation of $r = .47$ and the video observer ratings correlated at $r = .28$. The authors state that the quality of the videotapes may have been the reason for these especially low correlations.

A similar approach was implemented by de Jong and co-authors (de Jong et al., 2002) who investigated the effects of moral transgressions in dyads. As part of the experimental task, the two participants were asked to rate the blushing response of their counterpart on a single visual analogue scale; consequently, an evaluation of reliability was impossible. Also, Gerlach and colleagues (2001) evaluated blushing with a single question answered by one observer. Mulkens and co-authors also used a single VAS but had two confederates rate the participants' blushing reactions; however, reliabilities were not reported (Mulkens et al., 1997) or were found to be too low for further analyses ($r = .43$ and $r = .56$; Mulkens et al., 1999). Voncken and Bögels (2009) used two observer-rated items to assess the frequency and intensity of the participants' blushing response. These items were rated by four observers. Reported reliabilities are high ($r = .87$); however, it is not clear whether these values pertain to the internal consistency of the two items or to the inter-rater reliability.

In addition to single- or two-item VASs, items regarding observer-rated blushing are part of some broader social performance scales. For example, the item 'How often did the participant blush?' belongs to the 'anxious appearance' subscale of the Social Behaviour and Anxious Appearance rating scale (Voncken & Bögels, 2008). Also, the social skills rating scale developed by Rapee and Lim (1992) incorporates items regarding observer-rated blushing.

In summary, so far researchers have failed to develop a reliable and valid method for naïve observers to rate facial blushing in others. This is somewhat surprising since most people would be able to report that they know people who visibly blush and that they have observed individuals blushing numerous times in their lifetime. However, the problem may be that within a research context, often observations are not made in daylight but rather in artificially lighted research facilities, making it harder to detect visible facial colorations. Also, it may be advantageous to ask observers to indicate blushing whenever they detect it online rather than to ask them after a lengthy period of observation whether a subject had blushed or not. However, abandoning single-item measurements may also result in an increased reliability, although at the same time this may require a substantial increase of effort.

*Coloration comparison*

Only one study to date has assessed the blushing response by coloration comparison: to determine whether the peak blood flow or the peak temperature was more related to the visible blushing reaction, Shearn and colleagues (1990) gave observers pairs of three-second facial video segments that were taken before and during a blushing-eliciting task. In each of the pairs, one specific participant was shown during baseline and during the previously determined peak of blushing reaction, which was either the peak of the blood flow reaction or the peak of the temperature reaction. Observers were then asked to choose the video segment in which the participant was blushing more, yielding a dichotomous answering format. All twelve observers rated the blushing reaction of all participants; however, inter-rater reliabilities were not reported.

Potentially, this approach could be adapted for the aim of a *dimensional* rating, so that inter-individual differences between blushing reactions could be ranked. However, mathematically, this would involve pairing each participant's blushing reaction with every other one, quickly yielding an unfeasible number of comparisons. Although at first glance the approach of coloration comparison seems to enable a more valid judgment of a blushing reaction as compared to the naïve observer ratings, feasibility and validity problems are indeed difficult to solve.

## Conclusion

Although the number of articles focusing on blushing is still small, the breadth of methods developed to measure the blush is impressive. In this chapter, we have described methods to measure blushing physiologically, by self-report, using standardized questionnaires and through observation. We strongly believe that it is worthwhile to attempt to measure blushing covering at least the three different reaction systems whenever studying this interesting and, arguably, 'most human' of all emotional reactions. We hope our review will guide the readers of this chapter when having to choose what measures to use in their own research.

REFERENCES

Allen, J. A., Armstrong, J. E., & Roddie, I. C. (1973). The regional distribution of emotional sweating in man. *Journal of Physiology*, 235(3), 749–59.

American Psychiatric Association (2000). *Diagnostic and statistical manual of mental disorders*, 4th edn, text rev. Washington, DC: American Psychiatric Association.

Birbaumer, N., & Schmidt, R. F. (2010). *Biologische psychologie*, 7th edn. Heidelberg: Springer.

Bögels, S. M., Alberts, M., & de Jong, P. J. (1996). Self-consciousness, self-focused attention, blushing propensity and fear of blushing. *Personality and Individual Differences*, 21(4), 573–81.

Bögels, S. M., & Lamers, C. T. J. (2002). The causal role of self-awareness in blushing-anxious, socially-anxious and social phobics individuals. *Behaviour Research and Therapy*, 40(12), 1367–84.

Bögels, S. M., & Reith, W. (1999). Validity of two questionnaires to assess social fears: The Dutch Social Phobia and Anxiety Inventory and the Blushing, Trembling and Sweating Questionnaire. *Journal of Psychopathology and Behavioral Assessment*, 21(1), 51–66.

Bögels, S. M., Rijsemus, W., & de Jong, P. J. (2002). Self-focused attention and social anxiety: the effects of experimentally heightened self-awareness on fear, blushing, cognitions, and social skills. *Cognitive Therapy and Research*, 26(4), 461–72.

Buono, M. J., Tabor, B., & White, A. (2011). Localized beta-adrenergic receptor blockade does not affect sweating during exercise. *American Journal of Physiology – Regulatory Integrative and Comparative Physiology*, 300(5), R1148–51.

Castelfranchi, C., & Poggi, I. (1990). Blushing as a discourse: was Darwin wrong? In W. R. Crozier (Ed.), *Shyness and embarrassment: perspectives from social psychology*. Cambridge University Press, 230–51.

Challoner, A. V., & Ramsay, C. A. (1974). A photoelectric plethysmograph for the measurement of cutaneous blood flow. *Physics in Medicine and Biology*, 19(3), 317–28.

Chen, V., & Drummond, P. D. (2008). Fear of negative evaluation augments negative affect and somatic symptoms in social-evaluative situations. *Cognition and Emotion*, 22(1), 21–43.

Cook, M. R. (1974). Psychophysiology of peripheral vascular changes. In P. A. Obrist, A. H. Black, J. Brener, & L. V. DiCara (Eds.), *Cardiovascular* psychophysiology: current issues in response mechanisms, biofeedback and methodology. Chicago: Aldine, 60–84.

de Jong, P. J., & Peters, M. L. (2005). Do blushing phobics overestimate the undesirable communicative effects of their blushing? *Behaviour Research and Therapy*, **43**(6), 747–58.

de Jong, P. J., Peters, M., De Cremer, D., & Vranken, C. (2002). Blushing after a moral transgression in a prisoner's dilemma game: appeasing or revealing? *European Journal of Social Psychology*, **32**(5), 627–44.

Dijk, C., & de Jong, P. J. (2009). Fear of blushing: no overestimation of negative anticipated interpersonal effects, but a high-subjective probability of blushing. *Cognitive Therapy and Research*, **33**(1), 59–74.

Dijk, C., Voncken, M. J., & de Jong, P. J. (2009). I blush, therefore I will be judged negatively: influence of false blush feedback on anticipated others' judgments and facial coloration in high and low blushing-fearfuls. *Behaviour Research and Therapy*, **47**(7), 541–7.

Domschke, K., Stevens, S., Beck, B., Baffa, A., Hohoff, C., Deckert, J., & Gerlach, A. L. (2009). Blushing propensity in social anxiety disorder: influence of serotonin transporter gene variation. *Journal of Neural Transmission*, **116**(6), 663–6.

Drummond, P. D. (1997). The effect of adrenergic blockade on blushing and facial flushing. *Psychophysiology*, **34**(2), 163–8.

(1999). Facial flushing during provocation in women. *Psychophysiology*, **36**(3), 325–32.

(2001). The effect of true and false feedback on blushing in women. *Personality and Individual Differences*, **30**(8), 1329–43.

Drummond, P. D., Back, K., Harrison, J., Helgadottir, F. D., Lange, B., Lee, C., Leavy, K., Novatscou, C., Orner, A., Pham, H., Prance, J., Radford, D., & Wheatley, L. (2007). Blushing during social interactions in people with a fear of blushing. *Behaviour Research and Therapy*, **45**(7), 1601–8.

Drummond, P. D., Camacho, L., Formentin, N., Heffeman, T. D., Williams, F., & Zekas, T. E. (2003). The impact of verbal feedback about blushing on social discomfort and facial blood flow during embarrassing tasks. *Behaviour Research and Therapy*, **41**(4), 413–25.

Drummond, P. D., & Lance, J. W. (1981). Extra-cranial vascular reactivity in migraine and tension headache. *Cephalalgia*, **1**(3), 149–55.

(1987). Facial flushing and sweating mediated by the sympathetic nervous-system. *Brain*, **110**, 793–803.

Drummond, P. D., & Lim, H. K. (2000). The significance of blushing for fair- and dark-skinned people. *Personality and Individual Differences*, **29**(6), 1123–32.

Drummond, P. D., & Mirco, N. (2004). Staring at one side of the face increases blood flow on that side of the face. *Psychophysiology*, **41**(2), 281–7.

Edelmann, R. J., & Baker, S. R. (2002). Self-reported and actual physiological responses in social phobia. *British Journal of Clinical Psychology*, **41**, 1–14.

Fenigstein, A., Scheier, M. F., & Buss, A. H. (1975). Public and private self-consciousness: assessment and theory. *Journal of Consulting and Clinical Psychology*, **43**(4), 522–7.

Gerlach, A. L. (1998). *Blushing, embarrassment, and social phobia: physiological, behavioral and self-report assessment (dissertation Universität Marburg)*: Tectum Verlag Marburg, Edition Wissenschaft, Unterreihe Psychologie, Band 48.

Gerlach, A. L., Wilhelm, F. H., Gruber, K., & Roth, W. T. (2001). Blushing and physiological arousability in social phobia. *Journal of Abnormal Psychology*, 110(2), 247–58.

Gerlach, A. L., Wilhelm, F. H., & Roth, W. T. (2003). Embarrassment and social phobia: the role of parasympathetic activation. *Journal of Anxiety Disorders*, 17(2), 197–210.

Heinrichs, N., Rapee, R. M., Alden, L. E., Bögels, S., Hofmann, S. G., Oh, K. J., & Sakano, Y. (2006). Cultural differences in perceived social norms and social anxiety. *Behaviour Research and Therapy*, 44(8), 1187–97.

Hertzman, A. B. (1938). The blood supply of various skin areas as estimated by the photoelectric plethysmograph. *American Journal of Physiology*, 124, 323–40.

Hofmann, S. G., Moscovitch, D. A., & Kim, H. J. (2006). Autonomic correlates of social anxiety and embarrassment in shy and non-shy individuals. *International Journal of Psychophysiology*, 61(2), 134–42.

Hugdahl, K. (1981). The three-systems-model of fear and emotion – a critical examination. *Behaviour Research and Therapy*, 19(1), 75–85.

Katzman, M., Cornacchi, S., Coonerty-Femiano, A., Hughes, B., Vermani, M., Struzik, L., & Ross, B. M. (2003). Methyl nicotinate-induced vasodilation in generalized social phobia. *Neuropsychopharmacology*, 28(10), 1846–51.

Lang, P. J. (1993). *The three-systems approach to emotion*. Seattle: Hogrefe & Huber Publishers.

Lang, P. J., Levin, D. N., Miller, G. A., & Kozak, M. J. (1983). Fear behavior, fear imagery, and the psychophysiology of emotion – the problem of affective response integration. *Journal of Abnormal Psychology*, 92(3), 276–306.

Leary, M. R., & Meadows, S. (1991). Predictors, elicitors, and concomitants of social blushing. *Journal of Personality and Social Psychology*, 60(2), 254–62.

Mariauzouls, C. (1996). *Psychophysiologie von Scham und Erröten*. Munich: Ludwig-Maximilians-Universität München.

Mellander, S., Andersson, P. O., Afzelius, L. E., & Hellstrand, P. (1982). Neural beta-adrenergic dilatation of the facial vein in man: possible mechanism in emotional blushing. *Acta Physiologica Scandinavica*, 114(3), 393–9.

Mulkens, S., & Bögels, S. M. (1999). Learning history in fear of blushing. *Behaviour Research and Therapy*, 37(12), 1159–67.

Mulkens, S., Bögels, S. M., de Jong, P. J., & Louwers, J. (2001). Fear of blushing: effects of task concentration training versus exposure in vivo on fear and physiology. *Journal of Anxiety Disorders*, 15(5), 413–32.

Mulkens, S., de Jong, P. J., & Bögels, S. M. (1997). High blushing propensity: fearful preoccupation or facial coloration? *Personality and Individual Differences*, 22(6), 817–24.

Mulkens, S., de Jong, P. J., Dobbelaar, A., & Bögels, S. M. (1999). Fear of blushing: fearful preoccupation irrespective of facial coloration. *Behaviour Research and Therapy*, 37(11), 1119–28.

Nijboer, J. A., Dorlas, J. C., & Mahieu, H. F. (1981). Photoelectric plethysmography – some fundamental aspects of the reflection and transmission method. *Clinical Physics and Physiological Measurement*, 2(3), 205–15.

Pan, X., Banakou, D., & Slater, M. (2011). Computer based video and virtual environments in the study of the role of emotions in moral behavior. *Affective Computing and Intelligent Interaction*, 6975/2011, 52–61.

Poth, E., & Schandry, R. (1983). On the psychology and physiology of blushing – a review of pertinent literature. *Psychologische Beiträge*, 25(3–4), 494–502.

Rapee, R. M., & Lim, L. (1992). Discrepancy between self and observer ratings of performance in social phobics. *Journal of Abnormal Psychology*, 101(4), 728–31.

Sansen, L., Geuter, J., Reinhold, N., & Heinrichs, N. (2010). Kinder und Jugendliche in Bewertungssituationen: welche Reaktionen erwarten sie und welche zeigen sie? *Verhaltenstherapie mit Kindern und Jugendlichen*, 6, 17–29.

Schandry, R., & Poth, E. (1983). Eine experimentelle Untersuchung zur Psychologie und Physiologie des Errötens. *Psychologische Beiträge*, 25, 503–14.

Shearn, D., Bergman, E., Hill, K., Abel, A., & Hinds, L. (1990). Facial coloration and temperature responses in blushing. *Psychophysiology*, 27(6), 687–93.

(1992). Blushing as a function of audience size. *Psychophysiology*, 29(4), 431–6.

Stern, R. M., Ray, W. J., & Davis, C. M. (1980). *Psychophysiological recording*. Oxford University Press.

Stevens, S., Gerlach, A. L., & Rist, F. (2008). Effects of alcohol on ratings of emotional facial expressions in social phobics. *Journal of Anxiety Disorders*, 22(6), 940–8.

Turner, S. M., Beidel, D. C., Dancu, C. V., & Stanley, M. A. (1989). An empirically derived inventory to measure social fears and anxiety: the social phobia and anxiety inventory. *Psychological Assessment: A Journal of Consulting and Clinical Psychology*, 1(1), 35–40.

Vezhnevets, V., Sazonov, V., & Andreeva, A. (2003). A survey on pixel-based skin color detection techniques. In Proceedings of the 13th International Conference of Computer Graphics and Visualization Graphicon, Moscow, 27–9 May (pp. 85–92).

Voncken, M. J., & Bögels, S. M. (2008). Social performance deficits in social anxiety disorder: reality during conversation and biased perception during speech. *Journal of Anxiety Disorders*, 22(8), 1384–92.

(2009). Physiological blushing in social anxiety disorder patients with and without blushing complaints: two subtypes? *Biological Psychology*, 81(2), 86–94.

Vongsavan, N., & Matthews, B. (1993). Some aspects of the use of laser Doppler flow meters for recording tissue blood-flow. *Experimental Physiology*, 78(1), 1–14.

Weinman, J. (1967). Photoplethysmography. In P. H. Venables & I. Martin (Eds.), *A manual of psychophysiological methods*. Amsterdam: North-Holland, 185–217.

Weyrich, T., Matusik, W., Pfister, H., Bickel, B., Donner, C., Tu, C., McAndless, J., Lee, J., Ngan, A., Jensen, H. W., & Gross, M. (2006). Analysis of human faces using a measurement-based skin reflectance model. *ACM Transactions on Graphics*, **25**(3), 1013–24.

Yamada, T., & Watanabe, T. (2007). Virtual facial image synthesis with facial color enhancement and expression under emotional change of anger. Paper presented at the 16th IEEE International Conference on Robot & Human Interactive Communication, Korea, 26–9 August.

Zou, J. B., Hudson, J. L., & Rapee, R. M. (2007). The effect of attentional focus on social anxiety. *Behaviour Research and Therapy*, **45**(10), 2326–33.

*Part II*

Theoretical perspectives on the blush

# 4 Psychological theories of blushing

*Mark R. Leary and Kaitlin Toner*

Blushing is the uncontrollable experience of warmth, usually accompanied by reddening of the skin, on the face, neck, ears and upper chest that people sometimes experience in reaction to real or perceived evaluation or social attention. Physiologically, blushing reflects the vasodilatation of cutaneous blood vessels in the blush region. Dilation of these vessels causes an increase in blood volume in the affected area, which is experienced subjectively as warmth in the blush region and often perceived by others as a reddening or darkening of the skin, assuming that the individual's skin tone is light enough to allow the blush to be seen (Edelmann, 1987). Dark-skinned people – such as Blacks and Indians – show the same physiological responses when blushing as Whites but report that others often do not notice their blushing (Drummond & Lim, 2000; Simon & Shields, 1996).

In addition to these physical sensations, blushing is typically accompanied by a sense of self-consciousness or conspicuousness, as well as by emotions such as social anxiety, embarrassment, shame or fear, as might happen following a transgression or violation of social norms. However, not all emotional reactions that accompany blushing are negative. People may also blush while experiencing happiness or gratitude, such as when receiving a compliment or public recognition. Therefore, blushing cannot be tied exclusively to any particular emotion or even one valence of emotion. Rather, blushing seems to be experienced alongside a range of emotional reactions that are associated with social evaluation and self-consciousness.

Many of the first attempts to explain why people blush were couched in psychoanalytic terms (for a review, see Karch, 1971). Explanations for blushing that emerge from psychodynamic ideas point to a variety of presumed causes, including repressed incestual urges, shame conversion, exhibitionism, fear of castration, and unconscious hostility, but all such explanations incorporate some sort of inhibition of libidinal or aggressive desires (Karch, 1971; Leary *et al.*, 1992). For example, one explanation proposed that unacceptable sexual urges may cause blood to be shunted from the genital area to the face, thereby allowing a safe expression of the repressed desires. Similarly, blushes caused by unacceptable aggressive urges were theorized to result from a diversion of blood to the face in an imitation of red-faced rage.

Despite the efforts of psychoanalytic theorists to understand blushing, these theories have little empirical support and ignore numerous situations in which people blush that do not appear to involve sex or aggression. As a result of these conceptual and empirical difficulties, psychodynamic approaches have had virtually no impact on contemporary research on blushing. More recently, however, behavioural scientists operating from other perspectives have offered alternative explanations. In this chapter, we review and critique three major theoretical analyses of blushing that have dominated modern discussions of blushing – the remedial, undesired social attention, and exposure theories.

## Communicative and remedial theories

Most explanations of blushing make reference to people's concerns with others' evaluations of them. This perspective can be traced to Darwin (1872/1955), who viewed blushing as the result of concern with other people's appraisals. According to Darwin, 'thinking of what others think of us' causes the blush (p. 325). Interestingly, the father of evolutionary theory believed that blushing serves no useful function. Darwin wrote that blushing 'makes the blusher suffer and the beholder uncomfortable, without being of the least service to either of them' (p. 336). Instead, he viewed blushing as a by-product of self-directed attention, suggesting that focusing attention on any part of the body increases the blood flow to that part. Browne (1983) provided an excellent analysis of Darwin's view of blushing and its relationship to evolutionary theory.

Like Darwin, many contemporary theorists have suggested that blushing is a reaction to social evaluation. For example, Harris (1990) suggested that blushing arises from a state of acute negative public self-attention in which people are aware that they are projecting an image of themselves that is discrepant from their 'presumed or desired self-image' (p. 68). However, unlike Darwin, most contemporary theorists have suggested that blushing does serve an important function. Even before Darwin, Burgess (1839) proposed that blushing is a signal to other people that the individual recognizes that he or she has 'transgressed or violated those rules which should be held sacred' (p. 156). Along the same lines, MacCurdy (1930) suggested that blushing indicates that the person knows that he or she has violated particular social values and desires to be forgiven for the infraction, and Karch (1971) regarded blushing as a way in which people communicate that they are concerned that their image in other people's eyes has been lowered or damaged.

Castelfranchi and Poggi's (1990) seminal chapter on blushing conveyed this remedial view of blushing explicitly and stimulated a good deal of research on the communicative aspects of blushing. They wrote that people 'who are blushing are somehow saying that they know, care about and fear others' evaluations, and that they share those values deeply; they also communicate their sorrow over any possible faults or inadequacies on their part, thus performing an acknowledgement, a confession, and an apology aimed at inhibiting others' aggression or avoiding social ostracism' (p. 240). In contrast, people who fail to blush or otherwise appear distressed after breaking rules, behaving in inept or immoral ways, or performing other undesirable behaviours convey either that such actions are not unusual for them or that they are indifferent to the transgressions and other people's evaluations of them. Appearing distressed and contrite, however, conveys that the transgression is unusual, acknowledges that one supports social and moral rules, and shows that the person cares about other people's judgments.

Castelfranchi and Poggi (1990) also suggested that the involuntary nature of blushing is central to its remedial function. They noted that most face-saving behaviours that people use to repair a damaged social image – such as excuses, justifications and apologies – can be enacted deliberately, opening the possibility that people can pretend to be sorry for norm violations or other undesirable behaviours. In contrast, blushing cannot be faked. As a result, observers seem to regard it as a more authentic indicator of remorse or regret than verbal claims. Because it cannot be voluntarily produced, blushing unambiguously conveys that the person is sorry for whatever transpired and seeks others' forgiveness. In fact, because blushing can be elicited nonconsciously, other people may notice a blush before the blusher is aware of it. Research has shown that the facial coloration of blushing occurs a few seconds before the increase in cheek temperature is noticeable by the blusher (Shearn *et al.*, 1990).

The remedial function of blushing and other obvious signs of embarrassment or shame has been demonstrated in several studies. Specifically, blushing and other signs of social discomfiture (such as downcast eyes and nervous smiling) attenuate other people's negative reactions to misbehaviours, presumably because it signifies that the person recognizes that he or she has behaved inappropriately and regrets his or her actions. In this sense, blushing operates much like a nonverbal apology in which the person accepts responsibility for the undesired behaviour and asks others for forgiveness. This symbolic element of blushing extends beyond strictly human-to-human interactions: blushing also helps people to recognize shame in nonhuman computer avatars (de Melo et al., 2010).

In many cases, blushing leads others to forgive socially undesirable behaviours. Observers perceive people who blush after obvious transgressions as more sympathetic, trustworthy and socially skilled than people who do not blush after violating norms (Dijk, de Jong et al., 2009). These positive perceptions of blushers are found even in the absence of other nonverbal displays of embarrassment or shame (de Jong, 1999; Dijk, de Jong et al., 2009).

Interestingly, people seem to have an understanding that blushing and other expressions of embarrassment can repair their social image. Leary, Landel and Patton (1996) reasoned that people who are not perceived as embarrassed after behaving ineptly will want to convey their embarrassment to other people in alternative ways, whereas those who are obviously embarrassed will feel no need to do so. They led participants who had performed an embarrassing task to believe that the researcher did or did not know that they were embarrassed. Participants subsequently expressed greater embarrassment if the researcher did not already know that they were embarrassed than if she was aware of their embarrassment. In a second study, participants who thought that the researcher did not interpret their blushing as a sign of embarrassment presented themselves more positively to the researcher than participants who thought the researcher knew that they had blushed. Participants who were not perceived as blushing seemed to know that they needed to project a more favourable impression in some other way.

However, blushing does not always improve observers' impressions of the blusher. Whereas blushing seems to have remedial effects following an obvious transgression, it can backfire in ambiguous situations. When the person's responsibility for the undesired behaviour is not clear or when the severity of the infraction is in question, blushers are perceived to be less trustworthy than non-blushers (de Jong et al., 2003). This effect may occur because, in the absence of clear evidence linking the person to negative intentions or consequences, other people may interpret blushing as a sign of the person's guilt, whereas a non-blusher may be seen as innocent (de Jong et al., 2002).

For this reason, people probably do not want to be seen as blushing if they have not obviously behaved in an undesirable fashion. In the absence of a clear-cut predicament, others may interpret signs of embarrassment, including blushing, as evidence that the person has behaved in an undesirable manner. For example, people who are teased about private thoughts or actions may wish to conceal their embarrassment because it might appear to substantiate others' accusations. Because blushing implies that one has done something undesirable, merely being accused of blushing can cause people to blush, even if they were not blushing before the accusation. In short, people may wish for others to see them blush when they have performed a transgression but not when personal information has been exposed or when they are receiving negative attention (see Dijk & de Jong, 2009).

These potential negative implications of blushing may also explain why some people develop a pathological fear of blushing. People with a fear of blushing tend to overestimate the extent to which ambiguous mishaps are viewed as intentional, so their fear of blushing may be due to an assumption that other people will infer malicious intent from a blush (de Jong & Peters, 2005). Furthermore, people who fear blushing also rate the social costs of blushing higher (Dijk *et al.*, 2010; cf. de Jong *et al.*, 2006). Research also shows that people from collectivistic countries, which have stricter rules about appropriate social behaviour, report greater fear of blushing than people from individualistic countries, possibly because the ramifications of being viewed as guilty are greater (Heinrichs *et al.*, 2006). Together, this evidence suggests that blushing may serve a remedial function only when people have explicitly damaged their images. However, in the absence of a social predicament, blushing may cue observers to the possibility that the person has done something undesirable that they would not otherwise have detected.

People who fear blushing compound their anxiety by overestimating the degree to which they are blushing and the degree to which other people notice it (Dijk, Voncken *et al.*, 2009; Drummond, 2001). Blushing in reaction to accusations of blushing seems to happen most to people who have a higher general propensity to blush (Drummond *et al.*, 2003), possibly because they assume that blushing makes them appear guilty or because they have a stronger reaction to social attention. In either case, people with a fear of blushing may ironically blush in response to blushing! Along these lines, research shows that people who score high versus low in fear of blushing have similar onsets of blushing, but people with high fear of blushing have longer episodes (Drummond *et al.*, 2007).

As the most popular explanation of blushing, remedial theory has a good deal of support. Blushing tends to occur in situations in which people believe that they have conveyed an undesired impression of themselves to other people, and showing that one is embarrassed in such situations often improves the person's image. Furthermore, people seem to be aware that blushing can repair their public image and thus they resort to other face-work tactics when those who have witnessed their inept behaviour appear not to realize that they have blushed.

However, two facts are inconsistent with the remedial approach. First, in instances in which it is not otherwise obvious to others that the person has behaved in an undesirable way, blushing can convey culpability. Thus, blushing can damage rather than improve a person's image in the absence of an obvious misbehaviour. Second, the remedial approach does not easily account for instances in which people blush in the absence of a self-presentational predicament and particularly when other people clearly regard the person quite positively, as when people are complimented, receive special recognition or are singled out for their achievements.

## Undesired social attention theory

Although research evidence is mostly consistent with the notion that blushing can repair a person's image under certain circumstances, the remedial theory does not account easily for all instances in which people blush. In particular, positive attention can cause people to blush, as can merely being scrutinized. Furthermore, people do not blush every time they are worried about what others are thinking of them. Most situations in which people are concerned about others' impressions of them elicit social anxiety but not blushing (Leary & Kowalski, 1990), raising the question of why image-damaging events elicit blushing only occasionally.

To address the fact that remedial theory does not easily explain all blush-inducing situations or explain why some situations do not cause blushing when image repair is needed, Leary and colleagues (1992) proposed that blushing results not from a damaged social image but rather from undesired attention from other people, whether the undesired attention is associated with making a negative, positive or even neutral impression.

Although people often find attention from other people rewarding, under some circumstances being the focus of others' attention is not desired. For example, when people are worried that others are evaluating them negatively – and particularly when they have behaved in ways that others may view as incompetent, immoral or otherwise undesirable – they understandably find social attention discomfiting. According to the undesired attention theory, people do not blush in such situations because they have made a negative impression per se but rather because they are receiving undesired social attention.

Even when they are not projecting an undesired impression, people may find the attention they are receiving to be too intense: for example, because they are the object of many people's attention, observers are scrutinizing them very closely, or the attention lasts longer than feels comfortable. Along these lines, Shearn, Bergman, Hill and Abel (1992) found that blushing intensity was higher the greater the number of observers. And, although being complimented briefly might be desired, overwrought praise that goes on for too long might make the person blush, which may explain why overpraise more reliably induces blushing than a small amount of praise. When one regards the content, intensity and manner of praise as appropriate, the accompanying social attention is likely to be desired, and blushing is unlikely to occur. Furthermore, people sometimes overestimate the amount of attention that they are receiving from others. People sometimes experience a spotlight effect by which they think that other people are attending to their behaviour and appearance even when they are not (Gilovich et al., 2000). The spotlight effect may lead people to experience undesired social attention even when others are not paying much attention to them.

In the case of negative attention, undesired social attention theory and remedial theory make essentially the same predictions. However, undesired social attention theory more easily explains the effects of positive attention (e.g., compliments, praise and recognition) and even neutral attention (being visually scrutinized or stared at) than remedial theory. Certainly, one could argue that positive attention can trigger concerns about one's image when people worry that their reactions will create an undesirable impression if they react to the positive event incompetently or in a way that makes them seem conceited or smug. However, in our view, such an explanation must be stretched in many instances, such as when people blush as their friends sing 'Happy Birthday' or when they are lauded at their retirement dinner. We need not assume that praise necessarily raises concerns about one's social image. Rather, people sometimes regard the social attention that accompanies the praise as excessive and undesired even when they appreciate the accolades.

The undesired social attention theory also explains the effects of scrutiny and staring on blushing. According to the theory, excessive scrutiny and staring are often undesired, thereby triggering blushing. Research shows that intense visual attention, such as a fixed stare, is often intrinsically aversive and leads the target to want to escape the other's gaze (Ellsworth & Carlsmith, 1968, 1973; Ellsworth et al., 1972). Supporting this explanation, having strangers stare at one side of an actor's face results in increased blood flow to that side of the face (Drummond & Mirco, 2004). This staring-elicited blushing occurred regardless of whether the actor was performing an embarrassing or non-embarrassing task. Thus, blushing seemed to be caused by undesired attention rather than embarrassment. Of course, when social attention is desired, as when lovers look into one another's eyes for long periods of time, a steady gaze can induce pleasant emotions that are not accompanied by blushing (Argyle, 1967).

Blushing tends to be accompanied by other behaviours that also reflect reactions to undesired attention. For example, people who are blushing often desire to leave the situation or at least to withdraw socially while remaining physically present. In particular, they may lower their gaze to avoid eye contact with those who are giving them excessive attention, which may reflect a desire to disaffiliate and increase social distance (Exline & Winters, 1965). They may also hang their heads and engage in other acts of 'concealment' (see MacCurdy, 1930; Schneider, 1977).

Young children show gaze aversion in such situations starting at about 18 months of age (Lewis et al., 1991; Lewis et al., 1989). In one study, 2-year-old children showed gaze aversion when they danced in front of other people as well as when they were overpraised (Lewis et al., 1991, Study 2). Although the authors interpreted these effects in terms of embarrassment, they are also easily explained in terms of undesired social attention. There is a point in development – around 18 months – at which children begin to respond to excessive attention with blushing and gaze aversion.

Some writers have recommended that researchers 'assume that blushing means embarrassment even when the person refuses to admit it' (Buss, 1980, p. 238). However, if we disentangle the effects of making a negative impression from the effects of undesired social attention, it should be possible for people to blush in the absence of embarrassment. Embarrassment should occur only when people believe that others have formed an undesired impression of them (Goffman, 1959; Miller, 1986), but they should blush from undesired social attention regardless of its valence. Indeed, Leary and Meadows (1991) found that self-reported embarrassment was associated with only one variety of blush-inducing situation – those that involved self-presentational predicaments – and not with situations that did not involve damage to people's public impressions.

Presumably, blushing evolved as a social signal. As noted earlier, the remedial approaches assume that blushing communicates acknowledgment and regret about one's undesired behaviour. But what might blushing do with respect to undesired social attention? Although no direct evidence exists relevant to this point, Leary and colleagues (1992) suggested that blushing diverts others' attention from the blushing individual. Observers appear to be uncomfortable when looking at a person who is blushing and often break their gaze, change the topic or even help the blusher regain his or her composure. In some situations, observers may even empathically blush themselves (Shearn et al., 1999).

Overall, undesired social attention theory does a reasonably good job of accounting for situations in which people blush. People may blush when they receive excessive or undesired attention from other people, whether that attention is negative, positive or neutral. Furthermore, anecdotally, blushing seems to lead observers to decrease their attention to the blusher (unless they are intentionally trying to be cruel).

### Exposure theory

Exposure theory proposes that people blush when something that they desire to keep private is uncovered or threatened to be uncovered (Crozier, 2000, 2004, 2010; see also Crozier, Chapter 11, this volume). Unlike remedial theory and undesired social attention theory, exposure theory does not present blushing as having a communicative function but instead regards blushing as a reaction to the exposure of private, secret or taboo information. According to Crozier (2000), an event will elicit blushing when it 'brings into the open, or threatens to bring into the open' a topic that the person 'wishes to keep hidden or believes ought to be kept hidden' (p. 157). Importantly, the disclosed information need not be about the individual. People may blush when private information about others is revealed as well. For example, people may blush when another person recounts private details that the listener thinks should not be disclosed or when they accidentally see another person naked.

According to exposure theory, instances of blushing previously theorized to be caused by situations that damage people's public impressions are due instead to the revelation of private information: for example, regarding one's ineptitude or moral transgressions. Likewise, instances in which positive attention causes blushing (such as public praise) are due to the exposure of private thoughts, drawing into the open personal qualities that modesty dictates should be concealed (Crozier, 2001).

But why should merely imagining that information may be revealed cause blushing? One possibility is that people often believe (or at least fear) that other people are able to ascertain their secret thoughts. Research on the illusion of transparency shows that people overestimate the degree to which other people can understand their inner thoughts (Gilovich et al., 1998). Thus, people may worry about exposure of their unrevealed secrets partly because they believe that other people might already have an inkling of them. Exposure theory would predict that people who are prone to the illusion of transparency should be particularly likely to blush.

Exposure theory helps to explain some previously unaddressed instances of blushing. For example, people may blush when merely thinking a private and personal thought while in public even if no one else is privy to it if they want the thought to remain hidden. Crozier (2000) offered the example of a pregnant woman who wishes to keep her pregnancy a secret but involuntarily blushes when surrounded by other women who are talking about babies. One can also imagine an adolescent girl blushing when her friends are talking about a boy on whom she has a secret crush. In such cases, thinking a secret thought in a public venue can cause blushing even though the person has neither behaved in an undesired way nor is the target of undesired social attention.

Blushing in such situations seems to lack a useful interpersonal function. The person fervently desires that the secret thought remain hidden, yet the blush itself can potentially cue people into the blusher's secret and also lead the blusher to behave awkwardly during ongoing interactions. Blushing in such instances is certainly not remedial because no self-presentational predicament has occurred and, at least in Crozier's example, others would likely greet the news of the woman's pregnancy positively. And, contrary to undesired social attention theory, the blush does not deflect social attention and, in fact, might increase it.

Exposure theory appears to explain aspects of blushing quite well. Many instances in which people blush involve disclosure of things that they wish to conceal, whether those things are undesirable characteristics, shameful secrets, private body parts, or even positive but personal information. In the case of positive attention, people may certainly be concerned that their private thoughts – of self-satisfaction, dislike of receiving the attention, or pleasure at receiving acclaim instead of someone else – may be apparent to onlookers. Exposure theory explains instances of blushing that precede real or potential social attention in which private information might be revealed better than the remedial or undesired attention theories. Whether it also accounts better for other categories of factors that induce blushing, many of which also involve the exposure of private or taboo information, remains an open question.

The theory has difficulty explaining why people blush when purposefully disclosing positive information about themselves. For example, if the woman decided that she wanted to tell her friends that she was pregnant, we can imagine that she might blush while revealing the happy secret and receiving congratulations from the group.

Perhaps the biggest challenge for exposure theory involves explaining how this reaction evolved. People do not need to blush to know that they wish something to remain private, so it seems unlikely that blushing serves a private cuing or regulatory function. And, as noted, blushing often works against the best interests of a person who wishes to conceal some piece of private information. According to exposure theory

(Crozier, 2000), blushing communicates that the blusher recognizes that exposure of private information has occurred. Even when people are merely observers of a private action or secret revelation, blushing acknowledges that, in their view, the information should not have been revealed. But this cannot explain why people blush when information is entirely private or when they desire to reveal private information. Of course, not all aspects of human nature are functional, but most universal emotions and emotional displays appear to serve some personal or interpersonal function for the person.

## Overview and future directions

Each of the three modern theories of blushing – remedial, undesired social attention, and exposure – explains certain instances of blushing quite well but other instances only with difficulty. Remedial theory can account for blushing in response to events that damage people's social images and explains the interpersonal functions of blushing, but is less convincing when dealing with instances in which positive evaluations, mere scrutiny and private thoughts cause blushing. Undesired social attention theory can explain the effects of both negative and positive attention (when it is excessive and thus undesired) as well as mere scrutiny and staring, and offers a function of blushing in terms of diverting others' attention. But, it also does not easily explain why private thoughts that one wishes to conceal might lead to blushing. Exposure theory can explain a wide range of blush-inducing situations in which private information – whether undesirable or desirable information – that the person wishes not to disclose is either revealed or threatened to be revealed, and it can explain why secret knowledge can cause blushing when the possibility of disclosure is salient. However, exposure theory has more difficulty explaining why people blush when purposefully revealing positive information, and it does not easily explain why the capacity for blushing evolved in the first place.

Admittedly, each theory can be extended to cover the instances of blushing that seem to fall outside its range. For example, remedial theory can maintain that positive situations can create self-presentational predicaments and that even private thoughts can lead people to simulate mentally what might happen if the secret information were revealed. Similarly, undesired social attention theory could claim that people worry that revelation of private thoughts would elicit undesired attention, and exposure theory could insist that purposeful disclosures of positive information, such as a pregnancy, are made with some ambivalence.

However, each of these accommodations strikes us as a bit of a stretch, resulting in theories that are not particularly parsimonious.

At this point in time, we see no strong body of evidence that definitely supports one theory over the others. As noted, each theory has some degree of both conceptual and empirical support, and each also has difficulty explaining all instances of blushing. We have our preference – the undesired social attention theory – because, in our view, it most easily accounts for the primary causes identified by the other two perspectives. Events that require remedial actions to repair one's social image invariably involve undesired attention from other people, as does the undesired exposure of private information. Furthermore, the undesired social attention theory appears to explain blushing in response to positive, desired events and when people are merely stared at or scrutinized more easily than the other two approaches. Even so, experiments are needed that provide direct, head-to-head tests of the competing theories.

REFERENCES

Argyle, M. (1967). *The psychology of interpersonal behaviour.* Harmondsworth: Penguin.
Browne, J. (1983). Darwin and the expression of the emotions. In D. Kohn (Ed.), *The Darwinian heritage.* Princeton University Press, 307–26.
Burgess, T. (1839). *The physiology or mechanism of blushing.* London: J. Churchill.
Buss, A. H. (1980). *Self-consciousness and social anxiety.* New York: W. H. Freeman.
Castelfranchi, C., & Poggi, I. (1990). Blushing as a discourse: was Darwin wrong? In W. R. Crozier (Ed.), *Shyness and embarrassment: perspectives from social psychology.* New York: Cambridge University Press, 230–51.
Crozier, W. R. (2000). Blushing, social anxiety and exposure. In W. R. Crozier (Ed.), *Shyness: development, consolidation and change.* New York: Routledge, 154–70.
  (2001). Blushing and the exposed self: Darwin revisited. *Journal for the Theory of Social Behaviour,* 31, 61–72.
  (2004). Self-consciousness, exposure, and the blush. *Journal for the Theory of Social Behaviour,* 34, 1–17.
  (2010). The puzzle of blushing. *The Psychologist,* 23, 390–3.
Darwin, C. (1872/1955). *The expression of the emotions in man and animals.* New York: The Philosophical Library.
de Jong, P. J. (1999). Communicative and remedial effects of social blushing. *Journal of Nonverbal Behaviour,* 23, 197–217.
de Jong, P. J., & Peters, M. L. (2005). Do blushing phobics overestimate the undesirable communicative effects of their blushing? *Behaviour Research and Therapy,* 43, 747–58.
de Jong, P. J., Peters, M. L., & De Cremer, D. (2003). Blushing may signify guilt: revealing effects of blushing in ambiguous social situations. *Motivation and Emotion,* 27, 225–49.

de Jong, P. J., Peters, M., De Cremer, D., & Vranken, C. (2002). Blushing after a moral transgression in a prisoner's dilemma game: appeasing or revealing? *European Journal of Social Psychology*, 32, 627–44.

de Jong, P. J., Peters, M. L., Dijk, C., Nieuwenhuis, E., Kempe, H., & Oelerink, J. (2006). Fear of blushing: the role of the expected influence of displaying a blush on others' judgements. *Cognitive Therapy and Research*, 30, 623–34.

de Melo, C. M., Kenny, P., & Gratch, J. (2010). Influence of autonomic signals on perception of emotions in embodied agents. *Applied Artificial Intelligence*, 24, 494–509.

Dijk, C., & de Jong, P. J. (2009). Fear of blushing: no overestimation of negative anticipated interpersonal effects, but a high-subjective probability of blushing. *Cognitive Therapy and Research*, 33, 59–74.

Dijk, C., de Jong, P. J., Müller, E., & Boersma, W. (2010). Blushing-fearful individuals' judgmental biases and conditional cognitions: an internet inquiry. *Journal of Psychopathology and Behavioural Assessment*, 32, 264–70.

Dijk, C., de Jong, P. J., & Peters, M. L. (2009). The remedial value of blushing in the context of transgressions and mishaps. *Emotion*, 9, 287–91.

Dijk, C., Voncken, M. J., & de Jong, P. J. (2009). I blush, therefore I will be judged negatively: influence of false blush feedback on anticipated others' judgments and facial coloration in high and low blushing-fearfuls. *Behaviour Research and Therapy*, 47, 541–7.

Drummond, P. D. (2001). The effect of true and false feedback on blushing in women. *Personality and Individual Differences*, 30, 1329–43.

Drummond, P. D., Back, K., Harrison, J., Helgadottir, F., Lange, B., Lee, C., Leavy, K., Novatscou, A. O., Pham, H., Prance, J., Radford, D., & Wheatley, L. (2007). Blushing during social interactions in people with a fear of blushing. *Behaviour Research and Therapy*, 45, 1601–8.

Drummond, P. D., Camacho, L., Formentin, N., Heffernan, T. D., Williams, F., & Zekas, T. E. (2003). The impact of verbal feedback about blushing on social discomfort and facial blood flow during embarrassing tasks. *Behaviour Research and Therapy*, 41, 413–25.

Drummond, P. D., & Lim, H. (2000). The significance of blushing for fair- and dark-skinned people. *Personality and Individual Differences*, 29, 1123–32.

Drummond, P. D., & Mirco, N. (2004). Staring at one side of the face increases blood flow on that side of the face. *Psychophysiology*, 41, 281–7.

Edelmann, R. J. (1987). *The psychology of embarrassment*. Chichester: John Wiley & Sons.

Ellsworth, P. C., & Carlsmith, J. (1968). Effects of eye contact and verbal content on affective response to a dyadic interaction. *Journal of Personality and Social Psychology*, 10, 15–20.

(1973). Eye contact and gaze aversion in an aggressive encounter. *Journal of Personality and Social Psychology*, 28, 280–92.

Ellsworth, P. C., Carlsmith, J., & Henson, A. (1972). The stare as a stimulus to flight in human subjects: a series of field experiments. *Journal of Personality and Social Psychology*, 21, 302–11.

Exline, R. V., & Winters, L. C. (1965). Affective relations and mutual gaze in dyads. In S. S. Tomkins & C. Izard (Eds.), *Affect, cognition, and personality*. New York: Springer, 41–9.

Gilovich, T., Medvec, V., & Savitsky, K. (2000). The spotlight effect in social judgment: an egocentric bias in estimates of the salience of one's own actions and appearance. *Journal of Personality and Social Psychology*, **78**, 211–22.

Gilovich, T., Savitsky, K., & Medvec, V. H. (1998). The illusion of transparency: biased assessments of others' ability to read one's emotional states. *Journal of Personality and Social Psychology*, **75**, 332–46.

Goffman, E. (1959). *The presentation of self in everyday life*. New York: Doubleday/Anchor Books.

Harris, P. R. (1990). Shyness and embarrassment in psychological theory and ordinary language. In W. R. Crozier (Ed.), *Shyness and embarrassment: perspectives from social psychology*. New York: Cambridge University Press, 59–86.

Heinrichs, N., Rapee, R. M., Alden, L. E., Bögels, S., Hofmann, S. G., Oh, K., & Sakano, Y. (2006). Cultural differences in perceived social norms and social anxiety. *Behaviour Research and Therapy*, **44**, 1187–97.

Karch, F. E. (1971). Blushing. *Psychoanalytic Review*, **58**, 37–50.

Leary, M. R., Britt, T. W., Cutlip, W. D., & Templeton, J. L. (1992). Social blushing. *Psychological Bulletin*, **112**, 446–60.

Leary, M. R., & Kowalski, R. M. (1990). Impression management: a literature review and two-component model. *Psychological Bulletin*, **107**, 34–47.

Leary, M. R., Landel, J. L., & Patton, K. M. (1996). The motivated expression of embarrassment following a self-presentational predicament. *Journal of Personality*, **64**, 619–36.

Leary, M. R., & Meadows, S. (1991). Predictors, elicitors, and concomitants of social blushing. *Journal of Personality and Social Psychology*, **60**, 254–62.

Lewis, M., Stanger, C., Sullivan, M. W., & Barone, P. (1991). Changes in embarrassment as a function of age, sex and situation. *British Journal of Developmental Psychology*, **9**, 485–92.

Lewis, M., Sullivan, M. W., Stanger, C., & Weiss, M. (1989). Self-development and self-conscious emotions. *Child Development*, **60**, 146–56.

MacCurdy, J. T. (1930). The biological significance of blushing and shame. *British Journal of Psychology*, **21**, 174–82.

Miller, R. S. (1986). Embarrassment: causes and consequences. In W. H. Jones, J. M. Cheek & S. R. Briggs (Eds.), *Shyness: perspectives on research and treatment*. New York: Plenum Press, 295–311.

Schneider, C. D. (1977). *Shame, exposure, and privacy*. Boston: Beacon Press.

Shearn, D., Bergman, E., Hill, K., & Abel, A. (1990). Facial coloration and temperature responses in blushing. *Psychophysiology*, **27**, 687–93.

(1992). Blushing as a function of audience size. *Psychophysiology*, **29**, 431–6.

Shearn, D., Spellman, L., Meirick, J., & Stryker, K. (1999). Empathic blushing in friends and strangers. *Motivation and Emotion*, **23**, 307–16.

Simon, A., & Shields, S. (1996). Does complexion color affect the experience of blushing? *Journal of Social Behaviour and Personality*, **11**, 177–88.

# 5 Colours of the face: a comparative glance

*Jan A. R. A. M. van Hooff*

'Blushing is the most peculiar and the most human of all expressions.' This is the much cited first sentence of Chapter 13 of Darwin's (1872/1965) *The Expression of the Emotions in Man and Animals*. The text continues: 'Monkeys redden from passion, but it would require an overwhelming amount of evidence to make us believe that any animal could blush.' This implies – and this is elaborated more explicitly elsewhere in the chapter – that a very special kind of reddening is meant: namely, as an expression of 'mental states' consisting of 'shyness, shame, and modesty: the essential element in all being self-attention'. This, in turn, is supposed to imply a level of self-awareness that is generally taken not to exist in nonhuman species. Even more peculiar is the phenomenon that blushing acts as a signal to other humans about which the blusher feels embarrassed and which she or he would like to hide so badly. The latter, however, is impossible; the blush occurs as an uncontrollable response (e.g., Crozier, 2006, 2010).

This raises the question whether blushing is some unwelcome side-effect of our physiological and emotional functioning that is not only disagreeable for the actor, but also disadvantageous. Or must it be seen as a social display – that is, as an adaptive response – shaped in the course of our evolution to function in the regulation of social interactions? How, then, do we establish whether something that works as a signal has evolved into a communicative display? Does a comparative approach shed some light here? More specifically I would like to address the following issues:

- From signal to display: the evolution of structures and processes specifically intended for communication
- The adaptation of colour signals for purposes of social organization
- Blue and red skin colours in primates, the only taxon of mammals with this specialization and the only taxon of placental mammals where trichromatic colour vision has (re)appeared, enabling them to distinguish the hue 'red'
- Has the sensitivity for red evolved for ecological or for social reasons?

- Blushing has been interpreted as a display of guilt, functioning as an apology for moral transgressions. Is this analogous or even homologous to appeasement and reconciliation functions in nonhuman primates? Why blushing? Is it because it is an honest signal?
- Has there been an additional role for sexual selection?

## From signal to display: adaptation for communication

Animals must adjust their behaviour to that of other animals, whether friends or foes. These others are, first of all, their conspecifics, with which they share their habitat and which they encounter there in a variety of contexts. This is especially obvious for species where the individuals live together as members of a social organization. At times their interests may run in parallel. If so, it usually is advantageous to coordinate behaviours cooperatively in complementary or synchronous patterns. Sometimes, however, the individual interests may diverge or even conflict, requiring competitive or negotiating strategies. Depending on the nature of the species and the specific contexts in which the individuals encounter one another there will be a need for signals that inform conspecifics of the behavioural inclinations of the individual so as to make the other adjust appropriately.

The study of animal displays in terms of their message content, their function in social regulation, their derivation and their evolution has been a major subject of ethological research since the second half of the last century (e.g., Tinbergen, 1951, 1964). It has been found that there are three major sources from which displays have been derived.

The first is conflict between motivational systems: namely, when a situation arouses different behavioural tendencies at the same time, or when a behavioural tendency is thwarted. For example, if another individual intrudes into an animal's territory or private sphere this may simultaneously arouse aggressive behavioural tendencies and a tendency to flee. Incipient or intention movements of either one or both activated behaviours may stall or waver. This can result in ambivalent movements or postures in which elements of both attack and flight behaviours are mixed or alternated. The animal 'doesn't know what to do yet'. Depending on the way the other reacts to this signal, the pendulum might swing one way or the other, leading either to an attack or to flight, or – certainly better – to nothing if the adversary decides to leave without comment, thus settling the dispute without much further risky ado.

We find threat postures that can be understood in this way in the behavioural repertoire of many species. Similarly the postures and movements that make up courtship displays have been understood as the outcome of interacting aggressive, flight and/or sexual tendencies. A famous example of such ambivalence has been described as the 'zig-zag dance' of the male stickleback, a highly ritualized courtship display. With this dance a male lures a visiting female to the nest he has made and induces her to shed her eggs in there, which he then fertilizes. The dance consists of two rapidly alternating movements, a short dash towards the female – this 'zig' may occasionally result in attacking the female – and a movement in the direction of the nest opening – this 'zag' may turn into 'leading towards the nest'. When a female turns up she appears both as an intruder, eliciting aggressive responses, and as a potential mate, eliciting sexual responses. Components of both responses have been interlaced into a new behaviour pattern with a specific role in the courtship interaction, probing the inclinations of the other (Tinbergen, 1951, 1964).

Once a movement or posture is informative of an inclination or a characteristic of the sender, and when it is advantageous for the sender that the addressee takes notice of it, then natural selection is bound to go to work to favour variants of the signal that are more effective in releasing the 'desired' response. It may favour more conspicuous, distinct and unambiguous forms of the signal, thus shaping specialized communicative displays. In this process, termed 'ritualization', movements and postures are being exaggerated; they are getting stylized in that they assume typical intensities and frequencies (Morris, 1956) and often they are accentuated by specially evolved structures, such as plumes, crests, colour patterns and the like. Well-known examples of the latter are the gills and dewlaps of gallinaceous birds (Morris, 1957). When a male turkey is aroused the peripheral blood flow swells its wattle and gives it a bright red colour, an unmistakable signal for its companions. This 'blush', a ritualized autonomous response, is combined with other autonomous reactions, such as the raising of the feathers. These are thermoregulatory responses that have been ritualized in many bird species, one of the most extravagant forms being the tail-spreading of the male peacock. The turkey combines all this with a characteristic strutting walk in an impressive courtship display; a hen may be impressed and attracted: 'What a guy!' In mammals an analogous ritualization is found in the raising of the hairs, the bristling of the fur in excitement, and has been incorporated in displays of vigour and dominance.

### Colour signals

It is only a small frequency band of electromagnetic radiation that we call light. Its wavelengths are absorbed and reflected differentially by objects depending on their properties. This makes it a useful source of information for sensitive beings that orient in their environment and want to direct their behaviour selectively to relevant matter, whether these are lifeless phenomena or living things such as food species or conspecifics.

When it is advantageous for plants or animals to manipulate the attention of possible perceivers of colour signals then evolutionary selection pressures may adapt the colour patterns to the 'beneficial' end. The world must have become colourful when plants became dependent on animals that would help in the pollination process, and when flowers evolved to lure insects. Similarly, fruits evolved as rewards for those animal species that help in dispersing the seeds.

Contrasting and conspicuous colours can thus be evolutionarily 'intended' to draw the attention of certain receivers that are sensitive to the characteristic wave lengths.

## Changing colour and manipulating messages

Organisms can adopt certain patterns of coloration in different ways. Most frequently found are pigments in the skin, whether in the naked skin or in the scales, hairs or feathers that are formed in the skin. Take the sometimes dazzling colours of fish, reptiles such as lizards, and birds. As a rule, such pigment colours cannot easily be changed in the individual. However, in a number of taxa, such as the proverbial chameleons but also in other reptiles, in amphibians, fish and cephalopods (squids and octopuses), specialized structures exist, enabling the animal to modify its colour patterns. These *chromatophores* occur in a few types according to the hue of pigment granules they contain. The granules can be dispersed or concentrated within the chromatophore, thus changing the reflecting surface for a specific hue. Regulation is by hormones and neurotransmitters.

In contrast to the other vertebrate taxa – fish, amphibians, reptiles and birds – and also to many invertebrates, mammals are poor colour artists. To be sure, mammalian pelage occurs in a number of shades and hues, but the skin usually varies from pale to brownish or blackish, as determined by the amount of melanophores. But there are striking exceptions and these are to be found in the primates (Bradley & Mundy, 2008; Higham, 2009). A number of species – for example, many macaques and baboons – display strikingly red anal and genital areas, which may vary in intensity depending on conditions and situations (see section 'Red faces, red bottoms'). Some species have bright red faces: for example, the Japanese macaques (*Macaca fuscata*), the red-faced uakaris (*Cacajao* sp.) and some spider monkeys (*Ateles* sp.) in South America.

In addition, a number of primate species – for example, some guenons (*Cercopithecus* sp.) – show radiant blue colour strikes and patches in the skin of their faces, of their scrota and of their genital/anal regions. The mixture of reds and blues may yield brilliant violets and purples.

### Blue faces, blue scrota

The most bizarre facial coloration is found in the mandrill (*Mandrillus sphinx*), a baboon-like monkey of some West African forests. A bright red streak runs from between the eyebrows down over the middle of the nose to its tip where it broadens and ends in the region around the nostrils. This contrasts strongly with blue bulging ridges on either side of it.[1] Wickler (1967, 1968) noted the striking resemblance of this facial mask to the genital region of the male mandrill: the bright red shaft of the penis widening in the glans, on both sides surrounded by the blue scrotum. It is undoubtedly the most spectacular example of 'automimicry', a phenomenon seen in some other primate species as well, in which the appearance of the genital region is depicted on another part of the body.

The 'reds' and the 'blues' are similar in that neither is based on a specific pigment. Still, these colours differ fundamentally in how they are produced. Whereas the red colour is determined by the level of blood flow through the skin, the mechanism behind the blue colours has long been unclear. Recently Prum and Torres (2004) have shown that the blue is determined by an interference phenomenon known as coherent scattering. It is produced by arrays of minute collagen fibres arranged in parallel in the skin. Similarly arranged nanostructures explain the blue colours in the feathers of birds (Prum *et al.*, 1998, 1999) and in the scales of butterfly wings (for a review, see Ingram & Parker, 2008).

Whereas the red colour is variable, the blue colour was thought to remain stable after the collagen fibre arrangement had been formed. According to Setchell and Dixson (2001) the red and the structural blue become more saturated in males of high rank. These males have higher plasma testosterone levels and larger testes; they also have a higher mating success and produce more offspring. So the colours are a signal of quality. The authors reported that the blue colour remained when these males fell in rank, whereas the red faded. However, Prum and Torres (2004) refer to a well-documented case of a male that lost weight and also a lot of his structural blue after falling in rank. Such

---

[1] For a colour picture see http://www.sciencephoto.com/image/384814/530wm/ Z9100020-Mandrill-SPL.jpg

changes could be mediated by hormonal control of the thickness of the layers of collagen fibres in the dermis and consequently the colour saturation. A similar situation exists in some guenon monkey species: for instance, in the vervet monkey (*Cercopithecus aethiops*), where adult dominant males have a brilliant deep blue scrotum contrasting with a bright red penis and white belly hairs (the 'red-white-blue' display; Gerald, 1999; Isbell, 1995).

## Red faces, red bottoms

The most extreme 'ritualization' of facial reddening is found in the South American red uakari (*Cacajao rubicundus*). The whole of the face, the ears and the frontal part of the scalp of this monkey are of a bright and saturated red colour.[2] The upper dermis is densely suffused with capillary sinuses. In addition, the skin is richly innervated, indicative of neural regulation. In mature males the red area is expanded by an extensive baldness of the forehead and the frontal scalp (Perkins *et al.*, 1968). Similar extensive, richly innervated vascular beds have been found in the naked scalp and face and in the naked anal-genital region of the rhesus macaque, *Macaca mulatta* (Montagna *et al.*, 1964) and the stump-tail macaque, *Macaca speciosa* (Montagna *et al.*, 1966). The red colour is directly due to the venous blood in extensive sinusoidal arcades in the superficial dermis, because the colour disappears immediately and totally if the animals are exsanguinated.

There cannot be much doubt that these structures have evolved especially to carry important social signals. In several species redness varies with social status (especially in males) and with reproductive status (especially in females). Studies by Setchell and Dixson (2001) and Setchell, Smith, Wickings and Knapp (2008) found that when male mandrills rose in rank the level of circulating testosterone rose, their faces became redder, they fattened and their testicles grew bigger. Moreover, facial redness and androgen levels also rose even further when receptive females were present. When a male fell in rank the reverse occurred, though the effect was less pronounced: the red colour faded. In other words: facial redness is an honest signal of male quality and sexual motivation and, in rhesus monkeys, has appeared to reinforce female preferences (Waitt *et al.*, 2003).

Similar findings have been made in other species. The gelada baboon female *(Theropithecus gelada)* displays a conspicuous red genital-anal

---

[2] For a colour picture see http://www.flickr.com/photos/tark_mao/865311702/in/photostream

skin, which it also 'automimics' on a naked patch of the chest (Wickler, 1967). Remarkably, this is again mimicked by the male; the redness of the chest varies and appears to be a clear signal of male quality (Bergman et al., 2009).[3] In female rhesus monkeys estrogen is directly responsible for levels of vascularization and blood flow of the sexual skin. The resulting colour variations convey information that is of evident interest for males; the saturated red tells that ovulation is about to occur (Dubuc et al., 2009).

Analogous quality judgments appear to be made by humans (Re et al., 2011). High levels of oxygenated blood bring about a bright red coloration of the facial skin. A high level of oxygenation also reflects cardiovascular fitness. Conversely a bluish-red tint, due to deoxygenated blood, may indicate respiratory or coronary illness; nor is a pale skin a sign of good health. Facial redness appears to be perceived as a sign of health and influences male attractiveness to females. In women, higher estrogen levels cause increased vascularization and vasodilatation of the skin, making them more attractive to men. Red flushing of the skin of the face, neck and chest often accompanies sexual excitation. Lipsticks and other artificial means have long been used to accentuate the attractive red tint artificially (see Re et al., 2011).

## Colour perception as an adaptation: mono-, di-, tri- and tetrachromats

The above suggests that the respective species are able to distinguish hue differences in the reddish range of the spectrum (although in principle sensitivity to luminance differences might also explain the responses).

Seeing depends on the presence of light-sensitive pigments and a neural system that can process the information. With one pigment it is possible to perceive luminance differences. Spectral discrimination (i.e., *colour vision*) becomes possible if there is more than one type of pigment, each sensitive to a spectral band around a different maximum. A particular wavelength of light is then represented by a specific ratio of the degree to which each of these pigments is affected.

Birds and reptiles are mostly tetrachromats with fine discriminatory power over a broad spectral range. This is undoubtedly the ancestral vertebrate condition (Arrese et al., 2002). By contrast, almost all mammal taxa are dichromats, sensitive in the green to violet range, but unable to discriminate red (see Jacobs, 2009, for a review). This seemingly impoverished performance is thought to result from the fact that

---

[3] For a colour picture see http://4.bp.blogspot.com/UkbaN4g7vq0/T6piRRPB6dI/ AAAAAAAAKvg/0E2PSitBPmU/s1600/Gelada.jpg

early mammals were originally nocturnal in a time when a great diversity of reptiles, from small to gigantic, reigned during the day (Kemp, 2005). The early mammals would have been well off with a monochromatic system of very high sensitivity over a broad spectral range.

Even today most nocturnal prosimian primates, such as bushbabies (*Galago*), lorises (*Loris* and *Nycticebus*) and pottos (*Perodicticus*) have monochromatic vision. The exceptions are the tarsiers (*Tarsius*) and the aya-aye (*Daubentonia*), which have dichromatic vision. Moritz and Dominy (2010) argue that the distribution of this difference among prosimians provides evidence that the potential for spectral discrimination has been under selection pressure exerted by food choice. They investigated the radiance spectra of food consumed by monochromatic *Galagos* and dichromatic *Tarsius* under the irradiance conditions of twilight, of new moon and of full moon. They found that *Galago* should be able to find the food it thrives on solely by discriminating luminance contrasts, whereas for tarsiers the discrimination of chromatic cues would help them greatly to find the adequate foods in their habitats.

Trichromatic vision, providing the ability to distinguish reddish hues, has again evolved in only two mammalian taxa, the marsupials (Arrese et al., 2002) and most diurnal primates, the monkeys and apes. The catarrhine monkeys and apes of the old world are all trichromats. However, among the platyrrhine monkeys of the new world we find considerable polymorphism (Jacobs, 1993). Fully trichromatic platyrrhines have so far been found only in the genus *Alouatta* (howler monkeys). The other platyrrhines are dichromats or partial trichromats (within the species there is polymorphism; the males are dichromatic with trichromatism occurring often among females). Even the only truly nocturnal monkey *Aotus trivirgatus* is monochromatic.

## Why see red: to distinguish food or perceive emotions?

There is discussion about the possible evolutionary reason for the development of trichromatism. The traditional view is that it developed in iteration with the specialization on a frugivorous diet (Allen, 1879; Polyak, 1957). Regan and colleagues (1998) obtained support for this from showing that the species-specific chromatic sensitivity of *Alouatta seniculus* corresponds optimally with the chromaticity contrast of their fruits against the background of the foliage (*cf.* Regan *et al.*, 2001; Sumner & Mollon, 2000). And indeed, behavioural experiments with polymorphic callitrichid monkeys have shown that trichromats are better at detecting reddish objects against a greenish background than their dichromatic conspecifics (Caine, 2002; Smith *et al.*, 2003). However, a difference in feeding efficiency between the two morphs could not be established in natural populations of the spider monkeys *Ateles geoffroyi* (Hiramatsu *et al.*, 2008). In some cases trichromats were even at a disadvantage – for instance, when searching for insect prey – offering an explanation for the curious fact that the di-tri polymorphism is maintained in a number of species (Caine *et al.*, 2003; Melin *et al.*, 2009). A similar advantage of 'colour-vision deficiency' has also been demonstrated for humans (Saito *et al.*, 2006).

Recently Changizi, Zhang and Shimojo (2006) have proposed an alternative explanation: namely, that trichromatic vision evolved originally in primates for discriminating modulations in skin colour that are associated with sexual and emotional states (e.g., rage). Thus, these modulations can function as socio-sexual signals. They found that there are two dimensions of skin colour modulations, depending on the haemoglobin concentration in the skin and on the degree of oxygenation of the facial blood, oxygenated blood leading to a more reddish-purplish hue and deoxygenated blood to a more yellowish-greenish hue. They show that dichromats would be sensitive to only one of the variations – namely, of the haemoglobin concentration – and trichromats would be sensitive to both. A good discrimination of skin colour hues would only be possible on naked, hairless skins. The authors remarked that trichromatism in primates is associated with bare faces and have regarded this as a strong argument in favour of their hypothesis: roughly 20 per cent of the mono- and dichromats have hairless faces, whereas roughly 85 per cent of the polymorphs and full trichromats do, and, moreover, some of the polymorphic and full trichromat species have exaggerated red faces.

Clearly the findings that are in accordance with the one hypothesis do not falsify the other. In fact selection pressures associated with fruit detection, on the one hand, and with socio-sexual state discrimination, on the other hand, might have been operating alongside, reinforcing one another. The question is what has triggered it in the first place. The detection and selection of fruits may well have been at the roots of the development. For one thing, the other hypothesis does not explain why trichromatism has arisen precisely in a taxon with high frugivory and why other taxa of mammals, living diurnally in complex social organizations (rodents, canids, mongooses, meerkats, etc.) have not taken an analogous course. Obviously the dispute is not yet settled.

## Also short-term fluctuations in redness?

The studies reported above have shown that changes in the red hues of the face and other areas of naked skin, as well as in the blue hues, are informative about the state of the 'sender'. Moreover, the signals are noticed by 'receivers' and have an influence on their behaviours, yielding the selective pressures that have led to their ritualization: that is, they have been adapted, as elements of display. It has been suggested that not only long-term states, such as dominance status and reproductive state, are reflected, but also short-term motivational variations (moods), such as rage, are reflected in momentary colour fluctuations – not in the blue, but in the red. Changizi and colleagues (2006) even regard the ability to distinguish emotional states on the basis of subtle fluctuations in the redness of the face as the primary evolutionary reason for the (re) appearance of red perception in the primate branch of the mammals. However, well-documented observations showing that such motivation-dependent fluctuations in skin redness do exist are lacking. In part, this is certainly due to the fact that objective measurements of subtle colour variations in social groups under naturally varying light conditions are extremely difficult. Moreover, what we distinguish in physical measurements may be different from what our human colour sense, our visual pigments, distinguish, and that in turn may differ from what various primate species distinguish (Higham et al., 2010).

Our daily experiences tell us continuously that our emotions may let us go pale, redden, start sweating and so on. At the beginning of this chapter we asked whether these are useless and annoying physiological epiphenomena of our emotional (re)actions, or whether these have been adaptively tuned to convey social messages, analogous (but perhaps not homologous) to what has evolved in some other primate species. Evidence for an adaptive explanation comes from the fact that we are exceptional among hominids (the great apes) in having a distinct blush zone, a venous plexus of capillary loops in the dermis and an extensive network of veins in the subcutaneous layer in the area of the face, neck and shoulders. The appearance of these structures may, however, have been due to another adaptation. According to Rowell (1977) the human skin is rather unique: it possesses a neurogenic vasodilator system which reflexively responds to central body thermoreceptors, as well as tonically active vasoconstrictor nerve fibres, responsible for thermoregulatory reflexes which originate principally in cutaneous thermoreceptors and react to upright posture and exercise. It is very plausible that this vast, and highly responsive, thermoregulatory system has evolved, concomitant with a naked body and millions of sweat glands, in conjunction with the specialization of *Homo* as a bipedal long-distance endurance runner, requiring optimal dissipation of heat (Bramble & Lieberman, 2004). Thus, the momentous colour changes in the blush region may be particularly well suited for an instantaneous display of emotional changes and may indeed be a peculiarity of our species.

## Motivational conflict, arrested avoidance and submission

When an individual is attacked or feels threatened the natural response is to flee from or avoid the adversary. This has the dual effect of helping the individual to escape the harm and prevent further provocation. But often avoidance is impossible or undesirable. The latter is the case when both individuals are bonded as members of a social group and generally maintain mutually beneficial relationships. Then the stressful motivational conflict between the tendency to flee (with its concomitant sympathetic activation of the 'fight or flight' response) and the urge not to give up the relationship may result in displays of submission. The thwarted tendency to flee is manifest not only in the physiological autonomic preparations for fleeing but also in arrested incipient movements of fleeing, such as dodging and a crouched body posture oriented away from the adversary; it is manifested, moreover, in gaze avoidance and, at the same time, monitoring the position of the opponent with evasive glances. In primates this is often accompanied by a 'silent bared-teeth display' (van Hooff, 1967/2006). This is a ritualized expression of fear in which screaming is suppressed. Since the total compound display is the opposite of a threat display it signals that the actor is not willing to provoke the opponent, and it thus has an appeasing function (Preuschoft & van Hooff, 1997). Chance (1962) remarked that gaze aversion and withdrawal has an effect also on the subject itself, because it prevents the intimidated individual from receiving more disquieting stimuli. Thus, this 'cut-off' behaviour, as he called it, might not only reduce the unwanted attention from the partner, but it might also help the subject to resolve its motivational conflict and restore its emotional balance. Both these aspects can also be noticed in the compound display which is characterized by blushing.

## Conflict, reconciliation and maintaining beneficial relationships

An important determinant of the nature of the interactions between conspecifics is their long-term relationship. Recently there has been much research on the effect of agonistic confrontations between individuals that maintain mutually beneficial relationships. Confrontations, irritations and insults are bound to occur in animals that live in close relationship with one another, even if they are joined together by common interests and cooperation. Particularly in such relationships disturbances have appeared to be disquieting to the participants, obviously because they endanger the long-term bond which is of value to them. This has become a focus of scientific attention ever since, in the famous Burgers Zoo colony in Arnhem, the Netherlands, de Waal and van Roosmalen (1979) noted that, after a conflict with one another, chimpanzees had a higher than usual inclination to engage in a social-positive interaction with the antagonist. At first this seemed counter-intuitive, since, at the time, the traditional view was that aggression is a destructive phenomenon, damaging relationships (see Lorenz, 1963, for taking issue with this conventional view). De Waal and van Roosmalen deduced that these post-conflict affiliative contacts were to be interpreted functionally as reconciliations, restoring the damaged relationship, a conclusion that initially met with disbelief and scepticism ('We are talking of animals, aren't we!'). A number of subsequent studies have identified similar processes in other species, not only in primates: for example, long-tailed macaques (Aureli *et al.*, 1989) and baboons (Castles & Whiten, 1998; for reviews see Aureli *et al.*, 2002; van Hooff & Aureli, 1994), but also, remarkably, in goats (Schino, 1998) and in dogs (Cools *et al.*, 2008). The studies have corroborated the conclusion that these processes not only function to reduce uncertainty in the individuals involved, especially in those that have been subordinated (e.g., Silk *et al.*, 2000) but also that the animals felt uneasy with the disturbance of the relationship and sought to restore it (van Hooff & Aureli, 1994; de Waal, 1989; de Waal & Aureli, 2001). Individuals that maintained a mutually beneficial relationship indeed reconciled more frequently after conflicts than those with neutral or poor relationships (van Hooff, 2001; van Schaik & Aureli, 2000). Cords and Turnheer (1993) could even manipulate the reconciliation tendency experimentally. They took pairs of long-tailed macaques (*Macaca fascicularis*) out of their group and brought them into a situation in which they learned that they could get a reward if they acted cooperatively in coordinated fashion. After they had experienced their dependency on each other they were returned to their social group. Subsequently their rate of mutual reconciliation after conflicts rose by a factor of three; the value of their relationship had increased. In an experiment with a group of captive chimpanzees (*Pan troglodytes*) Koyama and Dunbar (1996) showed that these chimpanzees did anticipate possible conflicts and reacted to the tension this raised by increasing rates of grooming in the periods before expected feeding times. They did so with close associates, thus confirming their valued bonds (see Polizzi di Sorrentino *et al.*, 2010, for a similar process in capuchin monkeys).

## From 'normal' habits to (proto-)moral 'norms'

In social groups individuals have to manoeuvre within a context where there is tension between, on the one hand, conflicting and diverging interests and, on the other hand, parallel and complementary interests conducive to tolerance and cooperation, and even long-term investments in the interests of others: for instance, on the basis of mutuality. As we saw, animals do anticipate: in other words, expectations do govern their behaviour. What else to expect than the regular or the usual! The unusual may be fascinating and it may stimulate curiosity and exploratory behaviour, but often it also causes disquieting uncertainty. This also applies to regularities in the social sphere. Deviations frustrate expectations, and may release punitive actions. Consequently, the normal trusted procedures, to which the group members are accustomed, acquire a normative character. Normal becomes norm; 'This is how things go' becomes 'This is how things are expected (= ought) to go!' The regularities become rules, proto-moral rules, implicitly shared by the group members.

## Guilt and a moral conscience

Ever since Darwin the discussion has emphasized the uniqueness of the human blush, not only revealing, but also requiring, the faculties of self-consciousness and conscientiousness (Fessler, 2007). Two questions can be posed. First, does an inhibition of transgressing such (proto-)moral rules by nonhuman beings also reflect some primitive moral conscience? Is there evidence for a feeling of guilt if there has been a transgression? Second, are 'self-conscious emotions' indeed necessary to explain human blushing?

As to the first question, Horowitz (2009) discusses studies showing that a majority of dog owners do interpret the behaviour of their dog in this way; they feel that the distinct behaviour complex that is characterized by the 'guilty look' (askance look, evasive glancing, slinking back and cowering with ears back, tail between legs) indicates a 'bad conscience'. In an experiment Horowitz placed dogs in a situation where they could eat a forbidden treat, after the owners had left. When the owners reappeared the dogs did not behave differently, whether they had been obedient or not. However, they did show the 'guilty look' behaviour more frequently when the owners scolded them, and they did so regardless of whether they had eaten or not. In other words, Horowitz did not find evidence for an expression of guilt. She adds that her results do not indicate that domestic dogs do not experience guilt. It shows that what dog owners anthropomorphically interpret as an expression of guilt is to be explained differently. The 'guilty look' behaviour is similar to the submissive behaviour dogs and wolves show in interactions in which they preempt an expected reprimand; in other words, it reflects a tendency to flee (if you like, for fear of being punished) that is thwarted by the urge to stay with the pack leader and to maintain the affiliative relationship. In wolves two forms of submission can be distinguished: a passive form in which the facial expression and the cowering are combined with shrinking back in response to a threat, and an active form, in which the same elements are combined with approaching a dominant in a crouched position and often leading to licking the mouth corners of the partner (van Hooff & Wensing, 1987). Such submissive affiliation is also shown in reconciliation between dogs after a conflict. Then it is used especially in disturbed relations with closely bonded partners (Cools et al., 2008), similar to what has been found in nonhuman primates (see above).

Unease because of the disturbance of a valuable relationship and associating this with the behaviour that caused the social disturbance might well be within the cognitive grasp of highly social and cooperative animals (compare with the discussion about metacognitive abilities in some animals: that is, the suggestion that they may, to some extent, have access to their own psychological state – see, for instance, Call, 2010). Such an association may thus be responsible for maintaining and fine-tuning relationships of altruistic mutualism and partnership (e.g., de Waal, 1996, 2008). It is likely that such an association and a resulting moral sensitivity lies at the basis of the development of – though still being a far cry from – a moral conscience as we know it in our own species, with all its cognitive and emotional connotations and our capacity for self-conscious reflection on the contexts and consequences of our behaviour (e.g., Fessler, 2007). This undoubtedly has developed in connection with the cultural emancipation of cooperation in larger social units and not only with individuals that are literally those most familiar and nearest, but also with relative strangers. Thus, culturally enforced norms of cooperation have arisen, facilitated by the concordant development of an understanding of the needs and intentions of others. All this has reached unprecedented heights in humans. However, we may not be the only ones with such capacities; we see the beginnings of such 'theory of mind' (Call & Tomasello, 2008) and empathy in some socially developed mammals (e.g., de Waal, 2008).

## The social effects of blushing

A second question is: must we assume that 'self-consciousness' is a necessary factor for explaining human blushing? Not meeting the accepted standards in the face of social companions may require pacifying gestures. May not fear of negative treatment suffice, in analogy to the displays of submission and particularly those of reconciliation found in nonhuman species?

To understand the functionality of blushing, attention should be directed to the responses of those witnessing the blushing and their relationship with the blusher. To be sure, the blush does draw attention to the blusher, intensifying precisely what the blusher wants to escape from. However, it might be more interesting to know what the observers do subsequently.

Of course the blusher may be scathed or ridiculed, which is certainly not putting him or her at ease. However, it is plausible to assume that observers sympathetic to the blusher will either emphasize utterances of sympathy, when the blush was because of embarrassing praise, or act as if nothing had happened and stop playing up an issue if that issue provoked embarrassment, guilt or shame.

In this respect the blush clearly resembles the submissive gestures found in many species: for instance, the submissive 'silent bared-teeth display' that is shown by a number of primate species. As a result, actually or potentially threatening group members usually refrain from intruding further on the submitting individual, and leave it alone. Although systematic behavioural observations of the natural reactions to blushing by human companions are lacking, there are indications that the actual effect is often that the companions turn their attention away from the blusher and, if well-disposed, 'ignore' her or him. Often the blush is interpreted as a sign of guilt or shame (de Jong *et al.*, 2003) and as an apology for some action or utterance that could be seen as a breach of norms and could lead to negative appraisal (evidence reviewed by Crozier, 2006, 2010). In a series of experiments Dijk (2009) showed that participants judged a blushing actor after a transgression or mishap more favourably than one who did not blush. Blushing actors were also rated more trustworthy and honest than non-blushing ones. In spite of the belief by blushing participants that their blushing would have damaging consequences, it appeared to be an effective appeasing display. It derives its convincing nature from the fact that it is involuntary and cannot be feigned. This is in contrast with facial expressions and vocalizations that, at least in our species, can be manipulated in a dishonest way. In nonhuman primates these are emotional utterances that can be used in an intentional, voluntary manner only to a very limited extent. With the development of a symbolic referential communication system – namely, our language in the form of speech – the vocal and facial apparatus needed for this purpose, became, so to speak, liberated from its emotional chains and available for voluntary manipulation (van Hooff, 2012). Since then we have become good actors and have been looking for good lie detectors. But as Zahavi (1987) has argued, the conflicts that arise between signaller and receiver must lead to selection pressures for signals to be 'honest' in the long run: that is, resistant to cheating and bluffing (even though cheating might benefit an actor in the short run). And blushing qualifies as an honest signal.

Since Darwin (1872/1965) the emphasis in discussions about blushing has been on this 'guilt and excuse' context. But blushing also occurs in contexts where an individual is praised or drawn into the limelight (Leary & Meadows, 1991). A characteristic of these situations seems to be the unexpected exposure to the attention of others, especially in unusual and unfamiliar situations. Again this can be related to self-consciousness and self-esteem, but the reaction probably has much older roots. In many species, as in very young children, received attention is treated as something to worry about, especially if an already weak, vulnerable and subordinate position might be affected. It is uncomfortable if there exists an ambiguity about what the companion might be intending and, therefore, about the response required. A better signal, then, would be: 'Please, leave me alone ...' (i.e., the 'undesired attention theory' of Leary and Meadows, 1991).

'... what value were there in the love of the maiden, were it yielded without coy delay?' (Scott, 1832)

There is one more remarkable aspect of blushing. It is often assumed that women tend to blush more easily than men, although the evidence is not compelling. They do so more easily when they are young, and often in a context of courting advances (coyness blushing). Ethologists have noted that female reticence is generally found in socially monogamous species where female reproductive success depends on male help in caring for her and her (and his) offspring. This results in prolonged courtships. Female reserve wanes when the male convincingly demonstrates his commitment. It safeguards her from philandering males (Schuster & Sigmund, 1981) and appears to be an evolutionary stable strategy (McNamara et al., 2008; Wachtmeister & Enquist, 1999). The 'coyness blushing' behaviour can be seen as resulting from the arousal generated by the motivational conflict of withdrawal and attraction and could have been adapted as an element of human courtship by sexual selection. Although the message is 'Don't push me' or 'Wait a minute', a male is certainly not repelled by it; on the contrary, as the above quote from the writer Sir Walter Scott expresses!

## To conclude

Everywhere in nature colour is used as a meaningful signal indicative of certain characteristics of the coloured objects or organisms. If an organism derives an advantage from clearly advertising these characteristics, then natural selection is bound to go to work to elaborate the representative signals into displays. This process, known as ritualization, leads to more conspicuous, discrete and unmistakable signals. In the case of colour signals this often means higher saturation and greater contrast with the surroundings.

Everywhere in nature, and not only in animals, colour pigments have evolved for display. In the mammalian skin, colour variations are determined primarily by changes in the superficial blood flow and by structural properties leading to spectral interference patterns. We encounter specific adaptations of the cutaneous and subcutaneous blood circulation system in the skin of the face and the anal-genital area, especially in primates. These adaptations testify to the social significance of the colour variations of these structures. This is corroborated by behavioural studies. The existence of similar structures in the human skin, the pronounced character of the facial colour changes and the universality of the phenomenon of blushing (Edelmann, 1990) lend support to the notion that the human blush is an adaptive display. However, the comparatively instantaneous occurrences of colour changes that characterize the human blush may differ from colour signals in nonhuman primates, where observations of fast colour fluctuations are lacking.

To understand the message of the signal we have to understand the functionality of the physiological response. It has been interpreted as the manifestation of an activation of the fight or flight system (e.g., Salzen, 2010). Adrenaline and noradrenaline prepare the organism for an outburst of energetic action, increasing the blood flow in organs that are needed for the energetic explosion such as the muscles and reducing the supply of blood for general maintenance functions. When startled or caught by fear the skin becomes pale and peripheral blood is redirected to muscles. Reddening signals a high level of ambivalent arousal and has been interpreted as a thermoregulatory response in anticipation of a possible high level of activity. However, in view of the complexity of the underlying physiological processes of blood flow regulation, the original function of the blush response remains unclear (Crozier, 2010).

The blush proper forms part of a compound signal in which typical elements are turning away, avoiding visual contact, and, sometimes, nervous and apologetic smiling or laughter.

The question then arises, what is the adaptive significance of this display, particularly if it is often experienced as extremely disagreeable by the blusher (e.g., Jadresic, 2008)? Such disagreeableness in itself is no reason to regard a process as some sort of maladaptive side-effect. There are many evolved processes that are disagreeable to the individual involved from a proximate perspective, but are nevertheless highly adaptive from an ultimate perspective. The most obvious example is pain. It is based on especially evolved structures. It leads to a drastic reprogramming of behaviour patterns, in particular a suppression of behaviours that might aggravate the damage; the ultimate beneficial effect is that injured structures are spared (van Hooff *et al.*, 1993).

The ultimate beneficial effect of blushing may be comparable to that of the submissive displays that we see in many social species. They pacify the partner and stop further encroachments. It is also analogous to conciliatory behaviours generally found in species where individuals mend long-term valuable relationships that were harmed by some incident. Indeed, blushes after the revelation of a mishap or a breach of trust tend to be accepted as an honest apology and restore acceptance (e.g., Dijk, 2009; see also Chapter 12, this volume).

Self-conscious emotions and concern about the perception and the acceptance by others play an evident role (e.g., Leary & Meadows, 1991). However, in view of the comparative data the question remains whether an ability to form 'a theory of mind' – that is, a mental representation of the minds of others and a meta-representation of the self – is a *conditio sine qua non* for generating the display of blushing. This may tone down a bit the assertion, repeated ever since Darwin, that the blush is a uniquely human expression. Yes, perhaps in its appearance and certain aspects of its causation, but perhaps not in its function: safeguarding social bondedness and acceptance.

## REFERENCES

Allen, G. (1879). *The colour-sense: its origin and development – an essay in comparative psychology.* London: Truebner & Co.

Arrese, C. A., Hart, N. S., Thomas, N., Beazley, L. D., & Shand, J. (2002). Trichromacy in Australian marsupials. *Current Biology*, 12, 657–60.

Aureli F., Cords, M., & van Schaik, C. P. (2002). Conflict resolution following aggression in gregarious animals: a predictive framework. *Animal Behaviour*, 64, 325–43.

Aureli, F., van Schaik, C. P., & van Hooff, J. A. R. A. M. (1989). Functional aspects of reconciliation among captive long-tailed macaques (*Macaca fascicularis*). *American Journal of Primatology*, 19, 39–51.

Bergman, T. J., Ho, L., & Beehner, J. C. (2009). Chest color and social status in male geladas (*Theropithecus gelada*). *International Journal of Primatology*, **30**, 791–806.

Bradley, B. J., & Mundy, N. I. (2008). The primate palette: the evolution of primate coloration. *Evolutionary Anthropology*, **17**, 97–111.

Bramble, D. M., & Lieberman, D. E. (2004). Endurance running and the evolution of Homo. *Nature*, **432**, 345–52.

Caine, N. G. (2002). Seeing red: consequences of individual differences in color vision in callitrichid primates. In L. E. Miller (Ed.), *Eat or be eaten*. Cambridge University Press, 58–73.

Caine, N. G., Surridge, A. K., & Mundy, N. I. (2003). Dichromatic and trichromatic *Callithrix geoffroyi* differ in relative foraging ability for red-green color-camouflaged and non-camouflaged food. *International Journal of Primatology*, **24**, 1163–75.

Call, J. (2010). Do apes know they can be wrong? *Animal Cognition*, **13**, 689–700.

Call, J., & Tomasello, M. (2008). Does the chimpanzee have a theory of mind? 30 years later. *Trends in Cognitive Science*, **12**, 187–92.

Castles, D. L., & Whiten, A. (1998). Post-conflict behaviour of wild olive baboons. I. Reconciliation, redirection and consolation. *Ethology*, **104**, 126–47.

Chance, M. R. A. (1962). An interpretation of some agonistic postures: the role of 'cut-off' acts and postures. *Symposia of the Zoological Society of London*, **8**, 71–89.

Changizi, M. A., Zhang, Q., & Shimojo, S. (2006). Bare skin, blood and the evolution of primate colour vision. *Biology Letters*, **2**, 217–21.

Cools, A. K. A., Van Hout, A. J. -M., & Nelissen, M. H. J. (2008). Canine reconciliation and third-party-initiated postconflict affiliation: do peacemaking social mechanisms in dogs rival those of higher primates? *Ethology*, **114**, 53–63.

Cords, M., & Turnheer, S. (1993). Reconciling with valuable partners by long-tailed macaques. *Ethology*, **93**, 315–25.

Crozier, W. R. (2006). *Blushing and the social emotions: the self unmasked*. Basingstoke: Palgrave Macmillan.

(2010). The puzzle of blushing. *The Psychologist*, **23**, 390–3.

Darwin, C. (1872/1965). *The expression of the emotions in man and animals*. Chicago University Press.

de Jong, P. J. (1999). Communicative and remedial effects of social blushing. *Journal of Nonverbal Behavior*, **23**, 197–217.

de Jong, P. J., Peters, M. L., & De Cremer, D. (2003). Blushing may signify guilt: revealing effects of blushing in ambiguous situations. *Motivation and Emotion*, **27**, 225–49.

de Waal, F. B. M. (1989). *Peace making among primates*. Cambridge, MA: Harvard University Press.

(1996). *Good natured: the origins of right and wrong in humans and other animals*. Cambridge, MA: Harvard University Press.

(2008). Putting the altruism back into altruism: the evolution of empathy. *Annual Review of Psychology*, **59**, 279–300.

de Waal, F. B. M., & Aureli, F. (2001). Conflict resolution in primates. In P. Bateson & E. Alleva (Eds.), *Frontiers of life*. Vol. 4: *The living world*, Part 1: *Biology of behavior*. San Diego: Academic Press, 327–35.
de Waal, F. B. M., & van Roosmalen, A. (1979). Reconciliation and consolation among chimpanzees. *Behavioural Ecology and Sociobiology*, 5, 55–66.
Dijk, K. F. L. (2009). *To blush, or not blush: the interpersonal and clinical implications of the blush's signal value*. Doctoral thesis, University of Groningen.
Dubuc, C., Brent, L. J. N., Accamando, A. K., Gerald, M. S., MacLarnon, A., Semple, S., Heistermann, M., & Engelhardt, A. (2009). Sexual skin color contains information about the timing of the fertile phase in free-ranging rhesus macaques. *International Journal of Primatology*, 30, 777–89.
Edelmann, R. J. (1990). Embarrassment and blushing: a component-process model, some initial descriptive and cross-cultural data. In W. R. Crozier (Ed.), *Shyness and embarrassment: perspectives from social psychology*. Cambridge University Press, 205–29.
Fessler, D. M. T. (2007). From appeasement to conformity: evolutionary and cultural perspectives on shame, competition, and cooperation. In J. L. Tracy, R. W. Robins & J. P. Tangney (Eds.), *The self-conscious emotions: theory and research*. New York: Guilford Press, 174–93.
Gerald, M. S. (1999). *Scrotal color in vervet monkeys (Cercopithecus aethiops sabaeus): the signal functions and potential proximate mechanisms of color variation*. Los Angeles: University of California Press.
Higham, J. P. (2009). Primate coloration – an introduction to the special issue. *International Journal of Primatology*, 30, 749–51.
Higham, J. P., Brent, L. J. N., Dubuc, C., Accamando, A. K., Engelhardt, A., Gerald, M. S., Heistermann, M., & Stevens, M. (2010). Color signal information content and the eye of the beholder: a case study in the rhesus macaque. *Behavioral Ecology*, 21, 739–46.
Hiramatsu, C., Melin, A. D., Aureli, F., Schaffner, C. M., Vorobyev, M., Matsumoto, Y., & Kawamura, S. (2008). Importance of achromatic contrast in short-range fruit foraging of primates. *PLoS ONE*, 3(10): e3356.
Horowitz, A. (2009). Disambiguating the 'guilty look': salient prompts to familiar dog behaviour. *Behavioural Processes*, 81, 447–52.
Ingram, A. L., & Parker, A. R. (2008). A review of the diversity and evolution of photonic structures in butterflies, incorporating the work of John Huxley (The Natural History Museum, London, from 1961 to 1990). *Philosophical Transactions of the Royal Society B*, 363, 2465–80.
Isbell, L. A. (1995). Seasonal and social correlates of changes in hair, skin, and scrotal condition in vervet monkeys (*Cercopithecus aethiops*) of Amboseli National Park, Kenya. *American Journal of Primatology*, 36, 61–70.
Jacobs, G. H. (1993). The distribution and nature of colour vision among the mammals. *Biological Reviews*, 68, 413–71.
  (2009). Evolution of colour vision in mammals. *Philosophical Transactions of the Royal Society B*, 364, 2957–67.
Jadresic, E. (2008). *When blushing hurts: overcoming abnormal facial blushing*. Bloomington, IN: iUniverse.

Kemp, T. S. (2005). *The origin and evolution of mammals*. Oxford University Press.

Koyama, N. F., & Dunbar, R. I. M. (1996). Anticipation of conflict by chimpanzees. *Primates*, 37, 79–86.

Leary, M. R., & Meadows, S. (1991). Predictors, elicitors, and concomitants of social blushing. *Journal of Personality and Social Psychology*, 60, 254–62.

Lorenz, K. (1963). *Das sogenannte Böse: zur Naturgeschichte der Aggression*. Vienna: Borotha-Schoeler.

McNamara, J. M., Fromhage, L., Barta, Z., & Houston, A. I. (2008). The optimal coyness game. *Proceedings of the Royal Society B*, 276, 953–60.

Melin, A. D., Fedigan, L. M., Hiramatsu, C., & Kawamura, S. (2009). Fig foraging by dichromatic and trichromatic *Cebus capucinicus* in a tropical dry forest. *International Journal of Primatology*, 30, 753–75.

Montagna, W., Machida, H., & Perkins, E. (1966). The skin of primates XXVIII: the stump-tail macaque (*Macaca speciosa*). *American Journal of Physical Anthropology*, 24, 71–85.

Montagna, W., Yun, J. S., & Machida, H. (1964). The skin of primates XVIII: the skin of the rhesus monkey (*Macaca mulatta*). *American Journal of Physical Anthropology*, 22, 307–19.

Moritz, G. L., & Dominy, N. J. (2010). Selective advantages of mono- and dichromatic vision among nocturnal primates. *Journal of Vision*, 10(15), 1.

Morris, D. (1956). The feather postures of birds and the problem of the origin of social signals. *Behaviour*, 9, 75–113.

(1957). 'Typical Intensity' and its relation to the problem of ritualization. *Behaviour*, 11, 1–12.

Perkins, E., Arao, T., & Uno, H. (1968). The skin of primates XXXVIII: the skin of the red uacari (*Cacajao rubicundus*). *American Journal of Physical Anthropology*, 29, 57–79.

Polizzi di Sorrentino, E., Schino, G., Visalberghi, E., & Aureli, F. (2010). What time is it? Coping with expected feeding time in capuchin monkeys. *Animal Behaviour*, 80, 117–23.

Polyak, S. (1957). *The vertebrate visual system*. University of Chicago Press.

Preuschoft, S., & van Hooff, J. A. R. A. M. (1997). The social function of 'smile' and 'laughter': variations across primate species and societies. In U. Segerstråle & P. Molnár (Eds.), *Nonverbal communication: where nature meets culture*. Mahwah, NJ: Lawrence Erlbaum, 171–91.

Prum, R. O., & Torres, R. H. (2004). Structural coloration of mammalian skin: convergent evolution of coherently scattering dermal collagen arrays. *Journal of Experimental Biology*, 207, 2157–72.

Prum, R. O., Torres, R. H., Williamson, S., & Dyck, J. (1998). Coherent light scattering by blue feather barbs. *Nature*, 396, 28–9.

(1999). Two-dimensional Fourier analyses of the spongy medullary keratin of structurally coloured feather barbs. *Proceedings of the Royal Society London B*, 266, 13–22.

Re, D. E., Whitehead, R. D., Xiao, D., & Perrett, D. I. (2011). Oxygenated-blood colour change thresholds for perceived facial redness, health, and attractiveness. *PLoS ONE*, 6(3), e17859.

Regan, B. C., Julliot, C., Simmen, B., Viénot, F., Charles-Dominique, P., & Mollon, J. D. (1998). Frugivory and colour vision in *Alouatta seniculus*, a trichromatic platyrrhine monkey. *Vision Research*, **38**, 3321–7.

(2001). Fruits, foliage and the evolution of primate colour vision *Philosophical Transactions of the Royal Society B*, **356**, 229–83.

Rowell, L. B. (1977). Reflex control of the cutaneous vasculature. *Journal of Investigative Dermatology*, **69**, 154–66.

Saito, A., Hosokawa, A. M., & Hasegawa, T. (2006). Advantage of dichromats over trichromats in discrimination of color-camouflaged stimuli in humans. *Perceptual and Motor Skills*, **102**, 3–12.

Salzen, E. (2010). Letter: flushing and blushing. *The Psychologist*, **23**, 539.

Schino, G. (1998). Reconciliation in domestic goats. *Behaviour*, **135**, 343–56.

Schuster, P., & Sigmund, K. (1981). Coyness, philandering and stable strategies. *Animal Behaviour*, **29**, 186–92.

Scott, W. (1832). *Tales of the crusaders: the betrothed*. Boston: Samuel Parker.

Setchell, J. M., & Dixson, A. F. (2001). Changes in the secondary sexual adornments of male mandrills (*Mandrillus sphinx*) are associated with gain. *Hormones and Behavior*, **39**, 177–84.

Setchell, J. M., Smith, T., Wickings, E. J., & Knapp, L. A. (2008). Social correlates of testosterone and ornamentation in male mandrills. *Hormones and Behavior*, **54**, 365–72.

Silk, J. B., Kaldor, E., & Boyd, R. (2000). Cheap talk in conflict. *Animal Behaviour*, **59**, 423–32.

Smith, A. C., Buchanan-Smith, H. M., Surridge, A. K., Osorio, D., & Mundy, N. I. (2003). The effect of colour vision status on the detection and selection of fruits by tamarins (*Saguinus* spp.). *Journal of Experimental Biology*, **206**, 3159–65.

Sumner, P., & Mollon, J. D. (2000). Catarrhine photopigments are optimized for detecting targets against a foliage background. *Journal of Experimental Biology*, **203**, 1963–86.

Tinbergen, N. (1951). *The study of instinct*. Oxford: Clarendon.

(1964). The evolution of signalling devices. In W. Etkin (Ed.), *Social behaviour and organization among vertebrates*. University of Chicago Press, 206–30.

van Hooff, J. A. R. A. M. (1967/2006). The facial displays of catarrhine monkeys and apes. In D. Morris (Ed.), *Primate ethology*, new edn. New York: Aldine, 7–68.

(2001). Conflict, reconciliation and negotiation in non-human primates: the value of long-term relationships. In R. Noë, J. A. R. A. M. van Hooff & P. Hammerstein (Eds.), *Economics in nature: social dilemmas, mate choice, biological markets*. Cambridge University Press, 67–90.

(2012). Facial-vocal displays, gestures and language. In S. Pika & K. Liebal (Eds.), *Developments in primate gesture research*. Amsterdam: John Benjamins, 13–32.

van Hooff, J. A. R. A. M., & Aureli, F. (1994). Social homeostasis and the regulation of emotion. In S. H. M. van Goozen, N. E. van de Poll & J. A. Sergeant (Eds.), *Emotions: essays on emotion theory*. Hillsdale, NJ: Lawrence Erlbaum, 197–218.

van Hooff, J. A. R. A. M., Baumans, V., & Brain, P. F. (1993). Recognition of pain and distress. In L. F. M. van Zutphen, V. Baumans & A. C. Beynen (Eds.), *Principles of laboratory animal science*. Amsterdam: Elsevier, 255–66.

van Hooff, J. A. R. A. M., & Wensing, J. A. B. (1987). Dominance and its behavioral measures in a captive wolf pack. In H. Frank (Ed.), *Ecology and behavior of wolves*. Dordrecht: Junk, 219–52.

van Schaik, C. P., & Aureli, F. (2000). The natural history of valuable relationships in primates. In F. Aureli & F. B. M. de Waal (Eds.), *Natural conflict resolution*. Berkeley: University of California Press, 307–33.

Wachtmeister, C.-A., & Enquist, M. (1999). The evolution of female coyness – trading time for information. *Ethology*, **105**, 983–92.

Waitt, C., Little, A. C., Wolfensohn, S., Honess, P., Brown, A. P., Buchanan-Smith, H. M., & Perrett, D. I. (2003). Evidence from rhesus macaques suggests that male coloration plays a role in female primate mate choice. *Proceedings of the Royal Society B: Biological Sciences (Supplement)*, **270**, S144–6.

Wickler, W. (1967). Socio-sexual signals and their intra-specific imitation among primates. In D. Morris (Ed.), *Primate ethology*. London: Weidenfeld & Nicolson, 69–147.

  (1968). *Mimikry: Nachahmung und Täuschung in der Natur*. Munich: Kindler Verlag.

Zahavi, A. (1987). The theory of signal selection and some of its implications. In V. P. Delfino (Ed.), *International symposium on biological evolution*. Bari: Adriatica Editrice, 305–27.

# 6 Self-conscious emotional development

*Hedy Stegge*

> 'The young blush more freely than the old, but not during infancy.'
> (Darwin, 1872/1989, p. 310)

Given its recognition as a universal facial expression, it is remarkable that we know so little about the emergence of the blush in childhood and its development across the life span. This is all the more surprising, since Darwin had already introduced a developmental perspective on the phenomenon of blushing, arguing that 'the mental powers of infants are not as yet sufficiently developed to allow of their blushing' (p. 311). According to his writings, blushing could reliably be observed in children between the ages of 2 and 3 but not in younger ones and decreased in adulthood; it had to be actively stimulated in children born blind by making them aware of the fact that they were being observed. In order to understand the meaning of Darwin's early observations, we will take an emotion perspective on the social blush, trying to unravel the developmental functions of self-conscious affect and the mental capacities needed for its occurrence.

## A functionalist perspective on self-conscious affect

According to a functionalist perspective, emotions evolved to enable us to solve problems of adjustment in our external environment (Levenson, 1999). As humans are a highly social species, many of these problems concern our relationships with others. Therefore, our emotion system is designed in such a way that we are able to successfully navigate our social environment. Specifically, a unique class of emotions evolved that signal threats to social relationships: the self-conscious emotions. Self-conscious emotions monitor our ongoing interactions with others and mobilize us to (quickly) deal with interpersonal problems. As self-consciousness involves the process of looking at yourself through the eyes of another, self-conscious emotions can be considered *social self-feelings*.

Barrett (1995) argues that all emotions can be classified in terms of a set of three distinctive but related functions: a behavioural regulatory function, an internal regulatory function and a social regulatory function. Emotions that serve the same functions across contexts belong to the same emotion family. In her view, the self-conscious emotions of shame, embarrassment, humiliation, and feelings of abasement or shyness all belong to the emotion family of shame. Although these shame-variants may occur in slightly different contexts and can be expressed in slightly different ways (Keltner & Buswell, 1996), they are supposed to promote the same three adaptive functions. On a behavioural level, expressions of shame-related affect function to reduce exposure and distance the self from evaluating others. Internally, shame highlights societal rules, standards and values and helps the person to gain knowledge about the self. In interactions with others, shame signals deference or submission, communicates the self as small or inadequate, shows a commitment to social or moral values, and helps restore damaged relationships.

Across cultures and ages, shame-related affect is associated with blushing or reddening of the face (Casimir & Schnegg, 2002; Ferguson et al., 1991). So an important question would be how blushing helps shame to fulfil its adaptive functions. Whereas Darwin believed that blushing was merely a byproduct of social attention, more recent accounts emphasize its value as a communicative signal. For example, Leary, Britt, Cutlip and Templeton (1992) have argued that people usually respect the blushing person's need for privacy by politely turning away and showing consideration. Moreover, Castelfranchi and Poggi (1990) argued that blushing in response to social transgressions shows a commitment to social values and group norms, which functions to inhibit others' hostility or aggression and prevents social exclusion. In line with this view, empirical studies have shown that those who blush after having transgressed elicit sympathy, forgiveness and help in others (Dijk & de Jong, 2009; de Jong, 1999; see Chapter 12, this volume).

The blush can be considered an especially effective marker of shame-related affect. First, it cannot be voluntarily produced. As Seneca wrote: 'the Roman players hang down their heads, fix their eyes on the ground and keep them lowered, but are unable to blush in acting shame'. Its involuntary nature makes it a very convincing emotional signal, showing that someone is trustworthy and really cares about relationships (Frank, 1988). Second, blushing not only signals a need for privacy, but also a need for affiliation (Keltner & Anderson, 2000). In a sense, shame motivates us to both turn away from and towards the other. When displaying a shameful blush, we distance ourselves from the observing or evaluating other, while at the same time asking for his or her help in accomplishing the goal of social re-engagement. If, as Sartre (1943/2003) put it, the expression of shame is indeed an indication of a basic relatedness to others, the blush (as well as the smile) may occupy a special position in its nonverbal manifestation.

## *The developmental functions of shame-related affect*

Abe and Izard (1999) argue that because of their unique adaptive functions, emotions help a developing child achieve key developmental milestones. Shame is important in that it highlights standards of conduct and promotes self-understanding. This process starts at a very young age and continues across the life span. Toddlers and preschoolers show a rapid growth in their autonomy. Their strivings for independence ('I want to do it myself') quite often lead to emotional confrontations, which stimulate the child's emerging sense of self-awareness, the awareness of others, and the understanding of social rules. As Barrett (1995) argued, 'the shame experience highlights the "looking glass self" – the self as others see one (or as one must appear to others) and therefore causes one to step back from the self and to evaluate oneself' (p. 47). In middle childhood, shame plays an important role in the development of a trait-like self-concept and the internalization of social rules and behavioural standards (Ferguson & Stegge, 1995). Peer relationships become more important and the avoidance of shame becomes a powerful motive for children to conform in order to maintain peer acceptance. In adolescence, self-consciousness increases even further and the tendency to see the self as a social object cultivates a vulnerability for the emotion of shame. As adolescents are concerned with identity formation and experiment with different social roles, shame-related affect again becomes a major motivating force in their lives (Reimer, 1996).

The next sections will discuss self-conscious emotional development in more detail with an emphasis on two different periods. The first is the preschool period, during which self-consciousness emerges and shame-related affect appears. The second one is adolescence because self-consciousness reaches a high level in this developmental phase, and shame-related affect contributes significantly to one of life's most important developmental tasks: namely, identity formation. After having discussed developmental changes in the nature of shame-related affect, I will speculate about the developmental significance of the blush.

## The emergence of self-conscious affect

Although children already emotionally respond to others' attention during the first year of life (Reddy, 2003), the birth of 'true' self-consciousness is generally situated in the second half of the second year of life. It requires higher order representational skills: that is, a concept of the self as an object (Lewis, 1995, 2000, 2001; Mills, 2005). The standard paradigm to measure objective self-recognition is the mirror test (Amsterdam, 1972). When children younger than 15 months are placed in front of a mirror with a spot of rouge on their nose, they touch their mirror image as if they are interacting with another child. However, in the second half of their second year this mirror-directed behaviour gives way to mark-directed behaviour: children infer from the mirror image that they themselves have a mark, touch their own nose and are motivated to clean it. Because the children cannot see their own face directly, the situation requires them to compare the face in the mirror with a mental representation of their own face. Lewis names this the appearance of a meta-representation of the self, or 'the idea of Me' (Lewis et al., 1989; see also Harter, 2006). The child not only perceives the self as an actor (primary representation of the self), but also has constructed a secondary representation of the self: a mental model that can be situated in the past or the future, and also be manipulated in fantasy. Importantly, mirror self-recognition occurs together with other self-referential behaviours (Bretherton & Beegly, 1982; Thompson & Lagatutta, 2006). Two-year-olds start to refer to the self in verbal communication by the use of personal pronouns (I, or me), mental state words ('John sad'), and expressions of their own competence or characteristics ('Cindy big'). In addition, children capable of objective self-awareness have been shown to be able to construct mental models of others' intentions and plans and use these insights to engage in synchronized play (Asendorpf & Baudonnière, 1993).

As soon as the self has become an object to the self, shame-related affect is possible. Early forms occur when children are the centre of attention and focus on the appearance of the self. Two-year-old children capable of self-recognition show signs of embarrassment (coyness, smiling, gaze aversion, nervous movements) when looking in a mirror with an audience present, when asked to sing or dance, or when being (overly) complimented (Lewis et al., 1989). Lewis (1995) names this as exposure embarrassment. The presence of an audience is critical for its occurrence, but at this age there seems to be a concern with being observed rather than with being evaluated.

Between the ages of three and three and a half years, children develop the capacity to experience a cognitively more advanced form of shame-related affect, that could be defined as evaluative embarrassment, as they become able to judge the self vis-à-vis behavioural standards of conduct. This development starts with a number of different capacities or developmental sensitivities that gradually result in the development of a system of internal standards against which children come to evaluate their behaviours. The first ingredient concerns the development, at around the age of 2, of mental representations of how the world is supposed to be. Violations of a norm (e.g., broken or flawed objects) now become a source of distress, and children's attention is increasingly drawn to the connection between their behaviour and standards of conduct (Kagan, 1984). As children are very sensitive to the messages conveyed by the emotional expressions of important others, the continuous checking and rechecking of this information helps them to internalize social rules and expectations. A second ingredient concerns children's wish to be perceived as good and competent: their need for competence (Deci & Ryan, 1995). Children are not merely passive consumers of others' responses to their achievements, but actively try to engage them in a process of evaluation. Towards the end of the second year of life, they start to show mastery smiles and attract others' attention to good performances or new skills (Heckhausen, 1984; Kagan, 1984; Stipek, 1995). Similarly, when they fail at a competitive task, they show social avoidant behaviours (turning the head or the body away). Importantly, negative facial expressions (frowns) signalling negative judgments about the self in response to failure are only observed in children older than 3 years of age. Consistent with Lewis's suggestions, Stipek (1995) hypothesizes that this reflects a new milestone in the development of self-conscious affect. Whereas 2-year-olds are mainly concerned with others' approving or disapproving reactions, 3-year-olds seem to have developed the capacity for internalized negative self-evaluation and show evaluative shame-related affect (see also Lewis *et al.*, 1992; Lewis, 2003).

To summarize, emerging levels of self- and other-awareness enable some members of the emotion family of shame to occur at a relatively young age. Contrary to what was thought earlier, 2- and 3-year-olds already demonstrate a psychological understanding of themselves and others (Thompson, 2006). As soon as they are able to represent the self in consciousness, exposure-related embarrassment becomes possible. When, at about a year later, children are also able to engage in self-evaluative behaviour relative to their success or failure in reaching standards of conduct or performance, self-evaluative shame-related affect emerges. As children mature, the capacity for self-reflection, the development of more complex and flexible representational skills, and the engagement in shared conversations about the 'self-in-relationships' (Barrett, 1995) allow for more advanced forms of self-awareness and interpersonal understanding. As we will see in the next section, self-consciousness peaks in adolescence and the experience of shame-related affect becomes highly salient in this age period.

## The self-conscious adolescent

From a functionalist perspective, it is argued that whereas there is continuity in the functions of distinctive emotions, there are developmental transformations in their subjective experience and expression. Across age, shame-related affect involves a heightened degree of conscious self-awareness, as it is concerned with the self-in-relationships. With increasing age, the affective experience deepens as self-exposure becomes increasingly associated with self-*evaluation*, and children become more concerned about how they are viewed by their peers. The developmental task of identity formation creates an interesting paradox. Young people need to develop their own individuality while at the same time showing conformity to group norms to become a valued member of society and prevent social ostracism. Shame-related affect plays a role in these two (seemingly) contradictory goals of self-development (Lynd, 1958; Reimer, 1996; Thrane, 1979). We will now discuss self-conscious affect as it is related to the changing nature of adolescents' self-representations and their sensitivity to others' judgments of the self.

### *Changes in the nature of the self*

In middle childhood, self-evaluation becomes an important aspect of children's goal-structures (Lewis, 2003; Mascolo & Fischer, 1995). Children gradually develop differentiated and integrated representations of the self's skills and start to compare them with those of others (Harter, 2006). This results in self-conscious affect about concrete traits (e.g., being good or bad at sports). In adolescence, youths start to think about traits as enduring and pervasive qualities (Mills, 2005) and develop identity-related abstractions of a competent or incompetent person (Mascolo & Fischer, 1995). Their complex representational skills allow for comparisons with ideals or anti-ideals: the kind of person they do want or do not want to be. Shame-related affect becomes associated with personal flaws and inadequacies and reflects concerns with one's identity (Ferguson *et al.*, 1991; Thomaes, Bushman *et al.*, 2009). In addition, the development of meta-representational skills ('thinking about your own thinking') may further intensify the experience of self-conscious affect through a process of rumination and the engagement in persistent comparisons between different hypothetical self-constructs (actual vs ideal self, or hoped for vs dreaded self; Izard, 2002).

Adolescents' self-representations not only change as a result of cognitive maturation but also as a function of their changing environment, goals and concerns. As children grow older, they are confronted with a wide range of standards and expectations, and have ample opportunities for the experience of success or failure in different areas of functioning. Adolescents engage in self-assessments across a variety of domains relevant to their self-concept and develop views of their school performance, their social skills, their physical appearance, their athletic abilities and their moral conduct (Harter, 2006). Evaluations of the self in these different contexts are so salient because adolescents relate them to chances and opportunities later in life. As confrontations with physical changes, changes in body image, concerns about gender roles, and changing social relationships are common, self-conscious affective experiences in different areas of competence help shape the adolescent's orientation to current and future roles. They come to make their own choices regarding school, work, leisure settings and relationships, and develop their own independent world-views (Collins & Steinberg, 2006).

### Interpersonal sensitivity

Self appraisals are in large part a reflection of the views of important others on the self, and are therefore sometimes called the 'looking glass self' (Cooley, 1902/1983). In general, developments in social perspective-taking and role-taking abilities allow for a better and more nuanced understanding of the social world. However, in adolescence there is more to this story. Young people are so concerned with the question of who they are and how they are similar to or different from others, that they may become overly sensitive to others' evaluations. Elkind and Bowen (1979) have argued that adolescents show a unique form of egocentrism. As they are so preoccupied by themselves, their ability to see themselves as a social object (i.e., as being the focus of others' attention) may cause them to think that others are as preoccupied with them as they are themselves. They suffer from what Leary and Toner (Chapter 4, this volume) call the spotlight effect. In the process of identity formation, they may be extremely aware not only of their own behaviours, qualities and aspirations, but also of the feelings of others towards the self.

In adolescence, extra-familiar relationships become more and more important. Young people develop social contacts characterized by mutual influence, self-disclosure and support. Contrary to relations with parents and siblings, peer relations are initiated on a voluntary basis and whether or not they will continue depends on mutual gratification. Adolescents engage in different types of social relationships. They develop emotionally intimate friendships with peers, sexual relationships with romantic partners, and affiliations with different peer groups or cliques. Concerns with body image, romantic appeal and social acceptability are prominent and create ambiguity and uncertainties. In the process of finding new ways to fulfil the basic psychological need for relatedness, adolescents are concerned with both real and imagined audiences. They experiment with different peer groups and relationships, and anticipate the reactions of others in real and fantasized situations by projecting the self in the eyes of the other. As a result of this heightened sensitivity for peer evaluations, adolescents are vulnerable to the experience of self-conscious affect.

Adolescents struggle to develop their own identity and individuality. They need to coordinate and integrate multiple possible perspectives on the self in the ultimate search for an authentic self (Harter, 2006). Self-conscious affect plays a major and sometimes complicated role in this process, as it signals significant concerns and fosters personal choices and certain forms of interaction. Because of their newly acquired cognitive skills and the huge bodily and social changes they encounter, adolescents in particular may experience a tension between a sense of independence and a sense of interdependence. They need to find a new base of physical, academic and social self-esteem, and self-conscious affect is assumed to fulfil a dual role in this process. Intrapersonally, self-conscious affect becomes increasingly associated with self-evaluation. It functions to reveal personal flaws and inadequacies, contributes to the internalization of personal and societal standards, and identifies areas for improvement. Interpersonally, the expression of self-conscious affect signals a need for privacy, and communicates deference and a commitment to social or moral values. As blushing is commonly associated with shame-related affect, I will now speculate about the significance of the blush at different points in development.

## The developmental significance of the blush

Blushing is commonly understood as the nonverbal expression of self-conscious or self-evaluative affect. Its first occurrence is situated in early childhood, when children become aware of the self as the object of others' attention. However, at this young age, children seem to blush rather infrequently. Parents report a significant increase in children's blushing and embarrassment at the age of 5 or 6 (Buss et al., 1979).

This might suggest that for a blush to occur something more is needed than simply being the object of others' attention. Crozier (2004) argues that instances of blushing involve a clash of values. There is an unexpected change in one's perspective on the self caused by the awareness of another's possible point of view. Similarly, Taylor (1985) suggests that shame-related affect results from the perceived discrepancy between one's current state ('I am having a fascinating conversation with someone') and a possible detached observer description ('She is trying to get a date with an attractive guy'). Obviously, perceived negative evaluations by others provide one important class of situations where a clash of values occurs, since in these situations the person embodies an anti-ideal or an unwanted identity (Olthof *et al.*, 2000). However, blushing may also occur in situations in which there is a more general concern with the fact that something personal is revealed in the eyes of the other (see Crozier, Chapter 11, this volume). It is the process of looking at the self through the eyes of another person (and becoming aware of potential discrepancies or frictions) that elicits the self-conscious blush. Presumably, then, blushing might be expected to occur when children have developed the capacity to incorporate the relation between their own view on the self and the perspective of others into a representational system (Mascolo & Fischer, 1995; Rochat, 2003), thus somewhere between the ages of 5 and 7. This perspective also implies that blushing will be especially likely to occur as the developmental task of identity formation causes young people to be so consciously aware of and concerned with their own and others' views on the self that clashes of values will be commonly present. As Miller (1996) has argued, 'If God wanted to create a perfect recipe for embarrassment, the teen years might be it' (p. 87).

Unfortunately, empirical research on the frequency of blushing is very limited. Based on parental report, Buss and colleagues did not find a further increase in the frequency of blushing between the ages of 5 and 12 years. Shields, Mallory and Simon (1990) studied the frequency of blushing in 13–55-year-olds and found a negative relationship with age. More specifically, they showed that over half of the people younger than 25 years of age reported blushing more than once a week, while one third said they blushed daily. Above the age of 25, only a quarter said they blushed more than once a week and almost no one reported daily blushing.

*Self-exposure and self-evaluation*

As has already been argued, self-conscious affect has surprisingly early developmental roots. Two- and three-year-olds show the first signs of embarrassment as they start to become aware of the self as an object of others' attention. Lewis (1995) has labeled this 'exposure embarrassment', and Leary and Toner (Chapter 4, this volume) relate its occurrence to being the focus of others' attention. In their view, it is undesired social attention (positive or negative) that accounts for many instances of blushing. From a developmental perspective, this is an intriguing explanation, as we know that the regulation of interpersonal distance is crucial in early developing relationships. Babies already try to achieve optimal social distance in face-to-face interactions with their caretakers. They show distress and turn their head away when parents come too close or are overwhelming. When children have developed the capacity to see the self as a social object, instances of unwanted social attention (fixed stares, very close scrutinizing, being singled out for excessive praise) may trigger a more specific self-conscious emotional response, which can be interpreted as exposure embarrassment. As the expression of self-conscious affect may signal a need for privacy to which others will usually respond by withdrawing their attention (Leary et al., 1992), blushing or other signs of embarrassment provide children with additional resources to regulate social distance.

Self-conscious affect seems to be strongly related to exposure, to being present 'in the eye of the other', to the awareness of 'being seen'. Erikson (1963) very nicely captured this image, when he emphasized that shame-related affect emerges when 'one is visible and not ready to be visible' (p.252). Early embarrassment seems to be related to physical appearance, and occurs, for example, when a child is asked to dance or sing in front of an audience. With age, concerns with exposure expand to include the awareness of others' judgments of the self, resulting in the capacity to experience self-evaluative embarrassment. As children mature and representational skills increase, self-conscious affect can take the form of feelings of embarrassment or shame that reveal personal flaws and pose a threat to one's identity. In embarrassment, personal flaws are supposed to be apparent, whereas in shame they are thought to be real (Keltner & Buswell, 1996). In either case, blushing signals the awareness of the unwanted identity and prompts others to react with sympathy, kindness or forgiveness.

From a developmental perspective and consistent with the unwanted visual attention explanation of the blush, it might be argued that self-exposure is the primary elicitor of embarrassment in many situations. The person becomes aware of being 'seen'. With age, a concern with being seen physically may generalize to a concern with being seen in a metaphorical sense: that is, as a particular kind of person (Griffin, 1995). Yet another way in which exposure and evaluation become intertwined in the course of development involves the person's engagement in the emotion process per se. Since the capacity as well as the willingness to reflect on emotional experiences increase with age (Stegge & Meerum Terwogt, 2007), self-exposure may induce self-evaluation. When people find themselves in an embarrassing emotional state, they may look for an explanation for their uncomfortable feelings (Lewis, 1995). A negative evaluation of the self or the self's incompetence then easily comes to mind: 'I should have been more careful not to attract his attention'; 'I wish I were more assertive'; 'Others handle this situation much better than I do.' This mechanism would explain why in young children embarrassment may be a relatively transient feeling or state, whereas in adolescents exposure embarrassment may easily turn into evaluative embarrassment or shame with longer-lasting implications.

### The self-in-relationship

Exposure is intrinsically related to privacy issues and concerns the boundaries between the self and others (Crozier, 2001, 2004; Chapter 11, this volume). Early in development self-conscious affect may be primarily a body-related emotion. Young children are concerned with other people's attention to their physical appearance and overt behaviours. Boundary issues are limited to the physical and tangible world. As children mature, they become increasingly concerned with the privacy of their own thoughts, inner feelings or personal characteristics. The self-conscious individual observes the self as if from outside. Whereas young children's feelings of exposure are mainly directed to their physical presence, in adolescence these feelings may extend to secret parts of the self (Lewis, 1995, 2001). In their newly developing relationships, adolescents are very concerned with issues of disclosure. They need to find out what they want to share, what they want to keep to themselves, and with whom they do or do not want to share. In this process, they (or their relationship partners) will very likely make mistakes, and it thus might be expected that blushing in response to the revelation of personal matters is a relatively common phenomenon in adolescence.

Leary and Toner (Chapter 4, this volume) argue that exposure theory has difficulties in explaining the function of the blush as a response to personal disclosure. In their view, it is not very likely that blushing serves a private cueing or regulatory function. However, from a developmental perspective one would think otherwise. It is conceivable that blushing, at least in adolescence, helps the person deal with boundaries. In a rapidly changing and relatively unstable social environment, adolescents need to determine what is private and what is not. Blushing may reveal personal sensitivities, and help the adolescent deal with uneasy social distance as a result of inappropriate disclosure, either by the self or by others. At the individual level, this may help the adolescent stay within boundaries of appropriate behaviour (Keltner & Anderson, 2000). Moreover, it stimulates the development of shared relationship values and expectations. At the dyadic or group level, again the blush signals a need for privacy, diverts others' attention away from the self, asks for consideration and may prevent further intrusions.

Shame-related affect reflects a fundamental need for social connection. It evokes complementary emotions in others that help the person respond to the interpersonal problem. The experience of shame functions to prevent social exclusion and restore damaged relationships. When social transgressions are relatively mild, as in embarrassment, others may smile and discount their importance. When transgressions are more serious, others may sympathize with the transgressor, and offer help or forgiveness (Keltner *et al.*, 1997; Keltner & Haidt, 1999). In order to fulfil its adaptive interpersonal function, the expression of embarrassment or shame signals both submissiveness and affiliation. It might be that the blushing has acquired new uses because of its potential to remedy problematic social interactions and increase social affiliation. Examples can be found among adolescents who intentionally evoke embarrassment by acts of disclosure, flirtation or teasing (Keltner & Anderson, 2000).

## Some directions for future research

In order to gain more knowledge about the personal and social significance of the shameful blush, two different research approaches can be taken. First, it will be important to study children's awareness and understanding of blushing as an expression of self-conscious affect. Second, the occurrence of blushing as a function of contextual factors relevant to the experience of variants of self-conscious affect can be studied at different points in development.

### *Children's awareness and understanding of the blush*

According to a functionalist perspective the expression of an emotion conveys essential information to the self and others. Since the blush has generally been taken as a manifestation of shame-related affect, children's awareness and knowledge of this emotion signal is important. Ferguson and colleagues (1991) studied 7–11-year-old children's conception of shame, and found that across age children reliably associated the blush with feelings of embarrassment or shame. Moreover, studies that used scenario-based measures to assess self-conscious affect (shame, guilt and ruminative guilt) in children aged 5–12, showed that items referring to blushing were consistently part of the 'shame' subscale (Ferguson & Stegge, 1995; Ferguson et al., 2000). Similarly, Colonnesi, Engelhardt and Davies (2010) showed that 4–9-year-olds were able to reliably report blushing by means of a Shyness and Blushing Questionnaire consisting of facial rating scales. However, to what extent children's ratings on these questionnaires actually reflect the awareness and frequency of their own blushing in social situations is not clear.

To my knowledge no studies have specifically addressed the development of children's understanding of the function of the blush as an expression of shame. However, research on children's attributions of embarrassment and their reasoning about emotional expressions in potentially embarrassing situations provides us with some indirect evidence relevant to this issue.

Several studies have shown that the presence of an audience is important for embarrassment to occur (Denham, 1998). More specifically, empirical evidence has been found for a two-stage developmental theory of children's understanding of embarrassment. Children aged 5–8 were shown to report embarrassment mainly in the presence of a criticizing audience, whereas 11–13-year-olds also reported embarrassment in the presence of a passive or complimenting audience (Bennett, 1989). Colonnesi and colleagues (2010) studied 4–9-year-old children's attributions of embarrassment to characters who were the centre of attention in a school setting. They found that attributions of embarrassment using a nonverbal assessment procedure were very frequent when the audience reacted with criticism or mockery (90 per cent), somewhat less frequent when the audience remained silent (78 per cent), and even less frequent when the audience complimented the child (60 per cent). Thus, for pre-adolescent children, embarrassment seems to be more firmly related to negative than to positive social attention.

In another series of studies (Banerjee, 2000; Wattling & Banerjee, 2007) children's understanding of modesty was investigated. It was shown that it was only from the age of 8 years that children viewed modest responses to receiving praise more positively than immodest responses. This is a rather complex cognitive and social achievement as children need to understand that a deprecating presentation of the self can lead to enhanced social evaluation. Indeed, the increased appreciation of modesty proved to be related to concerns about others' opinions about the self, especially in situations with peers. Importantly, children's greater sensitivity to the interpersonal dynamics of these situations was also related to self-monitoring, suggesting that both self- and other-awareness are crucial factors in judging the accompanying emotional responses. More generally, Banerjee, Bennett and Luke (2010) showed that between the ages of 7 and 10 children increasingly recognize the self-presentational risks of interpersonal events that elicit social attention to the self.

In middle childhood, children increasingly rely on self-presentational motives for their emotional behaviour in social situations (Banerjee, 2002; Saarni, 1999). For example, they might be motivated to avoid expressions of fear, sadness or shame because this makes them vulnerable to others' criticism or ridicule. In adolescence, the deceptive masking of emotions becomes especially important. At this age, young people begin to develop complex representations involving emotions about emotions (Izard, 2002). For example, they might be anxious about being anxious, feel angry about feeling ashamed and so on. It might be expected that the fear of blushing becomes prominent in this age period. Adolescents have become quite good at regulating their emotional expressions, and emotions are increasingly used as social signals (Denham, 1998). A lack of ability to control certain involuntary responses might cause frustration and anxiety. Blushing may be especially painful and hard to deal with since personal control is already generally low in embarrassing or shameful situations and one is very much dependent on the help of others to solve the interpersonal problem. Moreover, people are often motivated to disguise shame-related affect from both the self and others. Blushing might thus reveal something about the self that the person is not ready to express yet (Crozier, Chapter 11, this volume; Scheff, 1988).

Together, these studies suggest that with increasing age, children come to acknowledge the interpersonal consequences of (expressions of) embarrassment in different social situations. Thus far, empirical research has mainly focused on developmental changes in children's attributions of embarrassment as a function of audience type, and evaluative or self-presentational concerns. An additional contribution to this literature could be made by examining children's reasoning about distinctive expressions of shame-related affect, since specific emotion signals may convey unique information to both the self and others. It would also be important to focus not only on the interpersonal consequences of expressions of shame-related affect, such as the blush, but also pay attention to its personal meaning.

## *Developmental changes in the occurrence of blushing*

Research on the development of shame-related affect in young children has relied heavily on behavioural signs of the emotion. For example, studies conducted by Lewis and colleagues used observational methods, in which shame was defined as 'body collapsed, corners of the mouth are downward/lower lip tucked between teeth, eyes lowered with gaze downward or askance, withdrawal from task situation' (Lewis et al., 1992, p. 632; cf. Lewis, 1995). Barrett, Zahn-Waxler and Cole (1993) studied 2-year-old children's responses to a moral transgression; namely, harming the experimenter's favourite doll. According to these authors, children prone to shame-like behaviours were inclined to avert their gaze, to physically avoid the experimenter, and to wait a long time before attempting to repair the doll. They were also more likely to smile while averting their gaze from the experimenter. Remarkably, in research with children this age, blushing is not part of the coding system used to assess shame, which might suggest that it occurs rather infrequently.

In older children and adolescents, the development of shame has mainly been studied by the use of self-report. Empirical research has provided valuable information on age differences in shame appraisals, individual differences in proneness to shame, and the experience of shame in daily life (e.g., Ferguson & Stegge, 1995; Ferguson et al., 1991; Ferguson et al., 1999; Ferguson et al., 2000; Olthof et al., 2000; Thomaes et al., 2011). In this work, developmental changes in the *expression* of shame have received hardly any attention. Nonetheless, it might be that particular components of the expression of shame will be present only in some members of the shame family and not in others, depending on the function these emotion signals serve both at the intrapersonal and at the interpersonal level. For example, it has been argued that shame-related affect will be accompanied by a smile when a relatively mild transgression has taken place, but not when the transgression is more serious (e.g., Barrett, 1995). Research in which both appraisal and behavioural components of the emotional experience are assessed may provide important additional information regarding the function of distinctive emotion signals, including the social blush.

Research on shame-related affect in different age groups is difficult for a variety of reasons. At a young age it is often quite hard to distinguish expressions of embarrassment or shame from basic emotions like sadness or fear, especially since young children cannot reliably and validly report on their emotional experiences. When children are somewhat older, they may have developed a whole range of different strategies to deal with shame (including denial or other defensive responses), which makes it difficult to unambiguously determine whether or not shame-related affect is present when only self-report is used. Observations of blushing may provide unique information on age-related changes in the experience of self-conscious affect, since blushing cannot voluntarily be controlled.

In previous studies, valid paradigms have been developed to elicit shame-related affect in young children (e.g., Barrett *et al.*, 1993; Lewis *et al.*, 1989, 1992; Stipek, 1995) and adolescents (Thomaes *et al.*, 2008). Relevant factors have been identified that seem to moderate the occurrence of shame-related responding in children, such as task difficulty, type of transgression (moral vs social-conventional transgressions), the nature of the audience (peers vs adults) or the nature of its responses (critical, neutral or supportive). It would be interesting to specifically assess the occurrence of blushing as a function of these diverging developmentally relevant situational elicitors. As it is important to know how emotion processes unfold within children's social relationships, artificial laboratory procedures should be complemented by naturalistic studies (Saarni, 1999). Intriguing possibilities to assess (infrequent) emotional responses in young children's own environment are found in research on guilt in toddlers (Zahn-Waxler & Radke-Yarrow, 1982; Zahn-Waxler *et al.*, 1992). In these studies, mothers were carefully trained to observe their children's responses to naturally occurring events. In addition, children's responses to simulated events elicited either by caretakers or investigators were observed. A similar approach could be taken in order to determine age-related changes in the situational elicitors of blushing. We could ask caretakers, for example, to observe children's responses to social attention when performing an act, to situations in which they are asked to do something that is too difficult, or to situations in which they transgress a norm, or receive praise or critical feedback. In adolescents, the procedure developed by Thomaes and colleagues (2011) to measure daily experiences of shame and anger could be extended to include blushing episodes.

To conclude, it might be expected that with age, more situations become capable of eliciting a blush, and blushing may serve useful functions at different points in development. Although empirical research has reliably identified common elicitors of blushing, the relation of the blush to the nature of the accompanying self-conscious feeling state has been largely unexplored. Developmentally oriented research on the function of the blush and its occurrence across the life span has the potential to further strengthen the conceptual and empirical basis of existing theories of blushing.

REFERENCES

Abe, J. A., & Izard, C. E. (1999). The developmental functions of emotions: an analysis in terms of differential emotions theory. *Cognition and Emotion*, **13**, 523–49.

Amsterdam, B. K. (1972). Mirror self-image reactions before age two. *Developmental Psychology*, 5, 297–305.
Asendorpf, J. B., & Baudonnière, P. (1993). Self-awareness and other-awareness: mirror self-recognition and synchronic imitation among unfamiliar peers. *Developmental Psychology*, 29, 88–95.
Banerjee, R. (2000). The development of an understanding of modesty. *British Journal of Developmental Psychology*, 18, 499–517.
   (2002). Audience effects on self-presentation in childhood. *Social Development*, 11, 487–507.
Banerjee, R., Bennett, M., & Luke, N. (2010). Upsetting others and provoking ridicule: children's reasoning about the self-presentational consequences of rule violation. *British Journal of Developmental Psychology*, 28, 941–7.
Barrett, K. C. (1995). A functionalist approach to shame and guilt. In J. P. Tangney & K. W. Fischer (Eds.), *Self-conscious emotions: the psychology of shame, guilt, embarrassment, and pride*. New York: Guilford Press, 25–63.
Barrett, K. C., Zahn-Waxler, C., & Cole. P. M. (1993). Avoiders versus amenders: implications for the investigation of guilt and shame during toddlerhood? *Cognition and Emotion*, 7, 481–505.
Bennett, M. (1989). Children's attribution of embarrassment. *British Journal of Developmental Psychology*, 7, 207–17.
Bretherton, I., & Beegly, M. (1982). Talking about internal states of mind: the acquisition of an explicit theory of mind. *Developmental Psychology*, 18, 906–21.
Buss, A. H., Iscoe, I., & Buss, E. H. (1979). The development of embarrassment. *Journal of Psychology*, 103, 227–30.
Casimir, M. J., & Schnegg, M. (2002). The evolution, ontogeny, and function of a moral emotion. In H. Keller, Y. H. Poortinga & A. Scholmerich (Eds.), *Between biology and culture: perspectives on ontogenetic development*. Cambridge University Press, 270–300.
Castelfranchi, C., & Poggi, I. (1990). Blushing as a discourse: was Darwin wrong? In W. R. Crozier (Ed.), *Shyness and embarrassment: Perspectives from social psychology*. Cambridge University Press, 230–51.
Collins, W. A., & Steinberg, L. (2006). Adolescent development in interpersonal context. In W. Damon & R. M. Lerner (Series Eds.) & N. Eisenberg (Vol. Ed.), *Handbook of child psychology*, 6th edn. Vol. 3: *Social, emotional, and personality development*. New York: John Wiley & Sons, 1003–67.
Colonnesi, C., Engelhard, I. M., & Bögels, S. M. (2010). Development in children's attribution of embarrassment and the relationship with theory of mind and shyness. *Cognition and Emotion*, 24, 514–21.
Cooley, C. H. (1902/1983). *Social organisation*. New Brunswick, NJ: Transaction.
Crozier, W. R. (2001). Blushing and the exposed self: Darwin revisited. *Journal for the Theory of Social Behaviour*, 31, 61–72.
   (2004). Self-consciousness, exposure, and the blush. *Journal for the Theory of Social Behaviour*, 34, 1–17.
Darwin, C. (1872/1989). *The expression of the emotions in man and animals.* New York University Press.
de Jong, P. J. (1999). Communicative and remedial effects of social blushing. *Journal of Nonverbal Behavior*, 23, 197–218.

Deci, E. L., & Ryan, R. M. (1995). Human autonomy: the basis for true self-esteem. In M. Kernis (Ed.), *Efficacy, agency, and self-esteem*. New York: Plenum Press, 31–49.

Denham, S. A. (1998). *Emotional development in young children*. London: Guilford Press.

Dijk, C., & de Jong, P. J. (2009). The remedial value of blushing in the context of transgressions and mishaps. *Emotion*, 9, 287–91.

Elkind, D., & Bowen, R. (1979). Adolescent egocentrism in early and late adolescence. *Adolescence*, 9, 101–16.

Erikson, E. (1963). *Childhood and society*. New York: Norton.

Ferguson, T. J., & Stegge, H. (1995). Emotional states and traits in children: the case of guilt and shame. In J. P. Tangney & K. W. Fischer (Eds.), *Self-conscious emotions: shame, guilt, embarrassment and pride*. New York: Guilford Press, 174–97.

Ferguson, T. J., Stegge, H., & Damhuis, I. (1991). Children's understanding of guilt and shame. *Child Development*, 62, 827–39.

Ferguson, T. J., Stegge, G. T. M., Eyre, H., Vollmer, R., & Ashbaker, M. (2000). Context effects and the (mal)adaptive nature of guilt and shame in children. *Genetic, Social and General Psychology Monographs*, 126, 319–45.

Ferguson, T. J., Stegge, H., Miller, E. R., & Olsen, M. E. (1999). Guilt, shame and symptoms in children. *Developmental Psychology*, 35, 347–57.

Frank, R. H. (1988). *Passions within reason: the strategic role of the emotions*. New York: Norton.

Griffin, S. (1995). A cognitive-developmental analysis of pride, shame, and embarrassment in middle childhood. In J. P. Tangney & K. W. Fischer (Eds.), *Self-conscious emotions: the psychology of shame, guilt, embarrassment, and pride*. New York: Guilford Press, 219–36.

Harter, S. (2006). The self. In W. Damon & R. M. Lerner (Series Eds.) & N. Eisenberg (Vol. Ed.), *Handbook of child psychology*. Vol. 3: *Social, emotional, and personality development*. New York: John Wiley & Sons, 505–70.

Heckhausen, H. (1984). Emergent achievement behavior: some early developments. In J. Nicholls (Ed.), *The development of achievement motivation*. Greenwich, CT: JAI Press, 1–32.

Izard, C. E. (2002). Translating emotion theory and research into preventive interventions. *Psychological Bulletin*, 128, 796–824.

Kagan, J. (1984). *The nature of the child*. New York: Basic Books.

Keltner, D. (1995). Signs of appeasement: evidence for the distinct displays of embarrassment, amusement, and shame. *Journal of Personality and Social Psychology*, 68, 441–54.

Keltner, D., & Anderson, C. (2000). Saving face for Darwin: the functions and uses of embarrassment. *Current Directions in Psychological Science*, 9, 187–92.

Keltner, D., & Buswell, B. N. (1996). Evidence for the distinctness of embarrassment, shame and guilt: a study of recalled antecedents and facial expressions of emotion. *Cognition and Emotion*, 10, 155–71.

Keltner, D., & Haidt, J. (1999). Social functions of emotions at four levels of analysis. *Cognition and Emotion*, 13, 505–21.

Keltner, D., Young, R. C., & Buswell, B. N. (1997). Appeasement in human emotion, social practice, and personality. *Aggressive Behavior*, **23**, 359–74.

Leary, M. R., Britt, T. W., Cutlip, W. D., & Templeton, J. L. (1992). Social blushing. *Psychological Bulletin*, **112**, 446–60.

Levenson, R. W. (1999). The intrapersonal functions of emotion. *Cognition and Emotion*, **13**, 481–504.

Lewis, M. (1995). Embarrassment: the emotion of self exposure and evaluation. In J. P. Tangney & K. W. Fischer (Eds.), *Self-conscious emotions: the psychology of shame, guilt, embarrassment, and pride*. New York: Guilford Press, 198–218.

(2000). The emergence of human emotions. In M. Lewis & J. Haviland-Jones (Eds.), *Handbook of emotions*, 2nd edn. New York: Guilford Press, 265–80.

(2001). Origins of the self-conscious child. In W. R. Crozier & L. E. Alden (Eds.), *International handbook of social anxiety*. Chichester: John Wiley & Sons, 101–18.

(2003). The role of the self in shame. *Social Research*, **70**, 1181–204.

Lewis, M., Alessandri, S. M., & Sullivan, M. W. (1992). Differences in shame and pride as a function of children's gender and task difficulty. *Child Development*, **63**, 630–8.

Lewis, M., Sullivan, M. W., Stanger, C., & Weiss, M. (1989). Self-development and self-conscious emotions. *Child Development*, **60**, 146–56.

Lynd, H. M. (1958). *On shame and the search for identity*. New York: Harcourt.

Mascolo, M. F., & Fischer, K. W. (1995). Developmental transformations in appraisals for pride, shame and guilt. In J. P. Tangney & K. W. Fischer (Eds.), *Self-conscious emotions: the psychology of shame, guilt, embarrassment, and pride*. New York: Guilford Press, 64–113.

Miller, R. S. (1996). *Embarrassment: poise and peril in everyday life*. New York: Guilford Press.

Mills, R. S. L. (2005). Taking stock of the developmental literature on shame. *Developmental Review*, **25**, 26–63.

Olthof, T., Schouten, A., Kuiper, H., Stegge, H., & Jennekens-Schinkel, A. (2000). Shame and guilt in children: differential situational antecedents and experiential correlates. *British Journal of Developmental Psychology*, **18**, 51–64.

Reddy, V. (2003). On being the object of attention: implications for self-other consciousness. *Trends in Cognitive Science*, **7**, 397–402.

Reimer, M. S. (1996). 'Sinking into the ground': the development and consequences of shame in adolescence. *Developmental Review*, **16**, 321–63.

Rochat, P. (2003). Five levels of awareness as they unfold in early life. *Consciousness and Cognition*, **12**, 717–31.

Saarni, C. (1999). *The development of emotional competence*. New York: Guilford Press.

Sartre, J.-P. (1943/2003). *Being and nothingness*. London: Routledge.

Scheff, T. J. (1988). Shame and conformity: the deference-emotion system. *American Sociological Review*, **53**, 395–406.

Shields, S. A., Mallory, M. E., & Simon, A. (1990). The experience and symptoms of blushing as a function of age and reported frequency of blushing. *Journal of Nonverbal Behavior*, **14**, 171–87.

Stegge, H., & Meerum Terwogt, M. (2007). Awareness and regulation of emotion in typical and atypical development. In J. Gross (Ed.), *Handbook of emotion regulation*. New York: Guilford Press, 269–86.

Stipek, D. J. (1995). The development of pride and shame in toddlers. In J. P. Tangney & K. W. Fischer (Eds.), *Self-conscious emotions: the psychology of shame, guilt, embarrassment, and pride*. New York: Guilford Press, 237–52.

Taylor, G. (1985). *Pride, shame, and guilt: emotions of self-assessment*. Oxford: Clarendon Press.

Thomaes, S., Bushman, B. J., Orobio de Castro, B., & Stegge, H. (2009). What makes narcissists bloom? A framework for research on the etiology and development of narcissism. *Development and Psychopathology*, 21, 1233–47.

Thomaes, S., Bushman, B. J., Stegge, H., & Olthof, T. (2008). Trumping shame by blasts of noise: narcissism, self-esteem, shame, and aggression in young adolescents. *Child Development*, 79, 1792–801.

Thomaes, S., Stegge, H., Olthof, T., Bushman, B. J., & Nezlek, J. B. (2011). Turning shame inside-out: 'humiliated fury' in young adolescents. *Emotion*, 11, 786–93.

Thompson, R. A. (2006). The development of the person: social understanding, relationships, self, conscience. In W. Damon & R. M. Lerner (Series Eds.) & N. Eisenberg (Vol. Ed.), *Handbook of child psychology*, 6th edn. Vol. 3: *Social, emotional, and personality development*. New York: John Wiley & Sons, 24–98.

Thompson, R. A., & Lagatutta, K. H. (2006). Feeling and understanding: early emotional development. In K. McCartney & D. Phillips (Ed.), *The Blackwell handbook of early childhood development*. Oxford: Blackwell, 317–37.

Thrane, G. (1979). Shame. *Journal for the Theory of Social Behaviour*, 9, 139–66.

Watling, D., & Banerjee, R. (2007). Children's understanding of modesty in front of peer and adult audiences. *Infant and Child Development*, 16, 227–36.

Zahn-Waxler, C., & Radke-Yarrow, M. (1982). The development of altruism: alternative research strategies. In N. Eisenberg-Berg (Ed.), *The development of prosocial behavior*. New York: Academic Press, 109–37.

Zahn-Waxler, C., Radke-Yarrow, M., Wagner, E., & Chapman, M. (1992). Development of concern for others. *Developmental Psychology*, 28, 126–36.

# 7 A biosocial perspective on embarrassment

*Ryan S. Darby and Christine R. Harris*

On the surface, embarrassment seems like a rather straightforward, and perhaps trivial, emotion. When people recount stories of their embarrassment, their social woes are often greeted with laughter and amusement. Television audiences tune in en masse to watch embarrassing protagonists such as Michael Scott (or David Brent) in *The Office*. Yet, in spite of this perceived levity, embarrassment is frequently dreaded. People will go to astounding lengths to avoid even the shadow of embarrassment. Important decisions such as whom to help, whether to use protection during intercourse, and even whether or not to visit the doctor are all affected by the mere threat of embarrassment. As the research examining embarrassment continues to evolve, it has become increasingly clear that embarrassment is a complex and powerful emotion. In this chapter, we examine this intriguing emotion by first reviewing its proposed causes and functions, including the nature of embarrassment's nonverbal displays. We will then examine the physiological and neural correlates of embarrassment. Finally, we will review how embarrassment affects cognitions and behaviour, particularly within the health domain, and whether it is distinct from a related emotion: namely, shame.

## Theories of embarrassment

The situations that give rise to embarrassment are diverse. Some of the more common types of elicitors are physical pratfalls (e.g., tripping), cognitive shortcomings (e.g., forgetting someone's name), and being teased (Miller, 1992). However, the presence of an audience, real or imagined, may be the most crucial situational cause of embarrassment. Embarrassment is not often felt when one is alone (Tangney *et al.*, 1996) and behaviours that are extremely embarrassing in public are less likely to evoke embarrassment in private. For example, defecating in public would cause most people to feel intense embarrassment, yet defecating in private is rarely an emotional experience. Spilling one's drink in public is generally regarded as embarrassing, yet spilling one's drink in private is merely a hassle. While this may seem like a fairly obvious point, it is nevertheless an important one. It seems that the cause of embarrassment is not merely one's actions, but rather engaging in those actions in front of an audience.

The two most prominent theories for the origins of embarrassment are the social evaluation model and the dramaturgic or awkward interaction account (for detailed discussion see Chapter 9 of this volume). The social evaluation model posits that embarrassment is caused by the threat of negative social evaluation (Modigliani, 1968; Miller, 1996). Accordingly, embarrassment arises when people perceive that the social image they want to project has been undermined and that others are forming negative impressions of them. The cognitive appraisals that the situation could result in damaged social esteem are key to eliciting embarrassment in this model (Miller, 1996). For example, a person who spills a drink at a dinner party is likely to become embarrassed. Based on the social evaluation account, this embarrassment arises from the spiller's perception that others are thinking more negatively of her ('What a klutz!'). While this theory has good explanatory power, as many embarrassing situations would seem to fit this account, it fails to adequately explain embarrassment that is caused by being the centre of attention. For example, the social evaluation model has a hard time accounting for why people feel embarrassment at having 'Happy Birthday' sung to them. It seems unlikely that this embarrassment is caused by evaluation threat, as the singers are likely not only friends but they are also in the midst of imparting well wishes to the embarrassed party.

The dramaturgic or awkward interaction account, on the other hand, proposes that embarrassment stems from a loss of social script (Silver et al., 1987). When a person does not know how to act and does not know what the social expectations are, he or she is likely to feel embarrassment (Goffman, 1956, 1967). Thus, it is the interruption of the smooth social functioning and not social evaluation that gives rise to embarrassment according to this model. In the 'Happy Birthday' example, embarrassment is therefore caused by not knowing what to do under the spotlight of positive well wishes.

There are several studies that have compared these two accounts and their ability to explain embarrassment (Miller, 1995, 1996; Parrott & Smith, 1991; Parrott et al., 1988). The general finding from these studies is that both theories are effective in explaining and predicting embarrassment. A likely explanation is that each theory accounts for a unique pathway to embarrassment. In fact, factor analyses of participants' ratings of embarrassing scenarios appear to support this conclusion.

These analyses demonstrate that embarrassing situations can be divided into three dimensions: committing a faux pas, being the centre of attention, and 'sticky situations' (e.g., asking for a loan to be repaid) (Sabini et al., 1999). While social evaluation apprehension seems best suited to explain faux-pas scenarios, the awkward-interaction model seems better suited to explain centre-of-attention scenarios. Sticky situations, on the other hand, may be a combination of the two. Interestingly, centre-of-attention scenarios seem to be one of the most prominent causes of blushing (Crozier, 2004).

From an evolutionary perspective, embarrassment probably arose because in our ancestral past it was likely an adaptive way to prevent social exclusion. Humankind has evolved to depend upon group living; successful members of a group presumably have greater inclusive fitness than lone individuals. For this reason, there is an adaptive benefit to remaining a group member in good standing and preventing social ostracism. Groups often create social conventions and rules to discourage behaviours that are counter to the group's welfare. Violations of these mores can result in loss of group membership (Gruter & Masters, 1986). To prevent social ostracism, embarrassment likely developed (1) as an appeasement gesture, (2) to deter social transgressions, and (3) to motivate amends and reparation for the social wrong (Harris, 2006; Keltner & Buswell, 1997).

There are several research findings that seem to support these proposed functions of embarrassment. The first is that experiencing embarrassment does seem to motivate embarrassed individuals to act prosocially (e.g., make amends). For example, in one classic study on embarrassment, participants were asked to perform either highly embarrassing tasks (e.g., singing the 'Star Spangled Banner' or dancing to a record) or mildly embarrassing tasks (e.g., count aloud to fifty or listen to a record) while being watched through a two-way mirror by a confederate (Apsler, 1975). Afterwards, the confederate approached all the participants and asked them to help with a class project by completing a questionnaire for a half-hour each day for as many days as they were willing. A control group had not performed any previous tasks but was still asked by the confederate to help with the class project. On average, participants who had engaged in the highly embarrassing acts volunteered to help the most number of days (14.9 days), followed by those who had performed the mildly embarrassing acts (8.7 days). The control group volunteered to help the least (5.0 days). A follow-up study further revealed that embarrassed individuals were more likely to help than non-embarrassed individuals, even when the person who was asking for help had not been a witness to the embarrassing act (Apsler, 1975).

Apparently, embarrassment produces a general motivation to act prosocially towards others, regardless of whether those others witnessed the social transgression.

This motivation to repair may even be evidenced in very basic psychological processes such as visual attention. In the only study, to our knowledge, that examined how embarrassment affects visual attention, researchers used an eye-tracker to follow the gazes of embarrassed people as they looked at still photographs of faces with angry, sad, happy or neutral expressions (Darby & Harris, 2010). They found that embarrassed individuals paid significantly more attention to the eyes in the photographs than did those who were not embarrassed and that embarrassed individuals paid significantly more attention to the eyes of angry expressions compared to neutral or happy expressions (Darby & Harris, 2010). Other researchers have noted that the eyes are especially critical in identifying complex emotions and emotional intensity (Baron-Cohen et al., 1997), as well as direction of attention (Hietanen, 1999). Therefore, it may be that embarrassed individuals are attempting to gather more information about their social surroundings than non-embarrassed individuals. Thus, although embarrassed individuals may signal submission and apology through blushing (de Jong, 1999), downward glances and gaze shifts (Harris, 2001; Keltner, 1995), it appears that they still actively scan their emotional surroundings, particularly by monitoring the eyes of others, as they attempt to repair their social transgressions.

Another line of evidence that appears to support functional accounts of embarrassment is that nonverbal displays of embarrassment seem to promote positive regard in witnesses of the social transgression in a variety of situations (Keltner et al., 1997; Semin & Manstead, 1982). For example, researchers showed participants several different versions of a man knocking over a store display of toilet paper (Semin & Manstead, 1982). In half of the recordings the man showed embarrassment, while in the other half he did not. The experimenters also manipulated whether or not the man was shown picking up the knocked-over display. Participants rating the different versions tended to rate the man as most likeable when he showed embarrassment, regardless of whether he picked up the display or not (Semin & Manstead, 1982). Even still pictures of embarrassment seem to produce positive feelings from viewers (Keltner et al., 1997). Research on the blush, which occurs often during embarrassment, similarly finds that blushing can ingratiate the blusher to an audience (de Jong, 1999; see Chapter 12, this volume).

However, there do seem to be some limitations in the extent to which displaying embarrassment wins over an audience. In one study assessing the relationship between helping behaviour and displays of embarrassment, researchers had a woman (a confederate) visit several college classes to request volunteers for a research study (Levin & Arluke, 1982). During the request, the woman displayed varying degrees of composure. In one condition, she remained calm. In another she dropped her papers and became embarrassed, but eventually recovered. In the final condition, she dropped her papers, became embarrassed, but never recovered; instead she wound up handing the volunteer forms to the teacher and fleeing the classroom. As with the toilet paper study discussed previously, showing some embarrassment seemed to ingratiate her with the audience (i.e., class members volunteered the most in this condition). Of note, the extreme embarrassment condition did not increase volunteering relative to the control condition. Thus, it seems that mild displays of embarrassment may act as an appeasement gesture to others and promote favour with them, but extreme displays of embarrassment may not be as efficacious.

### Nonverbal displays

Over the years a number of studies have examined the nonverbal displays that occur during embarrassment. The behaviours most commonly noted across studies are blushing, looking away or down, smiling, and increased body movement (Asendorpf, 1990; Edelmann & Hampson, 1979, 1981; Harris, 2001; Keltner, 1995; Shearn et al., 1990, 1992). Particularly fine-grained analyses of the displays of embarrassment, as well as their temporal dynamics, have been performed by Keltner (1995) and Asendorpf (1990).

Keltner (1995) used Ekman and Friesen's Facial Action Coding System (FACS; Ekman and Friesen, 1978) to code facial movements while participants experienced embarrassment and amusement. FACS catalogues distinct combinations of observable muscle movements into forty-four numbered appearance changes called 'action units'. Keltner's work found that the prototypical embarrassment expression includes frequent gaze shifts (particularly to the left), looking down, head movements and smiling, as well as attempts to inhibit or obscure the smile ('smile controls' such as pressing the lips together). People also commonly touched their faces when embarrassed. Temporal analyses found that embarrassment display onset was fairly fast and unfolded roughly over a four- to five-second period. Comparison of prototypical amusement and embarrassment displays revealed that embarrassment usually began with gazing down while amusement began with a smile, and that the smiles of embarrassment were more often accompanied and terminated by smile control attempts. Embarrassment was also more likely to end with a head movement. In addition, Keltner found that the first sideways gaze shift during embarrassment was to the left, in contrast to amusement which was to the right.

Research by Asendorpf (1990) focused on the temporal relationship between gaze aversion and smiling, revealing another difference between the smiles during embarrassment and those in non-embarrassed states. Asendorpf found that during embarrassed smiles (as rated by a variety of judges), gaze aversion typically took place one and half seconds before the offset of the smile's apex – the point during smiling when the lips are maximally turned up. Gaze aversion also occurred in non-embarrassed smiling but this was significantly more likely to happen after the smile apex offset, usually around a half second after. Asendorpf suggests that embarrassed smiles may be perceived as ambivalent because of the co-occurrence of gaze aversion (an avoidant behaviour) with peak smiling intensity (an approach behaviour).

## Bodily responses

### The psychophysiology of embarrassment

Like many other emotions, embarrassment is accompanied by activation of the sympathetic nervous system (SNS). For example, several studies have shown that embarrassment induces increases in skin conductance (sweat gland activity), indicating the involvement of the SNS (Gerlach et al., 2003; Hofmann et al., 2006; Shearn et al., 1990, 1992). Increased electrodermal activity was also found in a study on vicarious or empathetic embarrassment, which was elicited when observers watched someone with whom they had previously interacted engage in embarrassing acts (Miller, 1987).

Other research suggests that just as the facial and bodily displays of embarrassment unfold in a complex and rather distinct manner across time so may the changes in cardiovascular reactivity. In two studies in our lab (Harris, 2001), participants were videotaped as they sang the national anthem of the United States, the 'Star Spangled Banner' – a song that is particularly hard to sing due to the extensive vocal range needed to hit high and low notes coupled with some rather awkward phrasing of words. An a capella solo performance of this song by itself would be embarrassing for most, but the participants were even further embarrassed by having to watch, with the experimenter and two strangers, a 2-minute videotape of their vocal performance. Throughout this whole ordeal, continuous beat-to-beat readings of each participant's heart rate, systolic blood pressure and diastolic blood pressure were recorded. Participants' blood pressure rose substantially during the first minute of the video and continued to rise during the second minute, with an average increase of 16 mm for systolic blood pressure and 10 mm for diastolic blood pressure. This is an impressive increase given that no physical activity was involved – participants were simply sitting and watching themselves on video in the presence of an audience. Blood pressure remained significantly elevated even 5 minutes after the video had been turned off and the audience had left.

People's hearts also beat faster during the first minute of embarrassment in the Harris studies. However, unlike blood pressure, heart rate dropped back down to baseline (pre-embarrassment) levels during the second minute of the embarrassing episode. Interestingly, in both of the studies reported by Harris (2001), self-reports of the intensity of embarrassment were correlated with the increases in heart rate during the first minute of embarrassment but were not correlated with blood pressure changes. People can detect their own heart rate changes more easily than blood pressure changes (hence the common reference to hypertension as the 'silent killer') and so may more readily use heart rate when assessing the intensity of their feelings. This would fit with questionnaire studies that find that people report their heart rates increase during embarrassment (Edelmann et al., 1989; Edelmann, 1987).

The decoupling of heart rate and blood pressure as embarrassment unfolds is intriguing. Research on a number of emotions such as anger and fear suggests that heart rate and blood pressure generally increase and decrease together across many emotional states (e.g., Roberts & Weerts, 1982; Schwartz et al., 1981). Although caution should be exercised when comparing findings across studies, one suggestion is that the initial increase of heart rate and blood pressure followed by their decoupling, as heart rate returns to baseline and blood pressure continues to rise, may be unique to embarrassment. Hence, just as there is a complex and rather distinctive nonverbal display of embarrassment, there also may be a signature pattern of cardiovascular reactivity.

Some theorists have proposed that the parasympathetic nervous system may also play a role in embarrassment (Buss, 1980). Such a view would be consistent with early work suggesting that the anticipation of an embarrassing act (e.g., sucking on a pacifier) led to decreased heart rate relative to the anticipation of a fearful event (Buck et al., 1970) and with the finding in the Harris (2001) study that heart rate decreased as embarrassment continued over a 2-minute period. However, simply measuring heart rate activity cannot tell us which branch of the autonomic nervous system is producing changes since the heart is innervated by both the parasympathetic nervous system (engagement decreases heart rate) and the sympathetic nervous system (engagement increases heart rate). One way to determine whether the PNS is involved in physiological changes is by measuring respiratory sinus arrhythmia (RSA). Two studies have directly attempted to assess RSA activity but failed to find support for activation of the PNS during embarrassment (Gerlach et al., 2003; Hofmann et al., 2006). However, this work does not rule out that the PNS might affect other organs besides the heart during embarrassment.

Blushing frequently occurs during embarrassment and no description of embarrassment would be complete without considering the blush. However, given the number of other chapters in this book that specifically focus on blushing, we will keep our discussion of it relatively brief. We simply highlight a few of the more intriguing aspects of embarrassment and blushing and encourage readers to explore the remainder of the book for further information.

Some of the key research on the temporal dynamics of blushing during embarrassment has come from the work of Shearn and colleagues (Shearn et al., 1990, 1992). In this work, as in several embarrassment studies, participants watched themselves sing on a pre-recorded video in the presence of an audience. Cheek and ear coloration were measured using photoplethysmography, and cheek temperature was also taken. All three measures rose significantly more during the embarrassing video compared to a fearful video (the shower murder scene in the film *Psycho*). Furthermore, during embarrassment, the intensity of cheek coloration increased as the size of the audience expanded from one to four. Blushing during embarrassment began with a sharp increase of blood flow to the face, which was followed by a slower rise in temperature. The authors point out that the visibility of the blush is due to increases in blood flow, enabling others to detect it. However, people's awareness of their own blushing is likely due to increased facial temperature (i.e., feeling one's face getting hotter). From this, Shearn and colleagues make a keen inference – other people can likely see that we are blushing before we are conscious of it ourselves. These results suggest that the decoupling of temperature and blood flow may be due to activation of separate physiological mechanisms. The notion that several physiological mechanisms affect blushing is also supported by research by Drummond (1997). He found that blocking activation of facial beta-adrenergic receptors in the sympathetic nervous system does not completely eliminate blushing during singing, which suggests that the blush involves more than one vasodilator.

While there are still many questions about the physiological changes associated with embarrassment, such as the proposed role of the PNS, it does appear that embarrassment has some rather unique physical concomitants, which unfold in a complex manner over time.

### The neuroanatomy of embarrassment

While the neurological research specifically examining embarrassment is sparse, what there is seems to indicate that embarrassment is a cognitively complex emotion with widely distributed neural circuitry (Sturm et al., 2006). No one area of the brain has been found to be solely responsible for embarrassment, but there is converging evidence that embarrassment is tied to the regions of the brain that seem to be important to theory of mind and self-awareness (Beer, 2007). In a neuroimaging study of healthy adults, Berthoz and colleagues (Berthoz et al., 2002) found that reading stories of embarrassing situations or social transgressions was more likely than reading neutral stories to elicit activation in areas of the frontal and temporal lobes, specifically the medial prefrontal cortex, temporo-parietal region, the basal temporal cortex and the orbitofrontal cortex. These regions seem to be associated with tasks involving theory of mind and regulation of social behaviour (Berthoz et al., 2002; Frith & Frith, 1999; Gallagher & Frith, 2003).

While other emotions, such as fear or anger, likely also rely on distributed neural networks that could include the frontal and temporal lobes, research on patients with frontotemporal lobe degeneration (FTLD) indicates that damage to these regions seems to have a greater impact on embarrassment than other emotions (Sturm et al., 2006). FTLD is an uncommon degenerative disease in which portions of the frontal and temporal lobes of the brain atrophy, causing dementia and eventually death. Unlike Alzheimer's disease, another well-known form of dementia, the emotions and personality of the individual quickly erode during FTLD while the memory and spatial abilities initially remain intact (Levenson & Miller, 2007). FTLD patients often behave in socially inappropriate ways including overly aggressive behaviour, poor impulse control and disregard for social rules (Bozeat et al., 2000; Levenson & Miller, 2007; Neary et al., 1998; Rankin et al., 2005). Emotionally, they seem to have severe impairments in recognizing facial expressions of emotion, empathy, self-awareness, and self-conscious emotions (Neary et al., 1998; Rankin et al., 2005; Rosen et al., 2004; Snowden et al., 2001).

Important to this discussion of embarrassment and neuroanatomy, a recent study of patients with FTLD found evidence that frontotemporal decay seems to affect embarrassment before it affects other negative emotions such as fear and anger (Sturm et al., 2006). In this study, patients with FTLD and healthy control participants were unexpectedly subjected to a loud blast of white noise similar to a car backfiring. For control participants, this loud noise typically caused a startle response and negative affect (e.g., anger, fear, sadness) followed by obvious signs of embarrassment (e.g., smile suppression, gaze aversion, blushing). In FTLD patients, the loud noise effectively elicited the startle response and negative affect but only a small minority of FTLD patients showed any signs of embarrassment. One explanation for this finding is that since FTLD damages the regions of the brain associated with self-awareness and theory of mind, patients with FTLD are less capable of comparing their own behaviour to the standard held by others. Importantly, these findings demonstrate the significance of the frontal and temporal lobes in the embarrassment experience.

Two particular areas of the frontal lobes – the medial prefrontal cortex and the orbitofrontal region – may play especially important roles in embarrassment. Research on special populations with neuropsychological disorders or impairments indicates that deficits in these areas are associated with abnormally low rates of experiencing embarrassment. Autism, for example, is a neurodevelopmental disorder related to disruptions in social functioning and theory of mind (Baron-Cohen, 2000). Neuroimaging studies find that autistic individuals, compared to psychologically healthy controls, typically have less activation in the medial prefrontal cortex (Castelli *et al.*, 2002; Happé & Frith, 1996). This region of the brain, particularly the anterior paracingulate cortex, seems to be critical to self-awareness and understanding the mental states of others (Walter *et al.*, 2004). When it comes to experiencing embarrassment, some studies suggest that autistic individuals may experience less embarrassment and engage in more inappropriate social behaviours (Capps *et al.*, 1992; Kasari *et al.*, 2001). One suggestion is that the difficulties autistic people have with embarrassment may be due to deficits in theory of mind (Heerey *et al.*, 2003), which perhaps stem from abnormal neurodevelopment (Happé *et al.*, 1996). While this proposal is largely untested, one group of researchers has found that autistic individuals, compared to control participants, have more difficulty identifying self-conscious emotions (i.e., embarrassment and shame) than non-self-conscious emotions but that this difference disappears when theory of mind dissimilarities are statistically controlled (Heerey *et al.*, 2003). Thus, it appears that some of the difficulties autistic individuals have with embarrassment may be partially accounted for by their struggles with theory of mind. Whether this is due to disrupted development in the corresponding brain areas, however, is unclear.

Another special population that experiences difficulties with embarrassment is patients with orbitofrontal brain damage. One of the key findings to come from this line of research is that damage to the frontal lobes may impair the frequency of embarrassment, but it does not seem to actually prevent one from experiencing embarrassment. Similar to autistic individuals, people who experience orbitofrontal brain damage tend to engage in socially inappropriate behaviours and may have some difficulties understanding the feelings and emotional expressions of others (Blair & Cipolotti, 2000; Stone et al., 1998; Willis et al., 2010). Interestingly, when orbitofrontal patients are given paper-and-pencil tests of social norms, they are no worse at identifying appropriate social behaviours than healthy controls or patients with lateral prefrontal damage (Beer et al., 2006). However, when actually engaging in a task that requires upholding social norms, orbitofrontal patients will often violate the social norm and do so seemingly unaware that their violation was inappropriate. For example, in a series of studies testing the social ramifications of orbitofrontal brain damage, Beer and colleagues found that orbitofrontal patients, compared to healthy controls, disclosed more inappropriate information to strangers and tended to be overly familiar in their teasing of strangers (Beer et al., 2003; Beer et al., 2006). Though observers regarded these interactions as inappropriate, the patients did not show any embarrassment and actually reported more pride in their behaviours than the control participants (Beer et al., 2003). It seems that even though they are aware of the social norms, they often have difficulty applying this knowledge to their own behaviours.

It is important to note that despite these difficulties, orbitofrontal patients can, however, still experience embarrassment. Although the orbitofrontal patients in these studies did not initially report embarrassment, when shown video recordings of their inappropriate behaviour, they became significantly more embarrassed than control participants (Beer et al., 2006). A tentative summary of this line of research is that the damage to the orbitofrontal lobes most likely causes difficulties with embarrassment through diminished self-awareness, but if that self-awareness is increased (e.g., by showing them video of their behaviour) embarrassment can still occur.

Together, the work on these special populations and the neuroimaging of healthy controls converges on several general conclusions about the neuroanatomy of embarrassment. First, as stated by Sturm and colleagues (2006), 'self-conscious emotions rely on complicated, distributed brain networks' (p. 2509). Second, it appears that the frontal and temporal lobes are especially important to embarrassment, perhaps because of the need for theory of mind and self-awareness. Damage or poor development in these areas seems to hinder embarrassment more than other emotions. Third, as evidenced by orbitofrontal patients, damage to these areas causes difficulties with embarrassment, but does not prevent an individual from feeling embarrassment. Spontaneous embarrassment was less frequent but still possible. Thus, similar to physiological changes, the neural circuitry involved in embarrassment appears complicated and nuanced, but what else would one expect from such a complex emotion?

## Cognitive effects

In the past several years, there has been a growing interest in the effects that specific emotions can have on cognition, especially cognitions about risk. For example, fear has been found to increase risk perception and decrease risk taking while anger appears to have the opposite effect (Lerner & Keltner, 2001). But while other emotions, such as fear and anger, have been studied extensively, embarrassment has been relatively ignored in this literature until recently. To examine possible effects of embarrassment, Coffaro and Harris (2012) conducted five studies, in which embarrassment was induced via a variety of methods (including recall of embarrassing events, singing and appearing to stare at the crotches of swimmers in a picture). They found that relative to neutral conditions, embarrassment caused people to be more optimistic about their own futures and the futures of others. For example, embarrassed participants thought they were more likely to get a good job in the future, and that mortality from a variety of causes was lower for people in general. This optimistic bias is similar to that seen in anger, although unlike anger, experiencing embarrassment did not seem to influence risky decisions. When embarrassed participants were given gambling tasks or the Asian disease problem (Tversky & Kahneman, 1981), a task in which participants must decide between a risky and a certain choice option, they were no more likely than control participants to choose the risky but potentially more rewarding options. This pattern of risk perception and risk taking was replicated across several studies of embarrassment (Coffaro & Harris, 2012) and so appears robust.

Why does embarrassment elicit an optimistic bias? While the exact mechanism is unclear, Coffaro and Harris (2012) suggest that the increased optimism found during embarrassment might be due to people trying to regulate their negative emotion. They note that in their work participants were not given the opportunity to engage in the behaviours that embarrassment motivates (e.g., self-esteem restoration, appeasement, acknowledgment of embarrassment to others) and that under such circumstances participants may try to engage in mood repair through other means. Such an account is consistent with some other research that suggests that emotion regulation attempts can affect people's judgments and choice (Leith & Baumeister, 1996). One interesting possibility is that giving participants an opportunity to engage in social reparation might circumvent the optimistic bias created by embarrassment in the Coffaro and Harris work. Clearly, more work is needed to understand when and how experiencing embarrassment affects risk preferences, and in what way such effects differ from those of other emotional states.

## The irrationality of embarrassment: negative real-world consequences

Although, embarrassment can have positive effects on social functioning (e.g., amends making), it also can have serious personal and social costs. The desire to avoid even the potential of embarrassment leads people to engage, or fail to engage, in a wide range of behaviours that can be harmful not only to themselves but to others as well. For example, Sabini, Siepmann and Stein (2001) have proposed that the fear of embarrassment may be one of the major factors that contribute to the well-known psychological phenomenon of bystanders failing to help others who are potentially in need (the 'bystander' effect). In many such cases, Sabini and colleagues argue, observers are uncertain whether the situation is indeed an emergency. The bystanders fail to act because they fear looking foolish if they respond as if it were a crisis situation when it is not. Other research suggests that people are not only willing to put others' well-being at risk to avoid embarrassment, but they also are prepared to put their own health, and perhaps even their own lives, at risk. Such irrational behaviour can be readily seen in unsafe sexual practices. For example, several studies have noted that concern over embarrassment is one of the factors that contribute to unsafe sexual practices such as the failure to obtain and use condoms (Dahl *et al.*, 1997; Leary & Dobbins, 1983; Moore *et al.*, 2006).

### *Medical examinations*

A growing literature suggests that embarrassment's negative effects are particularly evident in the area of health and medical care. It is perhaps not surprising that embarrassment has been implicated as an impediment to having medically recommended examinations that involve the exposure or examination of private body parts. Embarrassment has been cited as a cause for delay or avoidance of many types of cancer screenings including pap smears, colonoscopies, breast examinations and mammograms, and testicle examinations (e.g., Consedine et al., 2004; Farraye et al., 2004; Gascoigne et al., 1999; Harewood et al., 2002; Shaw et al., 2001; Taylor et al., 2002).

Due to the correlational nature of most studies that link embarrassment with medical examination avoidance, one cannot conclude for certain that embarrassment is indeed playing a causal role in health-care neglect. However, one recent experiment in our laboratory (Harris & Coffaro, 2012) provides additional support for the proposition that embarrassment is a true barrier to medical examination. Women participants were randomly assigned to either recall an embarrassing medical examination or a neutral event. They then completed several measures regarding their perceptions of their risk of cervical cancer, their embarrassment over pap smears, and their intention to go in for future cervical cancer screenings. As expected, recall of an embarrassing event led women to experience greater embarrassment and to perceive that pap smears were generally more embarrassing, which in turn led these women to report that they were more likely to avoid or delay obtaining a future pap smear relative to women in a neutral state. Interestingly, embarrassment did not affect their perceptions of risk of cervical cancer.

## Medical embarrassment more generally

Most research on embarrassment has almost exclusively examined only one type of medical problem or situation in a single study (e.g., pap smears or breast screening) rather than looking at the more widespread effects that the embarrassment may play on various health-care decisions. Such research does not provide any indication of whether such phenomena are frequent or rare in the general population. Furthermore, until recently, virtually no attention had been paid to another, potentially equally important, way in which the potential for embarrassment may deter people from seeking needed medical care: prospective patients may anticipate embarrassment if they present what they judge to be worrisome symptoms and these are found to have a trivial cause.

To examine some of these issues, Harris (2006) had people complete an anonymous questionnaire over the internet, which included questions on embarrassment and health-care seeking. The sample primarily consisted of Caucasian adults from the United States and was demographically diverse with regards to age, education and income. Participants were asked whether embarrassment had led them to delay or avoid medical care across four types of medical situations that might pose embarrassment threats. These are described in Figure 7.1. Participants were also encouraged to provide information regarding their experiences including types of symptoms and issues involved.

Figure 7.1 shows the role that embarrassment played in different types of medical situations displayed by gender and whether people reported that embarrassment was an obstacle more than once in any given situation. The numbers presented here in the text are for the sample as a whole, collapsing across all medical situations and gender. Several interesting findings emerged. First, well over half (57 per cent) of the whole sample reported that embarrassment had led to delay or failure to seek medical care. Second, although 20 per cent of the sample reported that embarrassment was an obstacle to scheduling needed medical examinations, this was not the type of situation that produced the greatest medical delay or avoidance. Instead, the most prevalent form of medical embarrassment centred on the fear of being embarrassed if a symptom turned out to have a 'trivial cause'. Despite being worried about potentially serious symptoms, over one third of the sample (36 per cent) reported that they had failed or delayed seeking medical care in order to avoid looking silly or feeling embarrassed if the symptom turned out to have a trivial cause. The most common symptoms experienced in such situations were those that might indicate cardiac distress (e.g., chest pain). Such delays are particularly irrational given that thrombolytic agents and emergency angioplasty can greatly diminish the tissue damage produced by heart attacks, but require rapid treatment to be effective (Nallamothu & Bates, 2003). Given these data, it seems quite possible that delaying or failing to seek medical attention due to embarrassment threat may be a greater cause of avoidable mortality and morbidity than previous work focusing just on embarrassing medical examinations would suggest. Consistent with this proposition, there is at least some hint in the medical literature that potential embarrassment over a false alarm does deter at least some myocardial patients from seeking prompt treatment, although quantitative information on this point is lacking (Finnegan et al., 2000).

The Harris study (2006) also found that significantly more women than men reported that embarrassment had deterred or delayed them from seeking medical attention. One might wonder if this gender difference was due to women, particularly young women, facing more opportunities for embarrassing examinations (i.e., annual pap smears) than similar aged men. While this might explain some of the gender differences, it cannot explain all of them as the gender effect generalized to other types of situations. The differences between males and females can be seen in Figure 7.1. For each type of medical

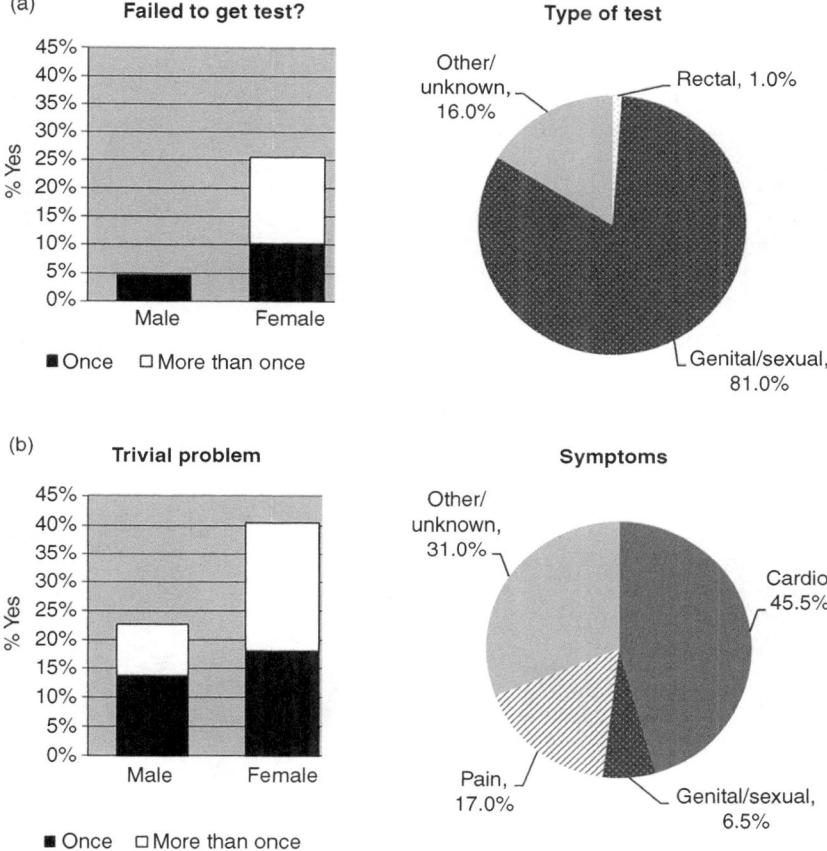

Figure 7.1 Embarrassment and delay or avoidance of medical care
(a) 'Have you ever failed to get a medically recommended examination (e.g., pap smear, colonoscopy) because you found the prospect of the examination so embarrassing?'
(b) 'Did you ever experience medical symptoms that you found worrisome, but delayed in seeking medical care (or failed to seek medical care altogether) because you anticipated feeling embarrassed if the problem turned out to be something trivial?'

situation, analyses of gender differences produced statistically significant results. Embarrassment was a greater deterrent for women when talking to a doctor or nurse and led them to avoid having a symptom checked out due to fear of looking silly if the symptom turned out to be of a trivial origin. In addition, people with lower

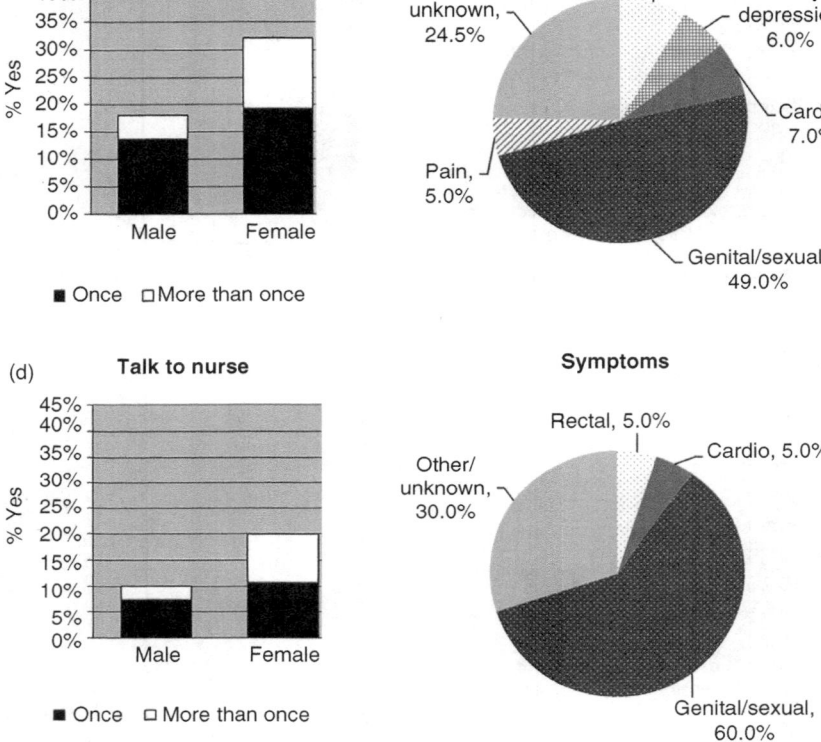

Figure 7.1 (cont.)
(c) 'Did you ever experience medical symptoms that you found worrisome, but delayed in seeking medical care (or failed to seek medical care altogether) because you felt embarrassed to talk about the symptom to a doctor?'
(d) 'Did you ever experience medical symptoms that you found worrisome, but delayed in seeking medical care (or failed to seek medical care altogether) because you felt embarrassed to describe your symptoms to a nurse in order to get an appointment with the doctor?'

incomes reported that fear of embarrassment was a greater deterrent to seeking medical care than those with higher incomes. Future health-related research should focus on special populations such as these as they seem to be the most affected and, perhaps, harmed by threat of embarrassment.

## Types of embarrassment

As mentioned previously, research outside the medical domain suggests there may be different forms of embarrassment – one that is aroused by awkward interactions and another that results from evaluation apprehension. Some recent work within the field of behavioural medicine also suggests that there may be at least two variants of medical embarrassment.

Noting the lack of an existing comprehensive medical embarrassment questionnaire, Consedine, Krivoshekova and Harris (2007) created a measure that included fifty-three questions that asked about people's tendencies towards medical embarrassment across a number of situations. This list included nine potentially separable categories (e.g., genital examinations, public exposure, concern over being viewed as a hypochondriac). However, factor analysis of data from young adults in the United States revealed that the items could be understood by two underlying factors. One was bodily embarrassment, which included feeling uncomfortable or awkward about the body or about being naked and examined. The other, more cognitive, factor tapped into concerns about being judged or negatively evaluated. Although the two types of embarrassment were correlated, they interacted with medical care visits differently, supporting the validity of separating the two constructs.

Evidence that bodily embarrassment and judgment-concern embarrassment are separate constructs has now emerged across three different samples, suggesting they are robust phenomena. These two factors were seen in both of the US samples examined in Consedine, Krivoshekova and Harris (2007), one made up of Caucasian and Asian participants and the other of Caucasian and African-American participants. Moreover, they also appeared in responses of Mexican participants residing in Mexico who completed a translated version of the same measure (Harris et al., 2012). Interestingly, in the Mexican sample, judgment concern was subdivided into two factors: a general concern over being judged and a second factor that might best be characterized as embarrassment specifically over a doctor's judgment.

With the one exception just noted, judgment-concern embarrassment did not appear to be affected by culture or by gender. In contrast, bodily embarrassment did show effects of culture and gender. Within the United States, African-Americans were less plagued by bodily embarrassment than European-Americans and both groups reported less of this type of embarrassment than Asian-Americans. Men also reported less susceptibility to bodily embarrassment than women in all of the four ethnicities studied to date.

In summary, embarrassment seems to play an important role in health behaviours. For many people, it appears to create a large barrier between themselves and the critical care they need. Research to date suggests that there may be variants of embarrassment. (i.e., bodily embarrassment vs fear of judgment) that may differentially affect behaviours and health-care-seeking outcomes.

## Embarrassment and shame: the same or different?

The appearance of different forms of embarrassment is reminiscent of another ongoing debate within psychology – are embarrassment and shame different forms of the same emotion or are they actually distinct emotions? The longstanding tradition in psychology, dating back to Darwin, has been to regard embarrassment as simply a less intense form of shame (see Keltner & Buswell, 1997, for review). After all, shame and embarrassment have similar functional accounts and, as Darwin noted, the blush occurs in breaches of etiquette as well as moral failings (Darwin, 1872/1999). Cross-cultural language researchers have also noted that in many cultures embarrassment is linguistically located close to shame and it is not uncommon for one word to be used for both constructs (Edelstein & Shaver, 2007; Haidt & Keltner, 1999; Lutz, 1982). Some theories of shame are remarkably similar to the negative evaluation model of embarrassment and posit that shame is produced by the exposure of a flaw or the loss of social esteem (Ausubel, 1955; Sabini, Garvey *et al.*, 2001; Smith *et al.*, 2002). Behaviourally, both may motivate one to make reparations for the transgression (Darby & Harris, 2012), and in a medical setting shame, like embarrassment, can create problem behaviours such as leading one to discontinue visits to a physician or lie about medical issues (Harris & Darby, 2009). In short, there are enough important similarities that some researchers question the extent to which these emotions are distinct from one another (Sabini, Garvey *et al.*, 2001).

Recently, however, the emotion field has begun to shift away from the view that shame and embarrassment reflect the same affective state. Diverse evidence ranging from differing phenomenological accounts to distinguishable nonverbal behaviours has led many researchers to conclude that embarrassment and shame are two distinct emotions (Keltner, 1995; Keltner & Buswell, 1997; Miller & Tangney, 1994; Tangney *et al.*, 1996). Some of the evidence offered for differentiating these two emotions comes from work examining the types of situations that give rise to them. Several studies have found that when people are asked to recall experiences in which they felt embarrassment and shame, embarrassing episodes tend to revolve around transgressions of social conventions (e.g., spilling one's coffee or burping in public), while shaming episodes tend to revolve around failures to meet personal standards (e.g., cheating in a test or on a spouse) (Miller & Tangney, 1994; Tangney et al., 1996). Relative to embarrassment, shame or guilt is also more likely to occur over harm done to another person (Keltner & Buswell, 1996).

In addition to having some different antecedent events, people's descriptions of the phenomenology or subjective experience of embarrassment seem to contrast with that of shame. When people feel embarrassed they often describe themselves as feeling awkward and out of sorts; whereas when they feel shame they often describe themselves as feeling immoral (Miller & Tangney, 1994). In multiple studies of the affective differences between these two emotions, participants report that embarrassment is tied to humour, amusement and startled surprise, while shame is tied to disgust, anger and sadness (Miller & Tangney, 1994; Tangney et al., 1996). Some studies also suggest that embarrassment is less intensely distressing than shame (Tangney et al., 1996; Darby & Harris, 2012). Consequently, some researchers describe the embarrassment experience as a fleeting feeling of having erred and shame as feeling that the whole self is bad (Tangney et al., 1996).

There are also several studies that suggest possible differences between the nonverbal displays of embarrassment and shame. One study of blind and seeing Olympians competing in Ju-Jitsu found that after defeat, the athletes, regardless of seeing ability, tended to slump their shoulders and narrow their chests while tilting their heads down and looking away from others (Tracy & Matsumoto, 2008). While this study did not obtain affective reports from the Olympians, failing a task is a common antecedent of shame but not of embarrassment (Keltner & Buswell, 1996). Other studies have similarly found that failure leads to frowns, body collapse and gaze aversion (Heckhausen, 1984; Lewis et al., 1992; Stipek et al., 1992). While there is the distinct possibility that the shoulder slump is due to disappointment and not shame, when people describe feeling ashamed they sometimes describe a physical response that includes slumping shoulders, putting one's head down and avoiding eye contact (Ablamowicz, 1992). Smiling and smile suppression, which often occur during embarrassment, are notably absent from these studies (Keltner & Harker, 1998; Lewis, 1993). One study found that others' perceptions of embarrassment were correlated with smile control attempts, but their perceptions of shame were not (Keltner, 1995). Taken together, these studies tentatively suggest that the prototypical shame expression may be characterized by head and eye movements down (Izard, 1977; Lewis *et al.*, 1992), with perhaps a slumping of the shoulders (Tracy *et al.*, 2009), and no smile or smile suppression attempts (Keltner, 1995).

While many of these behaviours are shared with embarrassment, people seem to be fairly adept at distinguishing the prototypical embarrassment display (i.e., gaze down, controlled smile, head turn, gaze shift, face touch) from the prototypical shame display (i.e., head and eyes downcast, no smile). When people are asked to label a display of embarrassment or shame, they rarely confuse one emotion with another, regardless of whether the emotion is presented as a still picture (Keltner & Buswell, 1996) or a video recording (Keltner, 1995). In fact, one study found that when people are shown still pictures of prototypical displays of embarrassment and shame, they tend to infer that the display is caused for reasons largely in line with the suggested distinct antecedents of these emotions (Keltner *et al.*, 1997). For example, for a shame display, people tend to infer that the person committed a moral wrong, such as hurting someone's feelings; for an embarrassment display, they tend to infer that the person made a social blunder, such as tripping in public. Further, when presented with a shame display, people reported that they are more likely to feel sympathy than amusement. For embarrassment, people reported the reverse (Keltner *et al.*, 1997). The blush is another display that may distinguish shame from embarrassment. While, to our knowledge, there is little work specifically addressing this distinction, blushing is often seen during embarrassment (Edelmann & Hampson, 1979) but has yet to be empirically linked with shame.

While there is not overwhelming evidence that embarrassment and shame reflect different underlying emotional states, it appears that the two emotions are distinguishable in terms of displays, subjective feelings and antecedents. Contrary to previous expectations, there is some evidence that these differences are not due to the intensity of the emotion (Tangney *et al.*, 1996). One general limitation of this line of research, and the work on embarrassment in general, is that it has almost exclusively been done with participants from the United States, Europe or Australia. Work with a wider range of cultures, particularly those from Asia and Africa, would greatly enhance our knowledge of the embarrassment experience, its concomitants and its relationship with other important emotions.

## Concluding remarks

Embarrassment affects everything from day-to-day interactions to important life decisions. Its role in decision making, especially in risky and health-related decisions, may be more profound than many had previously expected. Embarrassment's effects are complicated and nuanced, and there are different types of embarrassment that may differentially affect behaviour. In short, far from being the straightforward and trivial emotion that it appears to be at first blush, embarrassment is complex and powerful with far-reaching consequences.

REFERENCES

Ablamowicz, H. (1992). Shame as an interpersonal dimension of communication among doctoral students: an empirical phenomenological study. *Journal of Phenomenological Psychology*, 23, 30–49.

Apsler, R. (1975). Effects of embarrassment on behavior toward others. *Journal of Personality and Social Psychology*, 32, 145–53.

Asendorpf, J. (1990). The expression of shyness and embarrassment. In W. R. Crozier (Ed.), *Shyness and embarrassment: perspectives from social psychology*. Cambridge University Press, 87–118.

Ausubel, D. P. (1955). Relationships between shame and guilt in the socialization process. *Psychological Review*, 67, 378–90.

Baron-Cohen, S. (2000). Theory of mind and autism: a fifteen year review. In H. Tager-Flusberg, D. Cohen & S. Baron-Cohen (Eds.), *Understanding other minds: perspectives from autism and developmental cognitive neuroscience*. Oxford University Press, 1–20.

Baron-Cohen, S., Wheelwright, S., & Jolliffe, T. (1997). Is there a 'language of the eyes?' Evidence from normal adults, and adults with autism or Asperger syndrome. *Visual Cognition*, 4, 311–31.

Beer, J. S. (2007). Neural systems for self-conscious emotions and their underlying appraisals. In J. L. Tracy, R. W. Robins & J. P. Tangney (Eds.), *The self-conscious emotions: theory and research*. New York: Guilford Press, 53–67.

Beer, J. S., Heerey, E. H., Keltner, D., Scabini, D., & Knight, R. T. (2003). The regulatory function of self-conscious emotion: insights from patients with orbitofrontal damage. *Journal of Personality and Social Psychology*, 85, 594–604.

Beer, J. S., John, O. P., Scabini, D., & Knight, R. T. (2006). Orbitofrontal cortex and social behaviors: integrating self-monitoring and emotion-cognition interactions. *Journal of Cognitive Neuroscience*, 18, 871–9.

Berthoz, S., Armony, J. L., Blair, R. J. R., & Dolan, R. J. (2002). An fMRI study of intentional and unintentional (embarrassing) violations of social norms. *Brain*, 125, 1696–708.

Blair, R. J. R., & Cipolotti, L. (2000). Impaired social response reversal: a case of 'acquired sociopathy'. *Brain*, 6, 1122–41.

Bozeat, S., Gregory, C. A., Ralph, M. A. L., & Hodges, J. R. (2000). Which neuropsychiatric and behavioral features distinguish frontal and temporal variants of frontotemporal dementia from Alzheimer's disease? *Journal of Neurology, Neurosurgery, and Psychiatry*, 69, 178–86.

Buck, R. W., Parke, R. D., & Buck, M. (1970). Skin conductance, heart rate, and attention to the environment in two stressful situations. *Psychonomic Science*, 18, 95–6.

Buss, A. H. (1980). *Self-consciousness and social anxiety.* San Francisco: Freeman.

Capps, L., Yirmiya, N., & Sigman, M. (1992). Understanding of simple and complex emotions in non-retarded children with autism. *Journal of Child Psychology and Psychiatry,* 7, 1169–82.

Castelli, F., Frith, C., Happé, F., & Frith, U. (2002). Autism, Asperger syndrome and brain mechanisms for the attribution of mental states to animated shapes. *Brain,* 125, 1839–49.

Coffaro, F., & Harris, C. R. (2012). *Embarrassment and risk.* Manuscript submitted for publication.

Consedine, N. S., Krivoshekova, Y. S., & Harris, C. R. (2007). Bodily embarrassment and judgment concern as separable factors in the measurement of medical embarrassment: psychometric development and links to treatment-seeking outcomes. *British Journal of Health Psychology,* 12, 439–62.

Consedine, N. S., Magai, C., & Neuget, A. I. (2004). The contribution of emotional characteristics to breast cancer screening among women from six ethnic groups. *Preventive Medicine,* 38, 64–77.

Crozier, W. R. (2004). Self-consciousness, exposure, and the blush. *Journal for the Theory of Social Behaviour,* 34, 1–17.

Dahl, D. W., Gorn, G. J., & Weinberg, C. B. (1997). Condom carrying behavior among college students. *American Journal of Public Health,* 87, 1059–60.

Darby, R. S., & Harris, C. R. (2010). Embarrassment's effect on facial processing. *Cognition and Emotion,* 24, 1250–8.

(2012). *Predicting outcomes of the self-conscious emotions.* Manuscript in preparation.

Darwin, C. R. (1872/1999). *The expression of the emotions in man and animals.* Corrected 3rd edn with an introduction, afterword and commentaries by Paul Ekman. London: HarperCollins.

de Jong, P. J. (1999). Communicative and remedial effects of social blushing. *Journal of Nonverbal Behavior,* 23, 197–217.

Drummond, P. D. (1997). The effect of adrenergic blockade on blushing and facial flushing. *Psychophysiology,* 34, 163–8.

Edelmann, R. J. (1987). *The psychology of embarrassment.* Chichester: John Wiley & Sons.

Edelmann, R. J., Asendorpf, J., Contarello, A., Georgas, J., Zammuner, V., & Villanueva, C. (1989). Self-reported expression of embarrassment in five European cultures. *Journal of Cross-Cultural Psychology,* 20, 357–71.

Edelmann, R. J., & Hampson, S. E. (1979). Changes in non-verbal behaviour during embarrassment. *British Journal of Social and Clinical Psychology,* 18, 385–90.

(1981). Embarrassment in dyadic interaction. *Social Behavior and Personality,* 9, 171–7.

Edelstein, R. S., & Shaver, P. R. (2007). A cross-cultural examination of lexical studies of self-conscious emotions. In J. Tracy, R. Robins & J. Tangney (Eds.), *The self-conscious emotions: theory and research.* New York: Guilford Press, 91–113.

Ekman, P., & Friesen, W. (1978). *Facial action coding system: a technique for the measurement of facial movement.* Palo Alto, CA: Consulting Psychologists Press.

Farraye, F. A., Wong, M., Hurwitz, S., Puleo, E., Emmons, K., Wallace, M. B., & Fletcher, R. H. (2004). Barriers to endoscopic colorectal cancer screening: are women different from men? *American Journal of Gastroenterology*, **99**, 341–9.

Finnegan, J. R., Meischke, H., Zapka, J. G., Leviton, L., Meschack, A., Benjamin-Garner, R., Estabrook, B., Johnston Hall, N., Schaeffer, S., Smith, C., Weitzman, E. R., Raczunski, J., & Stone, E. (2000). Patient delay in seeking care for heart attack symptoms: findings from focus groups conducted in five US regions. *Preventive Medicine*, 31, 205–13.

Frith, C. D., & Frith, U. (1999). Interacting minds – a biological basis. *Science*, **286**, 1692–5.

Gallagher, H. L., & Frith, C. D. (2003). Functional imaging of 'theory of mind'. *Trends in Cognitive Science*, 7, 77–83.

Gascoigne, P., Mason, M. D., & Roberts, E. (1999). Factors affecting presentation and delay in patients with testicular cancer: results of a qualitative study. *Psycho-Oncology*, **8**, 144–55.

Gerlach, A. L., Wilhelm, F. H., & Roth, W. T. (2003). Embarrassment and social phobia: the role of parasympathetic activation. *Journal of Anxiety Disorders*, **17**, 197–210.

Goffman, E. (1956). Embarrassment and social organization. *American Journal of Sociology*, **62**, 264–71.

(1967). *Interaction ritual: essays on face-to-face behavior*. Garden City, NY: Anchor.

Gruter, M., & Masters, R. D. (1986). Ostracism: a social and biological phenomenon. *Ethology and Sociobiology*, 7, 149–58.

Haidt, J., & Keltner, D. (1999). Culture and facial expression: open-ended methods find more faces and a gradient of recognition. *Cognition and Emotion*, **13**, 225–66.

Happé, Â. F., Ehlers, S., Fletcher, P., Frith, U., Johansson, M., Gillberg, C., Dolan, R., Frackowiak, R., & Frith, C. (1996). 'Theory of mind' in the brain: evidence from a PET scan study of Asperger Syndrome. *Neuroreport*, 5, 197–201.

Happé, F., & Frith, U. (1996). The neuropsychology of autism. *Brain*, **199**, 1377–400.

Harewood, G. C., Wiersema, M. J., Melton, L. J. (2002). A prospective, controlled assessment of factors influencing acceptance of screening colonoscopy. *American Journal of Gastroenterology*, **97**, 3186–94.

Harris, C. R. (2001). Cardiovascular responses of embarrassment and effects of emotional suppression in a social setting. *Journal of Personality and Social Psychology*, **81**, 886–97.

(2006). Embarrassment: a form of social pain. *American Scientist*, **94**, 524–33.

Harris, C. R., & Coffaro, F. (2012). *When embarrassment kills: the effect of embarrassment on risk perceptions and behavioral intentions to get screened for cervical cancer.* Manuscript in preparation.

Harris, C. R., & Darby, R. S. (2009). Shame in physician–patient interactions: patient perspectives. *Basic and Applied Social Psychology*, **31**, 325–34.

Harris, C. R., Fernandez de Ortega, H., & Darby, R. S. (2012). *Three types of medical embarrassment in Mexico*. Manuscript in preparation.

Heckhausen, H. (1984). Emergent achievement behavior: some early developments. In J. Nicholls (Ed.), *Advances in movitation and* achievement, Vol 3: *The development of achievement motivation.* Greenwich, CT: JAI, 1–32.

Heerey, E. A., Keltner, D., & Capps, L. M. (2003). Making sense of self-conscious emotion: linking theory of mind and emotion in children with autism. *Emotion,* **3,** 394–400.

Hietanen, J. K. (1999). Does your gaze direction and head orientation shift my visual attention? *Neuroreport,* **10,** 3443–7.

Hofmann, S. G., Moscovitch, D. A., & Kim, H. J. (2006). Autonomic correlates of social anxiety and embarrassment in shy and non-shy individuals. *International Journal of Psychophysiology,* **61,** 134–42.

Izard, C. E. (1977). *Human emotions.* New York: Plenum Press.

Kasari, C., Chamberlain, G., & Bauminger, N. (2001). Social emotions and social relationships: can children with autism compensate? In J. A. Burack & T. Charman (Eds.), *The development of autism: perspectives from theory and research.* Mahwah, NJ: Erlbaum, 309–23.

Keltner, D. (1995). Signs of appeasement: evidence for the distinct displays of embarrassment, amusement, and shame. *Journal of Personality and Social Psychology,* **68,** 441–54.

Keltner, D., & Buswell, B. N. (1996). Evidence for the distinctness of embarrassment, shame, and guilt: a study of recalled antecedents and facial expressions. *Cognition and Emotion,* **10,** 155–71.

(1997). Embarrassment: its distinct form and appeasement functions. *Psychological Bulletin,* **122,** 250–70.

Keltner, D., & Harker, L. A. (1998). The forms and functions of the nonverbal signal of shame. In P. Gilbert & B. Andrews (Eds.), *Shame, interpersonal behaviour, psychopathology, and culture.* New York: Oxford University Press, 78–98.

Keltner, D., Young, R. C., & Buswell, B. N. (1997). Appeasement in human emotion, social practice, and personality. *Aggressive Behavior,* **23,** 359–74.

Leary, M. R., & Dobbins, S. E. (1983). Social anxiety, sexual behavior, and contraceptive use. *Journal of Personality and Social Psychology,* **45,** 1347–54.

Leith, K. P., & Baumeister, R. F. (1996). Why do bad moods increase self-defeating behavior? Emotion, risk taking, and self-regulation. *Journal of Personality and Social Psychology,* **71,** 1250–67.

Lerner, J. S., & Keltner, D. (2001). Fear, anger, and risk. *Journal of Personality and Social Psychology,* **81,** 146–59.

Levenson, R. W., & Miller, B. L. (2007). Loss of cells – loss of self: frontotemporal lobar degeneration and human emotion. *Current Directions in Psychological Science,* **16,** 289–94.

Levin, J., & Arluke, A. (1982). Embarrassment and helping behavior. *Psychological Reports,* **51,** 999–1002.

Lewis, M. (1993). Self-conscious emotions: embarrassment, pride, shame, and guilt. In M. Lewis & J. M. Haviland (Eds.), *Handbook of emotions.* New York: Guilford Press, 563–73.

Lewis, M., Alessandri, S. M., & Sullivan, M. W. (1992). Differences in shame and pride as a function of children's gender and task difficulty. *Child Development,* **63,** 630–8.

Lutz, C. A. (1982). The domain of emotion words in Ifaluk. *American Ethnologist,* **9,** 113–28.
Miller, R. S. (1987). Empathic embarrassment: situational and personal determinants of reactions to the embarrassment of another. *Journal of Personality and Social Psychology,* **53,** 1061–9.
  (1992). The nature and severity of self-reported embarrassing circumstances. *Personality and Social Psychology Bulletin,* **18,** 190–8.
  (1995). On the nature of embarrassability: shyness, social-evaluation, and social skill. *Journal of Personality,* **63,** 315–39.
  (1996). *Embarrassment: poise and peril in everyday life.* New York: Guilford Press.
Miller, R. S., & Tangney, J. P. (1994). Differentiating embarrassment from shame. *Journal of Social and Clinical Psychology,* **13,** 273–87.
Modigliani, A. (1968). Embarrassment and embarrassability. *Sociometry,* **31,** 313–26.
Moore, S. G., Dahl, D. W., Gorn, G. J., & Weinberg, C. B. (2006). Coping with condom embarrassment. *Psychology, Health and Medicine,* **11,** 70–9.
Nallamothu, B. K., & Bates, E. R. (2003). Percutaneous coronary intervention versus fibrinolytic therapy in acute myocardial infarction: is timing (almost) everything? *American Journal of Cardiology,* **92,** 824–6.
Neary, D., Snowden, J. S., Gustafson, L., Passant, U., Stuss, D., Black, S., Freedman, M., Kertesz, A., Robert, P. H., Albert, M., Boone, K., Miller, B. L., Cummings, J., & Benson, D. F. (1998). Frontotemporal lobar degeneration: a consensus on clinical diagnostic criteria. *Neurology,* **51,** 1546–54.
Parrott, W. G., Sabini, J., & Silver, M. (1988). The roles of self-esteem and social interaction in embarrassment. *Personality and Social Psychology Bulletin,* **14,** 191–202.
Parrott, W. G., & Smith, S. F. (1991). Embarrassment: actual vs typical cases and classical vs prototypical representations. *Cognition and Emotion,* **5,** 467–88.
Rankin, K. P., Kramer, J. H., & Miller, B. L. (2005). Patterns of cognitive and emotional empathy in frontotemporal lobar degeneration. *Cognitive and Behavioral Neurology,* **18,** 28–36.
Roberts, R. J., & Weerts, T. C. (1982). Cardiovascular responding during anger and fear imagery. *Psychological Reports,* **50,** 219–30.
Rosen, H. J., Narvaez, J. M., Hallam, B., Kramer, J., Wyss-Coray, C., Gearhart, R., Johnson, J. K., & Miller, B. L. (2004). Neuropsychological and functional measures of severity in Alzheimer disease, frontotemporal dementia, and semantic dementia. *Alzheimer Disease and Associated Disorders,* **18,** 202–7.
Sabini, J., Garvey, B., & Hall, A. L. (2001). Shame and embarrassment revisited. *Personality and Social Psychology Bulletin,* **27,** 104–17.
Sabini, J., Siepmann, M., & Stein, J. (2001). The really fundamental attribution error in social psychological research. *Psychological Inquiry,* **12,** 1–15.
Sabini, J., Siepmann, M., Stein, J., & Meyerowitz, M. (1999). Who is embarrassed by what? *Cognition and Emotion,* **14,** 213–40.
Schwartz, G. E., Weinberger, D. A., & Singer, J. A. (1981). Cardiovascular differentiation of happiness, sadness, anger, and fear following imagery and exercise. *Psychosomatic Medicine,* **43,** 343–64.

Semin, G. R., & Manstead, A. S. R. (1982). The social implications of embarrassment displays and restitution behaviour. *European Journal of Social Psychology*, **12**, 367–77.

Shaw, C., Tansey, R., Jackson, C., Hyde, C., & Allan, R. (2001). Barriers to help seeking in people with urinary symptoms. *Family Practice*, **18**, 48–52.

Shearn, D., Bergman, E., Hill, K., Abel, A., & Hinds, L. (1990). Facial coloration and temperature responses in blushing. *Psychophysiology*, **27**, 687–93.

(1992). Blushing as a function of audience size. *Psychophysiology*, **29**, 431–6.

Silver, M., Sabini, J., & Parrott, W. G. (1987). Embarrassment: a dramaturgic account. *Journal of the Theory of Social Behaviour*, **17**, 47–61.

Smith, R. H., Webster, J. M., Parrott, W. G., & Eyre, H. L. (2002). The role of public exposure in moral and nonmoral shame and guilt. *Journal of Personality and Social Psychology*, **83**, 138–59.

Snowden, J. S., Bathgate, D., Varma, A., Blackshaw, A., Gibbons, Z. C., & Neary, D. (2001). Distinct behavioural profiles in frontotemporal dementia and semantic dementia. *Journal of Neurology, Neurosurgery, and Psychiatry*, **70**, 323–32.

Stipek, D., Recchia, S., & McClintic, S. (1992). Self-evaluation in young children. *Monographs of the Society for Research in Child Development*, **57**, 1–84.

Stone, V. E., Baron-Cohen, S., & Knight, R. T. (1998). Frontal lobe contributions to theory of mind. *Journal of Cognitive Neuroscience*, **10**, 640–56.

Sturm, V. E., Rosen, H. J., Allison, S., Miller, B., & Levenson, R. W. (2006). Self-conscious emotion deficits in frontotemporal lobar degeneration. *Brain*, **129**, 2508–16.

Tangney, J. P., Miller, R. S., Flicker, L., & Barlow, D. H. (1996). Are shame, guilt, and embarrassment distinct emotions? *Journal of Personality and Social Psychology*, **70**, 1256–69.

Taylor, V. M., Jackson, J. C., Tu, S. P., Yasui, Y., Schwartz, S. M., Kuniyuki, A., Acorda, E., Lin, K., & Hislop, G. (2002). Cervical cancer screening among Chinese Americans. *Cancer Detection and Prevention*, **26**, 139–45.

Tracy, J. L., & Matsumoto, D. (2008). The spontaneous expression of pride and shame: evidence for biologically innate nonverbal displays. *PNAS*, **105**, 11655–60.

Tracy, J. L., Robins, R. W., & Schriber, R. A. (2009). Development of a FACS-verified set of basic and self-conscious emotion expressions. *Emotion*, **9**, 554–9.

Tversky, A., & Kahneman, D. (1981). The framing of decisions and the psychology of choice. *Science*, **211**, 453–8.

Walter, H., Adenzato, M., Ciaramidaro, A., Enrici, I., Pia, L., & Bara, B. G. (2004). Understanding intentions in social interaction: the role of the anterior paracingulate cortex. *Journal of Cognitive Neuroscience*, **16**, 1854–63.

Willis, M. L., Palermo, R., Burke, D., McGrillen, K., & Miller, L. (2010). Orbitofrontal cortex lesions result in abnormal social judgments to emotional faces. *Neuropsychologia*, **48**, 2182–7.

# 8 The affective neuroscience of human social anxiety

*Vladimir Miskovic and Louis A. Schmidt*

## Introduction

Psychologists and psychiatrists have long recognized that the varieties of human fears and phobias are not entirely arbitrary but rather seem circumscribed by a limited group of categories (Marks, 1969) including natural/situational triggers (e.g., darkness, heights), dangerous animals (e.g., snakes, spiders) and threatening conspecifics (American Psychiatric Association, 2000). Not surprisingly, these categories consistently emerge as stable factors in structural analyses of human fears (Arrindell *et al.*, 1991) and are also anticipated by ethological perspectives on animal behaviour (Öhman *et al.*, 1985). Taken together, the sum of these considerations suggests that phobic content is at least partially constrained by the evolution of core brain circuits that influence what qualifies as an 'emotionally competent stimulus'[1] (Damasio, 2003) capable of activating fear-related circuitry.

This chapter is devoted to a consideration of social anxiety, both in terms of its clinical and subsyndromal manifestations. A characteristic feature of social anxiety involves the fear and avoidance of interpersonal interactions, especially those with potential for scrutiny and evaluation. As with many other kinds of fear, the experience of social anxiety can range in intensity from relatively mild to severely disabling, producing responses that are increasingly dysfunctional in their effects (Rosen & Schulkin, 1998). Although some individuals with social anxiety may be

---

This research was supported by grants from the Natural Sciences and Engineering Research Council of Canada (NSERC) and the Social Science and Humanities Research Council of Canada (SSHRC) awarded to Louis Schmidt, and a Vanier doctoral scholarship from NSERC awarded to Vladimir Miskovic under the direction of Louis Schmidt.

[1] Damasio (2003) introduced the term 'emotionally competent stimulus' to indicate an object or event (actual or recalled/imagined) that is necessary and sufficient to engage specific brain circuits and trigger an emotional response. The notion of an emotionally competent stimulus was conceived as a (loose) analogy to antigen–antibody interactions in the immune system.

able to endure social interactions with a degree of discomfort and distress, for others the fears may be sufficiently powerful to induce active behavioural avoidance of almost all such encounters, resulting in marked disability and psychiatric impairment. A functional perspective suggests that the extreme manifestations of social anxiety represent the dysfunction of a behavioural system that evolved as a means of regulating dominance/submissiveness hierarchies in primate societies (Öhman, 1986, 2009).

We posit the existence of a general social anxiety spectrum that encompasses everything from shyness (moderate distress in some or most social situations) to a clinical diagnosis of social anxiety disorder (SAD). Such a dimensional framework is shared with previous evolutionary (Hermans & van Honk, 2006), developmental (Pérez-Edgar & Fox, 2005) and clinical (Hofmann et al., 2004) treatments of social anxiety and fearfulness. Although the notion of a continuum is not without some controversy (e.g., Heiser et al., 2009; Kagan, 1994), it accounts for the observation that the various phenomena being described are presumed to share many common neural, behavioural and cognitive correlates (Pérez-Edgar & Fox, 2005). A dimensional perspective on social fearfulness also encourages the integration of experimental findings from various laboratories. A growing number of research studies have recently emerged, that have considerably expanded our knowledge concerning the psychobiological correlates of social anxiety (see Fox, Henderson et al., 2005; Hermans & van Honk, 2006; Schmidt & Schulkin, 1999).[2] The aim of our chapter is to provide a systematic overview of this literature, with a special focus on central brain states.

The chapter is divided into four parts. First, we present an abridged summary of the neural circuitry that supports complex socioemotional functions, the dysregulation of which may contribute to social anxiety. Second, we chart the developmental precursors of adult social anxiety as reflected in a particular temperamental style of responding that emerges within the first months of post-natal life. Third, we review a series of studies, many of them from our own laboratory, concerning neural and cognitive activity during resting conditions and in response to either acute symptom activation or more subtle forms of affective challenge in socially anxious adults. Finally, we attempt to provide a

---

[2] The focus of this chapter is largely on studies conducted with human participants. Several promising animal models (e.g., subordination stress in nonhuman primates) of social anxiety are currently available, but those findings will not be reviewed here (see Mathew et al., 2001, for a brief summary).

preliminary framework for integrating important measures of peripheral physiology (such as the facial blush) into working neuroscience models of social anxiety.

## Functional neuroanatomy of emotion and its relation to social anxiety

This section briefly reviews the neurobiological substrates that underlie social behaviours (Adolphs, 2003). Dysfunctions in the regional and network activity of the brain systems outlined here contribute to the experience and expression of social anxiety.

Figure 8.1 presents midsagittal (a) and coronal (b) aspects of the human brain, highlighting many key regions that collectively help to mediate socioemotional functions. Given that the expression and regulation of fear[3] is a primary focus of this chapter, the amygdala represents a relevant starting point for further discussion. The amygdala is a complex of functionally distinct nuclei that reside deep within the temporal lobes of the human forebrain. Numerous lines of evidence indicate that the amygdala is implicated in fear learning and memory, rapid threat appraisals and emotional inhibition (Phelps & LeDoux, 2005). Due to its multifaceted roles, the amygdala is pivotal for understanding both normal and abnormal aspects of primate social cognition (Emery & Amaral, 2000).

A broad distinction can be made between the basolateral and central divisions of the amygdala. The basolateral division receives afferent connections from the thalamus, hippocampal formation and various regions of the cerebral cortex. Some of these connections convey highly processed and multimodal sensory information. In turn, the basolateral division reciprocates many of its incoming connections. For example, tract tracing in primates and *in vivo* diffusion tensor imaging in humans have revealed multiple reciprocal connections between the basal nucleus of the amygdala and cortical sensory areas, including all levels of the ventral ('object-based') visual pathway (Amaral, 2002; Catani *et al.*, 2003). A potential functional role of this re-entrant connectivity is to bias the perceptual representation of motivationally significant stimuli (e.g., threatening conspecific faces in the case of social anxiety). Another

---

[3] It is important to note that a fear state can be the final outcome of multiple causes or inducers (e.g., innate releasers vs aversively conditioned stimuli). The extent to which there is a common neurophysiological profile subserving all of these different kinds of fear states versus several distinct pathways is still a matter of some debate (Kagan & Schulkin, 1995) that awaits additional empirical evidence.

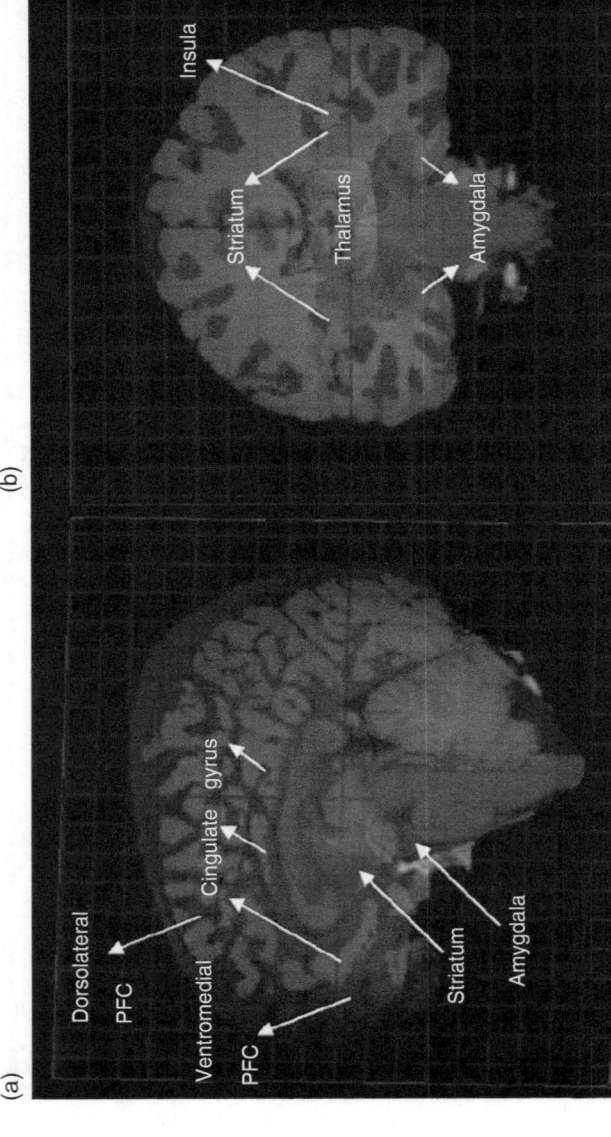

Figure 8.1 Midsagittal (a) and coronal (b) sections of the human brain highlighting some of the relevant neuroanatomy of affective function. Many of the regions outlined in the figure appear to be dysregulated in extreme cases of social anxiety. Not depicted in this image are the fibres connecting different regions, such as the numerous reciprocal connections between the amygdala and the posterior sensory cortices. The prefrontal cortex, along with the cingulate gyrus, also exerts important regulatory influences, via dense feedback projections, over the subcortical structures that mediate automatic aspects of emotional reactivity. The figure was generated using Brain Explorer 2 software provided by the Allen Brain Atlas Resources [Internet]. Seattle (WA): Allen Institute for Brain Science. ©2009. Available from: www.brain-map.org.

important source of output from the basolateral amygdala is to the central nucleus. The central nucleus interfaces, either directly or indirectly, with multiple downstream targets, including the lateral hypothalamus (which is involved in orchestrating wide-ranging autonomic and endocrine adjustments), the locus coeruleus and basal forebrain nuclei (which provide energizing noradrenergic and cholinergic inputs to the cerebral cortex) and periaqueductal grey (which is involved in highly stereotyped motor programmes such as freezing and flight). Collectively, these neural systems prepare the organism to cope with the source of threat by providing the metabolic support for motivated actions and simultaneously fostering a cognitive/perceptual framework for fear via relatively slow endocrine mechanisms and more rapidly via broadly distributed activations of the cerebral cortex.

A second major region that contributes to the neural instantiation of emotions necessary for social behaviours is the prefrontal cortex (PFC). The PFC is the most anterior region of the cerebral cortex and its primary function appears to be implementing complex behavioural goals by coordinating the flow of information in structures that receive and process sensory input and others that control motor output (Miller & Cohen, 2001). While debate continues concerning the precise role of the PFC in emotion (Davidson, 2002), it is well established that its function is important for representations of affective value as well as the capacity to exert regulatory control over limbic motivational reflexes. Much like the amygdala, the PFC is structurally and functionally heterogeneous in at least two ways, including in terms of (1) its ventromedial and dorsolateral sectors, and (2) hemispheric lateralization.

The ventromedial aspect lies on the underside of the PFC convexity and contains numerous reciprocal connections with the amygdala and other limbic centres. By contrast, the dorsolateral aspect encompasses more superior PFC regions and generally lacks direct connections with the 'lower' emotional regions, instead interfacing only through indirect pathways. There is steadily increasing evidence, derived from both human and nonhuman animal studies, that the PFC (in particular, the ventromedial sector) can dampen or inhibit the activation of fear-related circuits centred around the amygdala and its connections (Ochsner & Gross, 2007; Sotres-Bayon & Quirk, 2010). In human brains, the ventromedial PFC portion may be involved in outcome-based forms of fear regulation (e.g., as occurs following extinction of a conditioned fear response), while the dorsolateral system is more important for regulatory processes that involve a strategic reappraisal of stimuli, typically involving linguistic representations (Ochsner & Gross, 2007).

When considering hemispheric lateralization, there is evidence that the left PFC is an important component of a system that mediates appetitive approach tendencies (along with the consequent positive emotions), while the right PFC appears to form a major component of a circuit that instantiates defensive withdrawal and negative emotions (Fox, 1991). Interestingly, the left and right PFC sectors appear to be differentially associated with amygdalar glucose metabolism, such that the left PFC mediates an effective 'brake' over fear-related circuitry, while the right PFC is associated with its release (Davidson, 2002).

Given the important role that prefrontal and amygdala regions play in socioemotional functions, it is instructive to note that primate brain evolution has been accompanied by a conspicuous and correlated enlargement of these very structures (Barton & Aggleton, 2000; Bickart et al., 2011). This fact suggests that as the size and complexity of societies inhabited by anthropoid primates increased, there was a corresponding need to accommodate the heightened information-processing demands and the consequent neural infrastructure necessary to secure inhibitory control over motivational reflexes. The increased density of connections between the PFC and amygdala allowed for more refined, context-dependent modifications of emotional expressions – an important requirement for social interactions (Emery & Amaral, 2000).

The neural origins of social anxiety may be traced to dysfunctional patterns of prefrontal-amygdala interactions, resulting in activations of fear-related circuitry in inappropriate contexts or to a degree that seems disproportionate with respect to the eliciting situation. Dysregulation of amygdala function (in particular, that of its central component) has long been hypothesized to underlie high social anxiety (Kagan, 1994; Schmidt & Fox, 1999) – a prediction that has been largely borne out by functional neuroimaging studies (Freitas-Ferrari et al., 2010). However, whether amygdala dysregulation can be accounted for primarily on the basis of enhanced bottom-up (hyperexcitability intrinsic to amygdala circuits) or deficient top-down (neocortical) mechanisms (or some combination of the two; Liao, Qiu et al., 2010) remains to be determined.

Another brain region important in the context of social and affective processing is the insular cortex. Long considered to be part of the paralimbic cortex, the insula is located deep within the lateral sulcus and is implicated in a host of functions, involving interoceptive awareness, affective experience, physiological regulation and homeostasis as well as helping to detect salient environmental events (Craig, 2009; Denton, 2006; Menon & Uddin, 2010). A functional distinction is often drawn between the anterior and posterior insula, with the posterior aspect playing a larger role in physiological regulation and the anterior insula being important for representing affective experience and forming a putative salience network (Craig, 2010). The anterior insula exhibits connectivity with many of the regions that are involved in tracking the affective value of stimuli (e.g., amygdala, orbitofrontal cortex, nucleus accumbens, periaqueductal grey) as well as those involved in executive attention (e.g., anterior cingulate cortex), thereby forming an important integrative link between the value of stimuli, their relation to the organism and responses directed back into the external environment (Öngur & Price, 2000; Paulus & Stein, 2006).

Although the preceding section has reviewed some of the important structures and connections that are consistently implicated in socioemotional processes, there is no evidence for the simplistic notion that function *resides* directly within those structures. Rather, there is an increasing appreciation that psychological phenomena are the emergent products of dynamic and reciprocal interactions among interconnected neural elements. Accordingly, understanding the neural substrates of normal and pathological expressions of anxiety requires appreciation for a wide range of cortico-cortical and cortico-subcortical network interactions

## Developmental considerations

There is considerable interest in clarifying the developmental course and precursors to clinical manifestations of social anxiety, as anxiety disorders in general are increasingly being conceptualized as developmental in nature (Leonardo & Hen, 2008). Temperamental shyness (or behavioural inhibition)[4] constitutes the earliest appearing antecedent of subsequent social anxiety (Fox, Henderson et al., 2005). Temperamental shyness refers to an early appearing and extreme form of shyness which is observed in approximately 10–15 per cent of typically developing children (García Coll et al., 1984; Kagan et al., 1987). When followed longitudinally, those children who are classified as temperamentally shy show increased risk for development of anxiety disorders, especially SAD (Biederman et al., 2001; Hirshfeld-Becker et al., 2007; Schwartz et al., 1999).

The physiological and behavioural markers of temperamental shyness emerge within the first four months of post-natal life (Kagan & Snidman, 1991). These infant predictors include patterns of high motor activity (e.g., limb trashing, spastic back arching) and emotional distress (e.g.,

---

[4] This literature has often used the terms *shyness* and *behavioural inhibition* synonymously, sometimes to the detriment of conceptual clarity. The term 'temperamental shyness' is preferred here because it is more precise (i.e., specific to social fears), while the usage of 'behavioural inhibition' may be overly broad, potentially denoting a more generalized fear reaction (see Schmidt & Buss, 2010).

crying, fussing) in response to the presentation of novel sensory stimuli. Moreover, a subset of the highly motoric and easily aroused infants also exhibit elevated fetal heart rates and elevated heart rates during sleep, when held erect, within the first two weeks following birth (Kagan, 1994). A significant portion of infants selected for early temperamental shyness continue to display peripheral (Schmidt & Fox, 1998; Schmidt et al., 1997; Schmidt et al., 1999) and central (Calkins et al., 1996; Fox et al., 1994; Fox et al., 2001; Schmidt, 2008; Schmidt & Fox, 1994; Schmidt et al., 1999; Theall-Honey & Schmidt, 2006) markers associated with heightened limbic arousal across the life span. Behaviourally, these children exhibit quiet, restrained and overly cautious styles of responding to novel social situations (e.g., Rubin et al., 2002).

Heritability studies suggest that there is a considerable genetic contribution to social phobias (e.g., DiLalla et al., 1994; Kendler et al., 1999), although precise gene linkage attempts have been elusive thus far. Children of socially phobic parents are known to be at greater risk for psychopathology into adolescence and adulthood (Mancini et al., 1996), and they also show distinct patterns of frontal electroencephalographic (EEG) activity at rest when compared to children of healthy control parents (Campbell, M. J., et al., 2007; Miskovic, Campbell et al., 2011). As with the majority of complex phenotypic expressions, genes are continuously intertwined with environmental experiences to permit or restrict genomic potential in the sculpting of brain and behaviour (Fox, Nichols et al., 2005; Segalowitz & Schmidt, 2008). However, even a brief overview of the literature on temperamental shyness suggests the presence of biological constraints on the experience and expression of social anxiety – a subset of children enter the world predisposed to respond in fearful ways towards others.

## Adult studies

The neural correlates of social anxiety in adults can be profitably studied by recording brain activity under a variety of laboratory settings: (1) during periods of rest and relaxed wakefulness, (2) during cognitive-affective experiments (e.g., viewing of threatening faces) that are often designed to isolate specific components of information processing, and/or (3) during periods of acute symptom provocation induced by the anticipation of an actual or simulated social interaction that includes an evaluative dimension (e.g., anticipating or delivering a public speech). A large number of social anxiety studies employing one or more of the above paradigms are summarized in Table 8.1. Below, we provide a summary of selected findings.

Table 8.1 *A selected summary of studies on the neural correlates of social anxiety*

| Experiment type | Method | Sample characteristics | Sex ratio (F:M) | Findings (socially anxious relative to control) | Reference |
|---|---|---|---|---|---|
| Resting/ functional | fMRI | Medication-free patients with a diagnosis of social anxiety disorder | 4:13 | – decreased functional connectivity between frontal and occipital cortex<br>– decreased functional connectivity within frontal cortex | Ding *et al.* (2011) |
| Resting/ functional | fMRI | Medication-free patients with a diagnosis of social anxiety disorder, social anxiety disorder and panic disorder, panic disorder | 1:9 | – decreased functional coupling of left amygdala with medial prefrontal cortex and posterior cingulate<br>– reduced connectivity between medial prefrontal cortex and the anterior cingulate | Hahn *et al.* (2011) |
| Resting/ functional and structural | fMRI | Medication-free patients with a diagnosis of social anxiety disorder | 6:12 | – decreased grey matter volumes in the right posterior inferior temporal gyrus and right parahippocampal/ hippocampal gyrus<br>– increased functional connectivity between right posterior inferior temporal gyrus and left inferior occipital gyrus<br>– increased functional connectivity between right parahippocampal/ hippocampal formation and left middle temporal gyrus<br>– increased right medial prefrontal cortex volume<br>– greater structural connectivity in the genu of the corpus callosum | Liao *et al.* (2011) |

Table 8.1 (*cont.*)

| Experiment type | Method | Sample characteristics | Sex ratio (F:M) | Findings (socially anxious relative to control) | Reference |
|---|---|---|---|---|---|
| Resting/ functional | fMRI | Medication-free patients with a diagnosis of social anxiety disorder | 6:14 | – decreased connectivity in somatomotor and visual networks<br>– increased connectivity in a network including the medial prefrontal cortex | Liao, Chen *et al.* (2010) |
| Resting/ functional | fMRI | Medication-free patients with a diagnosis of social anxiety disorder | 6:16 | – decreased input from inferior temporal gyrus to amygdala<br>– increased bidirectional amygdala/ visual cortex connectivity | Liao, Qiu *et al.* (2010) |
| Resting/ functional | EEG | Patients with a diagnosis of social anxiety disorder | 11:12 | – greater resting left prefrontal activity associated with better response to cognitive behavioural therapy for SAD | Moscovitch *et al.* (2011) |
| Resting/ structural | DTI | Medication-free patients with a diagnosis of social anxiety disorder | 15:15 | – aberrant connectivity of a white matter tract connecting frontal cortex and amygdala | Phan *et al.* (2009) |
| Resting/ functional | EEG | Subsyndromal, selected for shyness and sociability | 20:0 | – greater relative right frontal EEG activity in high shy groups | Schmidt (1999) |
| Provocation | PET | Patients with a diagnosis of social anxiety disorder | 15:13 | – positive correlations between stress-induced cerebral blood flow in right supra genual anterior cingulate, right head of caudate nucleus, bilateral medial prefrontal cortex and high frequency heart rate variability | Ahs *et al.* (2009) |
| Provocation | PET | Patients with a diagnosis of social anxiety disorder | 7:5 | – positive correlations between stress-induced cortisol and blood flow in hypothalamus<br>– negative correlations between stress-induced cortisol and blood flow in the medial prefrontal cortex and motor/ premotor cortices | Ahs *et al.* (2006) |

| | | | | | |
|---|---|---|---|---|---|
| Provocation | EEG | Subsyndromal, selected for high social anxiety | 19:5 | – association between right frontal resting activity and shyness (when controlling for depression symptoms) | Beaton, Schmidt et al. (2008) |
| Provocation | EEG | Medication-free patients with a diagnosis of social anxiety disorder | 12:8 | – stress-induced increase in right-sided activation in the anterior temporal and lateral prefrontal scalp regions | Davidson et al. (2000) |
| Provocation | PET | Patients with a diagnosis of social anxiety disorder | 8:10 | – treatment associated reductions of stress-induced regional cerebral blood flow in bilateral amygdalae, hippocampus, periamygdaloid, rhinal and parahippocampal cortices<br>– attenuation of amygdalar-limbic activity associated with clinical improvements one year later | Furmark et al. (2002) |
| Provocation | fMRI | Adolescents with diagnosis of an anxiety disorder, associated with concerns of social evaluation | 10:4 | – greater amygdala activation, and positive functional connectivity with ventrolateral prefrontal cortex, when anticipating evaluation from peers previously rated as undesired for interaction | Guyer et al. (2008) |
| Provocation | fMRI | Medication-free patients with a diagnosis of social anxiety disorder | 0:8 | – greater stress-induced subcortical, limbic, and lateral paralimbic activity<br>– less cortical activity in the dorsal anterior cingulate/prefrontal cortex | Lorberbaum et al. (2004) |
| Provocation | EEG | Patients with a diagnosis of social anxiety disorder | 12:13 | – reduced EEG delta-beta coupling following group cognitive behavioural therapy for SAD | Miskovic, Moscovitch et al. (2011) |

Table 8.1 (*cont.*)

| Experiment type | Method | Sample characteristics | Sex ratio (F:M) | Findings (socially anxious relative to control) | Reference |
|---|---|---|---|---|---|
| Provocation | EEG | Subsyndromal, selected for high social anxiety | 19:5 | – increased EEG delta-beta coupling in the right midfrontal region | Miskovic *et al.* (2010) |
| Provocation | EEG | Subsyndromal, selected for shyness and sociability | 20:0 | – low sociable subjects displayed greater right midfrontal and great left parietal activity | Schmidt & Fox (1994) |
| Provocation | PET | Patients with a diagnosis of social anxiety disorder | 8:10 | – greater regional cerebral blood flow within the right dorsolateral prefrontal cortex, left inferior temporal cortex and left amygdaloid-hippocampal region during public speech anticipation | Tillfors *et al.* (2002) |
| Provocation | PET | Medication-free patients with a diagnosis of social anxiety disorder | 8:10 | – greater regional cerebral blood flow in the amygdaloid complex<br>– decreased cortical blood flow (orbitofrontal and insular cortex, temporal pole) | Tillfors *et al.* (2001) |
| Provocation | PET | Medication-free patients with a diagnosis of social anxiety disorder | 0:5 | – deactivations in the right lingual gyrus and right medial frontal gyrus | van Ameringen *et al.* (2004) |
| Affective processing (visual/faces) | fMRI | Medication-free (or stable dosage) patients with a diagnosis of social anxiety disorder | 8:3 | – increased anterior cingulate cortex activity during processing of disgust (vs neutral) faces | Amir *et al.* (2005) |
| Affective processing (visual/faces) | fMRI | Subsyndromal, selected for high shyness | 5:7 | – increased neural activation across a range of brain regions during implicit processing of emotional (vs neutral) faces | Beaton *et al.* (2010) |

| | | | | | |
|---|---|---|---|---|---|
| Affective processing (visual/faces) | fMRI | Subsyndromal, selected for high shyness | 5:7 | – less bilateral activation in the fusiform face area during processing of strangers' neutral faces, but greater activation during processing of personally familiar faces | Beaton et al. (2009) |
| Affective processing (visual/faces) | fMRI | Subsyndromal, selected for high shyness | 5:7 | – greater bilateral amygdala activation during the presentation of stranger faces<br>– greater left amygdala activation during processing of personally familiar faces | Beaton, Schmidt, Schulkin et al. (2008) |
| Affective processing (visual/faces) | fMRI | Patients with a diagnosis of social anxiety disorder | 0:7 | – increased amygdala activation during passive viewing of neutral faces | Birbaumer et al. (1998) |
| Affective processing (visual/faces) | fMRI | Adolescent and adult medication-free patients with a diagnosis of social anxiety disorder | 15:10 adults<br>7:7 adolescents | – increased activity in the rostral anterior cingulate cortex (during viewing of angry faces) and both amygdala/rostral anterior cingulate cortex (during viewing of fearful faces) in both adolescents and adults | Blair, Geraci, Korelitz et al. (2011) |
| Affective processing (visual/text) | fMRI | Medication-free patients with a diagnosis of social anxiety disorder | 7:8 | – increased medial PFC responses to others' criticism of self<br>– decreased medial PFC bold responses to own criticism of self | Blair, Geraci, Otero et al. (2011) |
| Affective processing (visual/text) | fMRI | Medication-free patients with a diagnosis of social anxiety disorder | 7:9 | – increased ventromedial prefrontal cortex activation when reading scenarios concerning unintentional social transgressions | Blair et al. (2010) |
| Affective processing (visual/faces) | fMRI | Medication-free patients with a diagnosis of social anxiety disorder | 8:9 | – increased amygdala activation for fearful (vs neutral) faces | Blair, Shaywitz et al. (2008) |

Table 8.1 (*cont.*)

| Experiment type | Method | Sample characteristics | Sex ratio (F:M) | Findings (socially anxious relative to control) | Reference |
|---|---|---|---|---|---|
| Affective processing (visual/text) | fMRI | Medication-free patients with a diagnosis of social anxiety disorder | 6:11 | – increased responses in regions of the medial PFC and amygdala during self- but not other-referential criticism | Blair, Geraci et al. (2008) |
| Affective processing (visual/scenes) | fMRI | Patients with a diagnosis of social anxiety disorder | 7:7 | – increased activity in upper midbrain/dorsal thalamus, amygdala, temporo-occipital and parietal regions during anticipation of negative and emotionally ambiguous images | Brühl et al. (2011) |
| Affective processing (visual/faces) | fMRI | Medication-free patients with a diagnosis of social anxiety disorder | 4:10 | – amygdala responses occurred later for fear, angry and happy faces | Campbell, D. W., et al. (2007) |
| Affective processing (visual/faces) | fMRI | Patients with a diagnosis of social anxiety disorder | 6:4 | – increased left amygdala activity during processing of neutral faces | Cooney et al. (2006) |
| Affective processing (visual/faces) | fMRI | Medication-free patients with a diagnosis of social anxiety disorder | 4:4 | – altered functional connectivity across brain regions within the core and the extended systems for face perception and the default mode network | Danti et al. (2010) |
| Affective processing (visual/faces) | fMRI | Medication-free patients with a diagnosis of social anxiety disorder | 6:4 | – increased right amygdala activation for angry (relative to neutral) schematic line drawing faces | Evans et al. (2008) |
| Affective processing (visual/faces) | PET | Medication-free patients with a diagnosis of social anxiety disorder | 20:14 | – increased left amygdala activation for angry (vs neutral) faces in both anxious and non-anxious groups<br>– serotonin transporter allelic variation explained more variance than clinical diagnosis | Furmark et al. (2005) |
| Affective processing (visual/faces) | fMRI | Medication-free patients with a diagnosis of social anxiety disorder | 4:4 | – increased activity in network of precuneus and posterior cingulate regions during viewing of faces (vs scrambled visual stimuli) | Gentili et al. (2009) |

| Domain | Method | Sample | Ratio | Findings | Reference |
|---|---|---|---|---|---|
| Affective processing (visual/faces) | fMRI | Medication-free patients with a diagnosis of social anxiety disorder | 4:4 | – increased activity in left amygdala, insula, bilateral superior temporal sulcus<br>– reduced activation in the left fusiform gyrus, left dorsolateral prefrontal cortex, and bilateral intraparietal sulcus during viewing of faces (vs scrambled visual stimuli) | Gentili et al. (2008) |
| Affective processing (visual/faces) | fMRI | Medication-free patients with a diagnosis of social anxiety disorder | 9:6 | – increased activity in multiple emotion-related regions (medial orbitofrontal cortex, subgenual anterior cingulate, bilateral hippocampal gyri) during viewing of harsh faces (relative to neutral scenes), but not physical threat scenes | Goldin et al. (2009) |
| Affective processing (visual/faces) | ERP | Individual differences in shyness (not pre-selected) | 19:22 | – reduced P1 amplitude for fearful relative to neutral expressions<br>– low shy individuals showed faster P1 latency for happy relative to other expressions and increased P1 amplitude for happy relative to neutral faces | Jetha et al. (2012) |
| Affective processing (visual/faces) | fMRI | Medication-free patients with a diagnosis of social anxiety disorder | N/A | – increased amygdala reactivity to threatening faces of moderate (50–60%) and high (90–100%) affective intensity | Klumpp et al. (2010) |

Table 8.1 (*cont.*)

| Experiment type | Method | Sample characteristics | Sex ratio (F:M) | Findings (socially anxious relative to control) | Reference |
|---|---|---|---|---|---|
| Affective processing (visual/faces) | ERP | Medication-free patients with a diagnosis of social anxiety disorder | 9:10 | – greater right-temporoparietal N170 component during angry face processing<br>– social fears associated with higher P1 amplitudes for angry faces | Kolassa & Miltner (2006) |
| Affective processing (visual/faces) | SSVEP | Subsyndromal, selected for high social anxiety | 7:7 | – sustained amplitude enhancement for occipital evoked potentials during viewing of emotional (relative to neutral) faces | McTeague *et al.* (2011) |
| Affective processing (visual/faces) | ERP | Subsyndromal, selected for high social anxiety | 15:6 | – negative face bias indicated by the P3b/late positive potential<br>– absence of positive face bias | Moser, Huppert *et al.* (2008) |
| Affective processing (visual/text) | ERP | Subsyndromal, selected for high social anxiety | 11:5 | – lack of a positive interpretation bias for ambiguous scenarios | Moser, Hajcak *et al.* (2008) |
| Affective processing (visual/faces) | ERP | Patients with a diagnosis of social anxiety disorder | 8:4 | – enhanced P1 amplitude for angry-neutral face pairs<br>– increased fusiform gyrus source activation for angry-neutral face pairs | Mueller *et al.* (2009) |
| Affective processing (visual/faces) | ERP | Subsyndromal, selected for high social anxiety | 10:8 | – increased early posterior negativity for fearful and angry facial expressions<br>– increased late positive potential for both emotional and neutral faces | Mühlberger *et al.* (2009) |
| Affective processing (visual/faces) | fMRI | Medication-free patients with a diagnosis of social anxiety disorder | 5:5 | – increased amygdala activation for harsh (vs happy) faces<br>– amygdala activation positively related to social anxiety severity | Phan *et al.* (2006) |

| Topic | Method | Sample | Ratio | Findings | Citation |
|---|---|---|---|---|---|
| Affective processing (visual/faces) | fMRI | Individual differences in social anxiety (not pre-selected) | 12:10 | – positive association between social anxiety and amygdala activation for fearful and happy faces, after controlling for fusiform activity | Pujol et al. (2009) |
| Affective processing (auditory) | fMRI | Medication-free patients with a diagnosis of social anxiety disorder | 6:6 | – increased orbitofrontal cortex activation in response to angry, compared to neutral, voices | Quadflieg et al. (2008) |
| Affective processing (visual/faces) | ERP | Subsyndromal, selected for fears of negative evaluation | N/A | – reduced N2b wave amplitude during detection of intensity changes in angry expressions | Rossignol et al. (2007) |
| Affective processing (visual/text) | fMRI | Medication-free patients with a diagnosis of social anxiety disorder | 10:9 | – increased amygdala and orbitofrontal cortex activation during implicit processing of phobia-related words<br>– insula activation correlated positively with symptom severity during explicit processing of phobia-related words | Schmidt et al. (2010) |
| Affective processing (visual/faces) | ERP | Individual differences in social anxiety (not pre-selected) | 12:9 | – social anxiety correlated positively with P3 amplitude for upright angry, but not happy, faces | Sewell et al. (2008) |
| Affective processing (visual/faces) | fMRI | Medication-free patients with a diagnosis of social anxiety disorder | 3:8 | – increased bilateral amygdala activation to negative (vs neutral) images<br>– amygdala activation positively related to social anxiety severity | Shah et al. (2009) |
| Affective processing (visual/faces) | fMRI | Medication-free patients with a diagnosis of social anxiety disorder | 5:10 | – increased activation of the left allocortex (amygdala, uncus, and parahippocampal gyrus) during viewing of contemptuous (vs happy) and angry (vs happy) faces | Stein et al. (2002) |
| Affective processing (visual/faces) | fMRI | Medication-free patients with a diagnosis of social anxiety disorder | 5:4 | – increased activation of extrastriate visual cortex regardless of facial expression | Straube et al. (2005) |

Table 8.1 (cont.)

| Experiment type | Method | Sample characteristics | Sex ratio (F:M) | Findings (socially anxious relative to control) | Reference |
|---|---|---|---|---|---|
| Affective processing (visual/faces) | fMRI | Medication-free patients with a diagnosis of social anxiety disorder | 6:4 | – angry (vs happy or neutral) faces produced more insular activation<br>– both angry and happy faces produce more amygdala activation | Straube et al. (2004) |
| Affective processing (visual/faces) | SSVEP | Subsyndromal, selected for high social anxiety | 15:2 | – increased insular responses to angry (vs neutral) faces in both explicit and implicit task modes<br>– greater amygdala, parahippocampal gyrus and extrastriate visual cortex activation to angry (vs neutral) faces during implicit task mode only | Wieser et al. (2011) |
| Affective processing (visual/faces) | fMRI | Medication-free patients with a diagnosis of social anxiety disorder | 6:5 | – angry (relative to neutral and happy) faces associated with electrocortical facilitation over visual regions across 3 secs of viewing | |
| | | | | – increased bilateral amygdala activation to high versus low intensity of emotional faces (angry, fearful, disgusted, sad, happy) | Yoon et al. (2007) |

Abbreviations: EEG, electroencephalogram; ERP, event-related potential; fMRI, functional magnetic resonance imaging; PET, positron emission tomography; SSVEP, steady state visual evoked potential.

## Resting activity

Because resting conditions are often employed for purposes of computing task reactivity difference scores, relatively few studies have directly examined the links between spontaneous brain activity and social anxiety. The most direct way to index spontaneous brain activity is by recording scalp potentials (EEG) during simple eyes open and closed conditions and performing spectral power analyses of the electrical signal. Studies from our laboratory (Beaton, Schmidt, Ashbaugh *et al.*, 2008; Schmidt, 1999) have noted a relation between social anxiety (in the non-clinical range) and greater relative electrophysiological activity of the right PFC region at rest. As already mentioned, such a pattern of frontal brain activity is associated with poor regulation of limbic arousal (see above section on functional neuroanatomy) and appears among temperamentally shy infants and children (see 'Developmental considerations'). Recently, Schmidt and colleagues (2012) have demonstrated that the pattern of resting frontal brain electrical activity remains stable across time in patients with SAD before they undergo treatment. It is interesting to note also that resting frontal EEG alpha asymmetry, involving greater left PFC activation at pre-treatment, predicts greater reductions in social anxiety among patients enlisted in cognitive behavioural therapy (Moscovitch *et al.*, 2011).

The past decade has heralded a 'paradigm shift' in the positron emission tomography (PET)/functional magnetic resonance imaging (fMRI) neuroimaging field, with a resurgence of interest in studying the functional significance of spontaneous brain activity in normal and pathological states (Zhang & Raichle, 2010). Large-scale brain networks typically exhibit organized patterns of connectivity at rest that appear to be selectively perturbed in patients with social phobia as reflected in decreased functional connectivity within some brain networks (somatomotor and visual), but increased connectivity in others (default mode and dorsal attention networks) (Liao, Chen *et al.*, 2010). A recent study employed sophisticated data-processing methods that rely on temporal precedence cues to infer directed interactions between distributed brain regions during relaxed wakefulness (Liao, Qiu *et al.*, 2010). The findings revealed that socially phobic patients exhibit increased influences deriving from the amygdala and impinging on the visual cortices as well as decreased regulatory influences from several neocortical regions, including the frontal cortex, to the amygdala.

## Threat-related cognitive-affective activation

Since angry facial expressions signal negative evaluation and represent prototypical stimuli for activating the social submissiveness system

(Öhman, 1986, 2009), numerous social anxiety studies have examined the neural correlates of threat-related processing using visual stimuli (see Staugaard, 2010, for a comprehensive review). Neuroimaging data indicate that adults with SAD show enhanced amygdala (and often insular) activity in response to hostile and contemptuous faces (Evans et al., 2008; Stein et al., 2002; Straube et al., 2004). Moreover, the magnitude of amygdala activation to threatening faces is positively related specifically to the severity of social – not generalized – anxiety (Phan et al., 2006). Event-related electrocortical studies have largely corroborated findings of increased reactivity to threatening faces among clinical and subsyndromal socially anxious populations (Kolassa & Miltner, 2006; Moser, Huppert et al., 2008; Mueller et al., 2009; Mühlberger et al., 2009; Wieser et al., 2011), with some uncertainty as to whether it is primarily the early or late stages of visual processing that are affected.

Cognitive studies of how socially anxious individuals process threatening faces have also been inconsistent in their findings, perhaps due to wide methodological variations in the experiments used, including factors such as the speed of stimulus exposure and type of facial stimuli (see Bögels & Mansell, 2004, for a review). As a result, Miskovic and Schmidt (2012a) have recently attempted to further characterize the nature of threat-related processing biases in social anxiety, by independently manipulating the temporal and energetic aspects of affective stimulus delivery in a visual dot probe experiment. The dot probe task involves the simultaneous presentation of two stimuli – for example, a threatening and neutral face – at spatially distinct locations. Immediately following stimulus offset, a simple geometric probe is shown in one of the two spatial positions. Threat-related attention biases can be inferred when reaction times are faster for probes occurring in the location previously occupied by the threatening stimulus compared to probes occurring in the opposite location. Our experiment systematically varied the presentation rate (100, 500, 1250 ms) of face stimuli in order to index both the relatively automatic aspects of information processing as well as more strategic components at the later durations. Independently of the temporal parameter, we also varied the affective quality of faces by using computer-assisted morphing procedures to create angry and happy expressions that were mild, moderate or strong in intensity. Our results showed that compared to the low anxious group, adults selected for high social anxiety exhibited increased vigilance for threatening faces that were rapidly (100 ms) displayed. No group differences in threat-related biases emerged during the more controlled phases of information processing, suggesting that social anxiety is marked mostly by initial hyper-reactivity. Interestingly, attentional vigilance in the high socially anxious group was enhanced even for faces that combined 50 per cent angry with 50 per cent neutral expressive features. This result suggests that high socially anxious individuals may be prone to detect threat even in ambiguous stimuli that others might categorize as relatively safe (see Klumpp et al., 2010, for recent neuroimaging evidence). Other evidence indicates that socially anxious individuals show hyper-reactivity of amygdala nuclei even in response to neutral faces. For example, an fMRI study from our group (Beaton, Schmidt, Schulkin et al., 2008) showed that adults selected for shyness and social anxiety exhibit greater amygdala activation when viewing strangers' neutral faces. Indeed, left amygdala activation in the high compared to the low shy group persisted when viewing personally familiar faces. The neural correlates of viewing strangers' faces also differed between high and low socially anxious adults at the level of the cerebral cortex within the putative fusiform face area (Beaton et al., 2009). Socially anxious adults displayed reduced fusiform responses to strangers' faces, which may indicate that anxious individuals actively averted their gaze when they encountered novel faces, possibly due to the increased anxiety they experienced as suggested by their simultaneously enhanced amygdala activity. Jetha and colleagues (2012) have provided evidence, derived from evoked brain responses, that subsyndromal socially anxious individuals display initial perceptual vigilance for expressive faces, followed by subsequent avoidance of them. Considered from a developmental perspective, avoidance and a corresponding lack of experience with faces may account for some of the deficits displayed by shy children in processing this category of stimuli (Brunet et al., 2010).

*Acute symptom provocation*

Experimental designs that involve anticipation of or direct confrontation with a feared event (e.g., public speaking in socially anxious populations) allow the researcher to examine the psychophysiological correlates of anxiety 'in the moment'. As previously mentioned (see above section on functional neuroanatomy), social anxiety is likely to involve reciprocal interactions between neocortical and subcortical affective structures. One way to study communication across different neuronal systems is by employing novel cross-frequency approaches to the analysis of EEG signals. For example, measuring the strength of correlations between the amount of spectral power residing in slow and fast EEG frequency bands provides some sensitivity to gross changes in the amount of cortical–subcortical interaction (Knyazev & Slobodskaya, 2003; Robinson, 1999;

Schutter et al., 2006). Slow neuronal oscillations (in the delta and theta range of frequencies) primarily reflect the arousal of phylogenetically older, subcortical regions while fast electrical rhythms (in the beta and gamma range) relate mostly to activities of the neocortex (Knyazev, 2007; Uhlhaas & Singer, 2006). When the amount of spectral power generated in the slow and fast frequency bands becomes positively correlated, it is hypothesized to reflect a state of increased cortical–subcortical communication and information transfer (Schutter et al., 2006) as well as heightened anxiety (see Schutter & Knyazev, 2012, for a recent review).

Miskovic and Schmidt (2009) and others (Schutter & van Honk, 2004, 2005; van Peer et al., 2008) have shown that EEG cross-frequency interactions are affected in predictable ways by natural and synthetic steroid hormones that are differentially associated with anxiogenic and anxiolytic properties. Converging evidence concerning the role that steroid hormones play in regulating cortical–subcortical interactions has come from the application of fMRI methodology (van Wingen et al., 2010), which has superior spatial resolution to EEG recordings derived from the scalp.

In a set of recent studies, Miskovic and colleagues (2010) demonstrated that when adults who are high in social anxiety anticipate the performance of a public speech, they show enhanced amounts of positively correlated power between the slow and fast EEG frequencies compared to low anxious participants. The neural signatures agree with self-report measures derived from the same participants, who indicate greater anticipatory anxiety concerning the public speech compared to their low anxious counterparts. Although speculative, the EEG results may indicate that part of the increased cortico–subcortical communication observed in high socially anxious individuals is associated with heightened bottom-up transmission of threat-related signals, conveyed by the subcortical regions to the neocortex (van Honk et al., 2010). Indeed, there is support for the suggestion that the degree of EEG delta-beta coupling is associated with increased attention for stimuli depicting social threat (Putman, 2011).

In a second study Miskovic and colleagues were able to replicate the finding of high delta-beta coupling both at rest and during speech anticipation in a clinical group of SAD patients (Miskovic, Moscovitch et al., 2011). Interestingly, a standardized course of group cognitive behavioural therapy was shown to produce significant decreases in correlated EEG power.

Other studies, employing nuclear and magnetic imaging, have shown that acute symptom provocation in social anxiety is associated with a combination of hyper-reactivity in limbic regions, consistently involving the amygdala, and hypo-activity of many neocortical regions (Guyer et al., 2008; Lorberbaum et al., 2004; Tillfors et al., 2001; Tillfors et al., 2002). The authors generally interpret their findings to imply that an evaluative interpersonal situation (e.g., public speaking) leads to engagement of phylogenetically older 'alarm' systems in socially phobic individuals, while non-anxious individuals engage a phylogenetically newer assembly of brain regions associated with higher-level cognitive/analytic processes, allowing them to remain calm and focused in the identical context. Treatment of social anxiety, either with cognitive behavioural therapy or selective serotonin reuptake inhibitors, is associated with a normalization of neural activity – namely, reductions in limbic/amygdalar blood flow during speech anticipation (Furmark et al., 2002).

*Summary*

It is worth noting at the outset that most of the neural correlates of social anxiety reviewed above appear generally similar regardless of whether the study samples involved clinically diagnosed patients or adults selected from the extremes of the normal population, providing some support for our dimensional framework.

Across the majority of studies reviewed in this section the most consistent neural correlate of social anxiety involves amygdala hyperexcitability, accompanied by over-responsiveness to social threat cues at multiple levels of information processing. Unfortunately, the resolution of contemporary PET and low-field fMRI imaging precludes the possibility of discriminating activations in individual amygdaloid nuclei (e.g., basolateral vs central divisions) and testing more refined theoretical hypotheses. Studies of human social anxiety are therefore confined, for the time being, to broad statements about the excitability of a functionally heterogeneous complex of amygdaloid nuclei.

Exaggerated neural activity is also commonly observed in the insula region (Etkin & Wager, 2007) and the orbitofrontal cortex. In addition to increased activity of regionally isolated structures, social anxiety seems to be related to atypical patterns of connectivity in several brain networks. While heightened amygdala responses may explain sensitization of perceptual and attentional systems for signals of external threat (e.g., a threatening facial expression), aberrations in other brain networks (e.g., anterior insula and orbitofrontal cortex) may be related to the distortions in self-image and bodily awareness that are also common in extreme cases of social anxiety. Some (e.g., Paulus & Stein, 2006) have theorized that the anterior insula of anxious individuals generates exaggerated prediction signals about aversive interoceptive states and that cognitive and behavioural correlates of anxiety represent subsequent coping mechanisms activated to reduce the discrepancy between predicted and observed bodily states. We turn to a further consideration of neural correlates underlying altered self-perceptions in the remainder of the chapter, with some suggestions for how to begin integrating measures of the brain and peripheral physiology in future studies.

## Future directions: integrating the brain and periphery in studies of social anxiety

Most contemporary cognitive models of social anxiety (Clark & McManus, 2002; Heinrichs & Hofmann, 2001) emphasize biases in the processing of self-relevant information as contributing to the onset and maintenance of social anxiety. One prediction to be derived from these models is that the perception of bodily arousal (e.g., facial blushing, increased sweating, heart palpitations and voice quiver) reinforces a negative self-image leading to further increases in the intensity of social anxiety. Clinical neuroscience might inform cognitive models of social anxiety by helping to delineate the neural networks that underlie bodily and interoceptive awareness and their dysregulation in social anxiety.[5] However, most neuroscience research on social anxiety has treated brain and peripheral measures as relatively independent outcomes. We have previously emphasized the potential utility of integrating measures of brain and peripheral physiology in a unified framework for the study of emotion and individual differences (Miskovic & Schmidt, 2012b). Here, we would like to extend part of this framework to the study of social anxiety, with a special focus on the blush in light of previous work highlighting its unique sensitivity to trait differences in shyness (Hofmann et al., 2006).

The facial blush has long been linked to the experience and expression of social anxiety (Darwin, 1872/1965). Neuroethological models of the blush suggest that this vascular response represents an appeasement display, meant to signal awareness of social submissiveness in dominance hierarchies (Stein & Bouwer, 1997). Accordingly, extreme manifestations

---

[5] Dysfunction here can refer to abnormalities in the intensity of evoked visceral and somatic responses and/or disruptions in the neural processing of these signals, resulting in the *mis*perception of heightened arousal.

of social anxiety might be properly understood as habitual deployments of false appeasement alarms. When viewed from this perspective, the blushing response in social anxiety holds promise for permitting novel insights into the positive feedback loops interposed between the information-processing deficits related to external cues of social threat and those that relate to biases in self-image. There are presently several useful avenues for integrating measures of the facial blush within predominant affective neuroscience models of social anxiety.

The first approach involves employing the facial blush as an online marker of social anxiety since it appears to possess greater specificity when compared to other autonomic and peripheral indices (Hofmann et al., 2006). The inclusion of a plethysmograph transducer in a standard electrocortical or neuroimaging experimental set-up would allow researchers to segment neural time series data into discrete epochs associated with blushing episodes. Such analyses could yield evidence concerning the patterns of regional brain activity and brain connectivity associated with discrete changes in the submissiveness–dominance hierarchy presumed to underlie the expression of social anxiety (Öhman, 2009). Moreover, if combined with additional self-report measures, researchers could begin to discover the neural correlates of negative self-perception in social anxiety.

In addition, there is a challenge for neuroscientific models to shed further light on the nature of distortions in bodily state that are experienced by individuals with high social anxiety. There is an increasing understanding of the neural networks that underlie awareness of visceral and somatic states in healthy individuals (Craig, 2009; Critchley et al., 2004). One of the interesting findings to emerge from this field of inquiry has been that the anterior insula and the orbitofrontal cortex constitute vital structures for continuous monitoring of the body and representations of bodily responses. In addition to receiving information from the internal viscera, the insula receives input from skin receptors. It is interesting to recall that the insula is both hyperactivated (Etkin & Wager, 2007) and more weakly connected to regions important for executive functions (Klumpp et al., 2012) among patients with SAD. Whether the perceptual feedback from blushing relies on similar neural pathways centred on the insula or whether it primarily relies on cutaneous sensations delivered to the somatosensory cortices remains to be answered in the future. Such knowledge will be able to advance neuroscientific models of social anxiety, while potentially introducing important revisions to previously advanced cognitive theories of self-relevant biases (Clark & McManus, 2002; Heinrichs & Hofmann, 2001).

## Final summary and conclusions

The perspective we have adopted is that the experience and expression of social anxiety exists on a continuum of severity from moderate distress to incapacitating fear. As this chapter illustrates, fruitful research on the psychophysiology of social anxiety involves the integration of many separate experimental paradigms and methods derived from both basic and clinical research. Converging evidence from cortical electrophysiology, magnetic and nuclear imaging, as well as measures of peripheral reactivity, helps to direct and constrain theoretical frameworks. Future research will likely carry an increasing emphasis on novel methodological measures (e.g., cross-frequency EEG analyses) and theoretical frameworks (e.g., central/peripheral integration) that permit researchers to make inferences about dynamic, system-wide interactions that underlie the experience and expression of social anxiety. A unified neuroscientific approach to investigating the bases of social anxiety may hold some hope for building pathophysiological models with sufficient depth to propose improvements in diagnosis, prognosis and treatment of pathological social fear.

## REFERENCES

Adolphs, R. (2003). Cognitive neuroscience of social behaviour. *Nature Reviews Neuroscience*, **4**, 165–78.

Ahs, F., Furmark, T., Michelgard, A., Langstrom, B., Appel, L., Wolf, O. T., Kirschbaum, C., & Fredrikson, M. (2006). Hypothalamic blood flow correlates positively with stress-induced cortisol levels in subjects with social anxiety disorder. *Psychosomatic Medicine*, **68**, 859–62.

Ahs, F., Sollers, J. J., Furmark, T., Fredrikson, M., & Thayer, J. F. (2009). High-frequency heart rate variability and cortico-striatal activity in men and women with social phobia. *NeuroImage*, **47**, 815–20.

Amaral, D. G. (2002). The primate amygdala and the neurobiology of social behavior: implications for understanding social anxiety. *Biological Psychiatry*, **51**, 11–17.

American Psychiatric Association (2000). *Diagnostic and statistical manual of mental disorders*, 4th edn, text rev. Washington, DC: American Psychiatric Association.

Amir, N., Klumpp, H., Elias, J., Bedwell, J. S., Yanasak, N., & Miller, L. S. (2005). Increased activation of the anterior cingulate cortex during processing of disgust faces in individuals with social phobia. *Biological Psychiatry*, **57**, 975–81.

Arrindell, W. A., Pickersgill, M. J., Merckelbach, H., Ardon, M. A., & Cornet, F. C. (1991). Phobic dimensions: III. Factor analytic approaches to the study of common phobic fears: an updated review of findings obtained with adult subjects. *Advances in Behaviour Research and Therapy*, **13**, 73–130.

Barton, R. A., & Aggleton, J. (2000). Primate evolution and the amygdala. In J. Aggleton (Ed.), *The amygdala: a functional analysis*. Oxford University Press, 480–508.

Beaton, E. A., Schmidt, L. A., Ashbaugh, A. R., Santesso, D. L., Antony, M. M., & McCabe, R. E. (2008). Resting and reactive frontal brain electrical activity (EEG) among a non-clinical sample of socially anxious adults: does concurrent depressive mood matter? *Neuropsychiatric Disease and Treatment*, 4, 187–92.

Beaton, E. A., Schmidt, L. A., Schulkin, J., Antony, M. M., Swinson, R. P., & Hall, G. B. (2008). Different neural responses to stranger and personally familiar faces in shy and bold adults. *Behavioral Neuroscience*, 122, 704–9.

(2009). Different fusiform activity to stranger and personally familiar faces in shy and social adults. *Social Neuroscience*, 4, 308–16.

Beaton, E. A., Schmidt, L. A., Schulkin, J., & Hall, G. B. (2010). Neural correlates of implicit processing of facial emotions in shy adults. *Personality and Individual Differences*, 49, 755–61.

Bickart, K. C., Wright, C. I., Dautoff, R. J., Dickerson, B. C., & Feldman-Barrett, L. (2011). Amygdala volume and social network size in humans. *Nature Neuroscience*, 14, 163–4.

Biederman, J., Hirshfeld-Becker, D. R., Rosenbaum, J. F., Perenick, S. G., Wood, J., & Faraone, S. V. (2001). Further evidence of association between behavioral inhibition and social anxiety in children. *American Journal of Psychiatry*, 158, 1673–9.

Birbaumer, N., Grodd, W., Diedrich, O., Klose, U., Erb, M., Lotze, M., Schneider, F., Weiss, U., & Flor, H. (1998). fMRI reveals amygdala activation to human faces in social phobics. *NeuroReport*, 9, 1223–6.

Blair, K., Geraci, M., DeVido, J., McCaffrey, D., Chen, G., Vythilingam, M., Ng, P., Hollon, N., Jones, M., Blair, R. J. & Pine, D. S. (2008). Neural response to self- and other referential praise and criticism in generalized social phobia. *Archives of General Psychiatry*, 65, 1176–84.

Blair, K. S., Geraci, M., Hollon, N., Otero, M., DeVido, J., Majestic, K., Jacobs, M., Blair, R. J. R., & Pine, D. S. (2010). Social norm processing in adult social phobia: atypically increased ventromedial frontal cortex responsiveness to unintentional (embarrassing) transgressions. *American Journal of Psychiatry*, 167, 1526–32.

Blair, K. S., Geraci, M., Korelitz, K., Otero, M., Towbin, K., Ernst, M., Leibenluft, E., Blair, R. J. R., & Pine, D. S. (2011). The pathology of social phobia is independent of developmental changes in face processing. *American Journal of Psychiatry*, 168, 1202–9.

Blair, K. S., Geraci, M., Otero, M., Majestic, C., Odenheimer, S., Jacobs, S., Jacobs, M., Blair, R. J., & Pine, D. S. (2011). Atypical modulation of medial prefrontal cortex to self-referential comments in generalized social phobia. *Psychiatry Research: Neuroimaging*, 193, 38–45.

Blair, K., Shaywitz, J., Smith, B. W., Rhodes, R., Geraci, M., Jones, M., McCaffrey, D., Vythilingam, M., Finger, E., Mondillo, K., Jacobs, M., Charney, D. S., Blair, R. J. R., Drevets, W. C., & Pine, D. S. (2008). Response to emotional expression in generalized social phobia and generalized anxiety disorder: evidence for separate disorders. *American Journal of Psychiatry*, **165**, 1193–202.

Bögels, S. M., & Mansell, W. (2004). Attention processes in the maintenance and treatment of social phobia: hypervigilance, avoidance, and self-focused attention. *Clinical Psychology Review*, **24**, 827–56.

Brühl, A. B., Rufer, M., Delsignore, A., Kaffenberger, T., Jäncke, L., & Herwig, U. (2011). Neural correlates of altered general emotion processing in social anxiety disorder. *Brain Research*, **1378**, 72–83.

Brunet, P. M., Mondloch, C. J., & Schmidt, L. A. (2010). Shy children are less sensitive to some cues to facial recognition. *Child Psychiatry and Human Development*, **41**, 1–14.

Calkins, S. D., Fox, N. A., & Marshall, T. R. (1996). Behavioral and physiological antecedents of inhibited and uninhibited behavior. *Child Development*, **67**, 523–40.

Campbell, D. W., Sareen, J., Paulus, M. P., Goldin, P. R., Stein, M. B., & Reiss, J. P. (2007). Time-varying amygdala response to emotional faces in generalized social phobia. *Biological Psychiatry*, **62**, 455–63.

Campbell, M. J., Schmidt, L. A., Santesso, D. L., Van Ameringen, M., Mancini, C. L., & Oakman, J. M. (2007). Behavioral and psychophysiological characteristics of children of parents with social phobia: a pilot study. *International Journal of Neuroscience*, **117**, 605–16.

Catani, M., Jones, D. K., Donato, R., & Ffytche, D. H. (2003). Occipito-temporal connections in the human brain. *Brain*, **126**, 2093–107.

Clark, D. M., & McManus, F. (2002). Information processing in social phobia. *Biological Psychiatry*, **51**, 92–100.

Cooney, R. E., Atlas, L. Y., Joorman, J., Eugene, F., & Gotlib, I. H. (2006). Amygdala activation in the processing of neutral faces in social anxiety disorder: is neutral really neutral? *Psychiatry Research*, **148**, 55–9.

Craig, A. D. (2009). How do you feel – now? The anterior insula and human awareness. *Nature Reviews Neuroscience*, **10**, 59–70.

(2010). The sentient self. *Brain Structure and Function*, **214**, 563–77.

Critchley, H. D., Wiens, S., Rotshtein, P., Öhman, A., & Dolan, R. J. (2004). Neural systems supporting interoceptive awareness. *Nature Neuroscience*, **7**, 189–95.

Damasio, A. (2003). *Looking for Spinoza: joy, sorrow and the feeling brain*. New York: Harcourt.

Danti, S., Ricciardi, E., Gentili, C., Gobbini, M. I., Petrini, P., & Guazzelli, M. (2010). Is social phobia a mis-communication disorder? Brain functional connectivity during face perception differs between patients with social phobia and healthy control subjects. *Frontiers in Systems Neuroscience*, **22**, 152.

Darwin, C. (1872/1965). *The expression of the emotions in man and animals*. Chicago University Press.

Davidson, R. J. (2002). Anxiety and affective style: role of prefrontal cortex and amygdala. *Biological Psychiatry*, **51**, 68–80.

Davidson, R. J., Marshall, J. R., Tomarken, A. J., & Henriques, J. B. (2000). While a phobic waits: regional brain electrical and autonomic activity in social phobics during anticipation of public speaking. *Biological Psychiatry*, **47**, 85–95.

Denton, D. (2006). *The primordial emotions: the dawning of consciousness*. New York: Oxford University Press.
DiLalla, L. F., Kagan, J., & Reznick, J. S. (1994). Genetic etiology of behavioral inhibition among two-year-old children. *Infant Behavior and Development*, 17, 401–8.
Ding, J., Chen, H., Qiu, C., Liao, W., Warwick, J. M., Duan, X., Zhang, W., & Gong, Q. (2011). Disrupted functional connectivity in social anxiety disorder: a resting-state fMRI study. *Magnetic Resonance Imaging*, 29, 701–11.
Emery, N. J., & Amaral, D. G. (2000). The role of the amygdala in primate social cognition. In R. D. Lane & L. Nadel (Eds.), *Cognitive neuroscience of emotion*. New York: Oxford University Press, 156–91.
Etkin, A., & Wager, T. D. (2007). Functional neuroimaging of anxiety: a meta-analysis of emotional processing in PTSD, social anxiety disorder, and specific phobia. *American Journal of Psychiatry*, 164, 1476–88.
Evans, K. C., Wright, C. I., Wedig, M. M., Gold, A. L., Pollack, M. H., & Rauch, S. L. (2008). A functional MRI study of amygdala responses to angry schematic faces in social anxiety disorder. *Depression and Anxiety*, 25, 496–505.
Fox, N. A. (1991). If it's not left, it's right: electroencephalograph asymmetry and the development of emotion. *American Psychologist*, 46, 863–72.
Fox, N. A., Calkins, S. D., & Bell, M. A. (1994). Neural plasticity and development in the first two years of life: evidence from cognitive and socioemotional domains of research. *Development and Psychopathology*, 6, 677–96.
Fox, N. A., Henderson, H. A., Marshall, P. J., Nichols, K. E., & Ghera, M. M. (2005). Behavioral inhibition: linking biology and behavior within a developmental framework. *Annual Review of Psychology*, 56, 235–62.
Fox, N. A., Henderson, H. A., Rubin, K. H., Calkins, S. D., & Schmidt, L. A. (2001). Continuity and discontinuity of behavioral inhibition and exuberance: psychophysiological and behavioral influences across the first four years of life. *Child Development*, 72, 1–21.
Fox, N. A., Nichols, K. E., Henderson, H. A., Rubin, K. H., Schmidt, L. A., Hamer, D. H., Ernst, M., & Pine, D. S. (2005). Evidence for a gene environment interaction in predicting behavioral inhibition in middle childhood. *Psychological Science*, 16, 921–6.
Freitas-Ferrari, M. C., Hallak, J. E., Trzesniak, C., Filho, A. S., Machado-de-Sousa, J. P., Chagas, M. H., Nardi, A. E., & Crippa, J. A. (2010). Neuroimaging in social anxiety disorder: a systematic review of the literature. *Progress in Neuropsychopharmacology and Biological Psychiatry*, 34, 565–80.
Furmark, T., Henningsson, S., Appel, L., Åhs, F., Linnman, C., Pissiota, A., Faria, V., Oreland, L., Bani, M., Pich, E. M., Eriksson, E., & Fredrikson, M. (2005). Genotype over-diagnosis in amygdala responsiveness: affective processing in social anxiety disorder. *Journal of Psychiatry and Neuroscience*, 34, 30–40.
Furmark, T., Tillfors, M., Marteinsdottir, I., Fischer, H., Pissiota, A., Langstrom, B., & Fredrikson, M. (2002). Common changes in cerebral blood flow in

patients with social phobia treated with citalopram or cognitive-behavioral therapy. *Archives of General Psychiatry*, 59, 425–33.

García Coll, C., Kagan, J., & Reznick, J. S. (1984). Behavioral inhibition in young children. *Child Development*, 55, 1005–19.

Gentili, C., Gobbini, M., Ricciardi, E., Vanello, N., Pietrini, P., Haxby, J. V., & Guazzelli, M. (2008). Differential modulation of neural activity throughout the distributed neural system for face perception in patients with social phobia and healthy subjects. *Brain Research Bulletin*, 77, 286–92.

Gentili, C., Ricciardi, E., Gobbini, M., Santarelli, M. F., Haxby, J. V., Pietrini, P., & Guazzelli, M. (2009). Beyond amygdala: default mode network activity differences between patients with social phobia and healthy controls. *Brain Research Bulletin*, 79, 409–13.

Goldin, P. R., Manber, T., Hakimi, S., Canli, T., & Gross, J. J. (2009). Neural bases of social anxiety disorder: emotional reactivity and cognitive regulation during social and physical threat. *Archives of General Psychiatry*, 66, 170–80.

Guyer, A. E., Lau, J. Y., McClure-Tone, E. B., Parrish, J., Shiffrin, N. D., Reynolds, R. C., Chen, G., Blair, R. J., Leibenluft, E., Fox, N. A., Ernst, M., Pine, D. S., & Nelson, E. E. (2008). Amygdala and ventrolateral prefrontal cortex function during anticipated peer evaluation in pediatric social anxiety. *Archives of General Psychiatry*, 65, 1303–12.

Hahn, A., Stein, P., Windischberger, C., Weissenbacher, A., Spindelegger, C., Moser, E., Kasper, S., & Lanzenberger, R. (2011). Reduced resting-state functional connectivity between amygdala and orbitofrontal cortex in social anxiety disorder. *NeuroImage*, 56, 881–90.

Heinrichs, N., & Hoffmann, S. G. (2001). Information processing in social phobia: a critical review. *Clinical Psychology Review*, 21, 751–70.

Heiser, N. A., Turner, S. M., Beidel, D. C., & Roberson-Nay, R. (2009). Differentiating social phobia from shyness. *Journal of Anxiety Disorders*, 23, 469–76.

Hermans, E. J., & van Honk, J. (2006). Toward a framework for defective emotion processing in social phobia. *Cognitive Neuropsychiatry*, 11, 307–31.

Hirshfeld-Becker, D. R., Biederman, J., Henin, A., Faraone, S. V., Davis, S., Harrington, K., & Rosenbaum, J. F. (2007). Behavioral inhibition in preschool children at risk is a specific predictor of middle childhood social anxiety: a five-year follow-up. *Journal of Developmental and Behavioral Pediatrics*, 28, 225–33.

Hofmann, S. G., Heinrichs, N., & Moscovitch, D. A. (2004). The nature and expression of social phobia: toward a new classification. *Clinical Psychology Review*, 24, 769–97.

Hofmann, S. G., Moscovitch, D. A., & Kim, H. -J. (2006). Autonomic correlates of social anxiety and embarrassment in shy and non-shy individuals. *International Journal of Psychophysiology*, 61, 134–42.

Jetha, M. K., Zheng, X., Schmidt, L. A., & Segalowitz, S. J. (2012). Shyness and the first 100 milliseconds of emotional face processing. *Social Neuroscience*, 7, 74–89.

Kagan, J. (1994). *Galen's prophecy: temperament in human nature*. New York: Basic Books.
Kagan, J., Reznick, J. S., & Snidman, N. (1987). The physiology and psychology of behavioral inhibition in children. *Child Development*, 58, 1459–73.
Kagan, J., & Schulkin, J. (1995). On the concepts of fear. *Harvard Review of Psychiatry*, 3, 231–4.
Kagan, J., & Snidman, N. (1991). Infant predictors of inhibited and uninhibited profiles. *Psychological Science*, 2, 40–4.
Kendler, K. S., Karkowski, L. M., & Prescott, C. A. (1999). Fears and phobias: reliability and heritability. *Psychological Medicine*, 29, 539–53.
Klumpp, H., Angstadt, M., Nathan, P. J., & Phan, K. L. (2010). Amygdala reactivity to faces at varying intensities of threat in generalized social phobia: an event-related functional MRI study. *Psychiatry Research*, 183, 167–9.
Klumpp, H., Angstadt, M., & Phan, K. L. (2012). Insula reactivity and connectivity to anterior cingulate cortex when processing threat in generalized social anxiety disorder. *Biological Psychology*, 89, 273–6.
Knyazev, G. G. (2007). Motivation, emotion, and their inhibitory control mirrored in brain oscillations. *Neuroscience and Biobehavioral Reviews*, 31, 377–95.
Knyazev, G. G., & Slobodskaya, H. R. (2003). Personality trait of behavioral inhibition is associated with oscillatory systems reciprocal relationships. *International Journal of Psychophysiology*, 48, 247–61.
Kolassa, I., & Miltner, W. H. R. (2006). Psychophysiological correlates of face processing in social phobia. *Brain Research*, 1118, 130–41.
Leonardo, E. D., & Hen, R. (2008). Anxiety as a developmental disorder. *Neuropsychopharmacology Reviews*, 33, 134–40.
Liao, W., Chen, H., Feng, Y., Mantini, D., Gentili, C., Pan, Z., Ding, J., Duan, X., Qiu, C., Lui, S., Gong, Q., & Zhang, W. (2010). Selective aberrant functional connectivity of resting state networks in social anxiety disorder. *NeuroImage*, 52, 1549–58.
Liao, W., Qiu, C., Gentili, C., Walter, M., Pan, Z., Ding, J., Zhang, W., Gong, Q., & Chen, H. (2010). Altered effective connectivity network of the amygdala in social anxiety disorder: a resting-state fMRI study. *PLoS One*, 5, e15238.
Liao, W., Xu, Q., Mantini, D., Ding, J., Machado-de-Sousa, J. P., Hallak, J. E. C., Trzesniak, C., Qiu, C., Zeng, L., Zhang, W., Crippa, J. A., Gong, Q., & Chen, H. (2011). Altered gray matter morphometry and resting-state functional and structural connectivity in social anxiety disorder. *Brain Research*, 1388, 167–77.
Lorberbaum, J. P., Kose, S., Johnson, M. R., Arana, G. W., Sullivan, L. K., Hamner, M. B., Ballenger, J. C., Lydiard, R. B., Brodrick, P. S., Bohning, D. E., & George, M. S. (2004). Neural correlates of speech anticipatory anxiety in generalized social phobia. *NeuroReport*, 15, 2701–5.
McTeague, L. M., Shumen, J. R., Wieser, M. J., Lang, P. J., & Keil, A. (2011). Social vision: sustained perceptual enhancement of affective facial cues in social anxiety. *NeuroImage*, 54, 1615–24.
Mancini, C., van Ameringen, M., Szatmari, P., Fugere, C., & Boyle, M. (1996). A high-risk pilot study of the children of adults with social phobia. *Journal of the American Academy of Child and Adolescent Psychiatry*, 35, 1511–7.

Marks, I. M. (1969). *Fears and phobias.* Oxford: Academic Press.
Mathew, S. J., Coplan, J. D., & Gorman, J. M. (2001). Neurobiological mechanisms of social anxiety disorder. *American Journal of Psychiatry*, **158**, 1558–67.
Menon, V., & Uddin, L. Q. (2010). Saliency, switching, attention and control: a network model of insula function. *Brain Structure and Function*, **214**, 655–67.
Miller, E. K., & Cohen, J. D. (2001). An integrative theory of prefrontal cortex function. *Annual Review of Neuroscience*, **24**, 167–202.
Miskovic, V., Ashbaugh, A. R., Santesso, D. L., McCabe, R. E., Antony, M. M., & Schmidt, L. A. (2010). Frontal brain oscillations and social anxiety: a cross-frequency spectral analysis during baseline and speech anticipation. *Biological Psychology*, **83**, 125–32.
Miskovic, V., Campbell, M. J., Santesso, D. L., Van Ameringen, M., Mancini, C., & Schmidt, L. A. (2011). Frontal brain oscillatory coupling in children of parents with social phobia: a pilot study. *The Journal of Neuropsychiatry and Clinical Neurosciences*, **23**, 111–14.
Miskovic, V., Moscovitch, D. L., Santesso, D. L., McCabe, R. E., Antony, M. M., & Schmidt, L. A. (2011). Changes in EEG cross-frequency coupling during cognitive behavioral therapy for social anxiety disorder. *Psychological Science*, **22**, 507–16.
Miskovic, V., & Schmidt, L. A. (2009). Frontal brain oscillatory coupling among men who vary in salivary testosterone levels. *Neuroscience Letters*, **464**, 239–42.
  (2012a). Early information processing biases in social anxiety. *Cognition and Emotion*, **26**, 176–85.
  (2012b). New directions in the study of individual differences in temperament: a brain–body approach to understanding fearful and fearless children. In T. A. Dennis, K. A. Buss & P. D. Hastings (Eds.), *Physiological measures of emotion from a developmental perspective: state of the science.* Monographs of the Society for Research in Child Development, **77**, 28–38.
Moscovitch, D. A., Santesso, D. L., Miskovic, V., McCabe, R. E., Antony, M. M., & Schmidt, L. A. (2011). Frontal EEG asymmetry in response to cognitive behavioral therapy in patients with social anxiety disorder. *Biological Psychology*, **87**, 379–85.
Moser, J. S., Hajcak, G., Huppert, J. D., Foa, E. B., & Simons, R. F. (2008). Interpretation bias in social anxiety as revealed by event-related brain potentials. *Emotion*, **8**, 693–700.
Moser, J. S., Huppert, J. D., Duval, E., & Simons, R. F. (2008). Face processing biases in social anxiety: an electrophysiological study. *Biological Psychology*, **78**, 93–103.
Mueller, E. M., Hofmann, S. G., Santesso, D. L., Meuret, A. E., Bitran, S., & Pizzagalli, D. A. (2009). Electrophysiological evidence of attentional biases in social anxiety disorder. *Psychological Medicine*, **39**, 1141–52.
Mühlberger, A., Wieser, M. J., Herrmann, M. J., Weyers, P., Troger, C., & Pauli, P. (2009). Early cortical processing of natural and artificial emotional faces

differs between lower and higher socially anxious persons. *Journal of Neural Transmission*, 116, 735–46.
Ochsner, K. N., & Gross, J. J. (2007). The neural architecture of emotion regulation. In J. J. Gross (Ed.), *The handbook of emotion regulation*. New York: Guilford Press, 87–109.
Öhman, A. (1986). Face the beast and fear the face: animal and social fears as prototypes for evolutionary analyses of emotion. *Psychophysiology*, 23, 123–45.
  (2009). Of snakes and faces: an evolutionary perspective on the psychology of fear. *Scandinavian Journal of Psychology*, 50, 543–52.
Öhman, A., Dimberg, U., & Öst, L.-G. (1985). Animal and social phobias: biological constraints on learned fear responses. In S. Reiss & R. R. Bootzin (Eds.), *Theoretical issues in behavior therapy*. Orlando, FL: Academic Press, 123–78.
Öngur, D., & Price, J. L. (2000). The organization of networks within the orbital and medial prefrontal cortex of rats, monkeys and humans. *Cerebral Cortex*, 10, 206–19.
Paulus, M. P., & Stein, M. B. (2006). An insular view of anxiety. *Biological Psychiatry*, 60, 383–7.
Pérez-Edgar, K., & Fox, N. A. (2005). Temperament and anxiety disorders. *Child and Adolescent Psychiatric Clinics of North America*, 14, 681–706.
Phan, K. L., Fitzgerald, D. A., Nathan, P. J., & Tancer, M. E. (2006). Association between amygdala hyperactivity to harsh faces and severity of social anxiety in generalized social phobia. *Biological Psychiatry*, 59, 424–9.
Phan, K. L., Orlichenko, A., Boyd, E., Angstadt, M., Coccaro, E. F., Liberzon, I., & Arfanakis, K. (2009). Preliminary evidence of white matter abnormality in the uncinate fasciculus in generalized social anxiety disorder. *Biological Psychiatry*, 66, 691–4.
Phelps, E. A., & LeDoux, J. E. (2005). Contributions of the amygdala to emotion processing: from animal models to human behavior. *Neuron*, 48, 175–87.
Pujol, J., Harrison, B. J., Ortiz, H., Deus, J., Soriano-Mas, C., Lopez-Sola, M., Yucel, M., Perich, X., & Cardoner, N. (2009). Influence of fusiform gyrus on amygdala response to emotional faces in the non-clinical range of social anxiety. *Psychological Medicine*, 39, 1177–87.
Putman, P. (2011). Resting state EEG delta-beta coherence in relation to anxiety, behavioral inhibition, and selective attentional processing of threatening stimuli. *International Journal of Psychophysiology*, 80, 63–8.
Quadflieg, S., Mohr, A., Mentzel, H. J., Miltner, W. H., & Straube, T. (2008). Modulation of the neural network involved in the processing of anger prosody: the role of task-relevance and social phobia. *Biological Psychology*, 78, 129–37.
Robinson, D. L. (1999). The technical, neurological and psychological significance of 'alpha', 'delta' and 'theta' waves confounded in EEG evoked potentials: a study of peak latencies. *Clinical Neurophysiology*, 110, 1427–34.
Rosen, J. B., & Schulkin, J. (1998). From normal fear to pathological anxiety. *Psychological Review*, 105, 325–50.
Rossignol, M., Anselme, C., Vermeulen, N., Philippot, P., & Campanella, S. (2007). Categorical perception of anger and disgust facial expression is

affected by non-clinical social anxiety: an ERP study. *Brain Research*, **1132**, 166–76.
Rubin, K. H., Burgess, K. B., & Hastings, P. D. (2002). Stability and social-behavioral consequences of toddlers' inhibited temperament and parenting behaviors. *Child Development*, **73**, 483–95.
Schmidt, L. A. (1999). Frontal brain electrical activity in shyness and sociability. *Psychological Science*, **10**, 316–20.
  (2008). Patterns of second-by-second resting frontal brain (EEG) asymmetry and their relation to heart rate and temperament in 9-month-old human infants. *Personality and Individual Differences*, **44**, 216–25.
Schmidt, L. A., & Buss, A. H. (2010). Understanding shyness: four questions and four decades of research. In K. H. Rubin & R. J. Coplan (Eds.), *The development of shyness and social withdrawal*. New York: Guilford Press, 23–41.
Schmidt, L. A., & Fox, N. A. (1994). Patterns of cortical electrophysiology and autonomic activity in adults' shyness and sociability. *Biological Psychology*, **38**, 183–98.
  (1998). Fear-potentiated startle responses in temperamentally different human infants. *Developmental Psychobiology*, **32**, 113–20.
  (1999). Conceptual, biological, and behavioral distinctions among different categories of shy children. In L. A. Schmidt & J. Schulkin (Eds.), *Extreme fear, shyness and social phobia: origins, biological mechanisms and clinical outcomes*. New York: Oxford University Press, 47–66.
Schmidt, L. A., Fox, N. A., Rubin, K. H., Sternberg, E. M., Gold, P. W., & Smith, C. C. (1997). Behavioral and neuroendocrine responses in shy children. *Developmental Psychobiology*, **30**, 127–40.
Schmidt, L. A., Fox, N. A., Schulkin, J. & Gold, P. W. (1999). Behavioral and psychophysiological correlates of self-presentation in temperamentally shy children. *Developmental Psychobiology*, **35**, 119–35.
Schmidt, L. A., Santesso, D. L., Miskovic, V., Mathewson, K. J., McCabe, R. E., Antony, M. M., & Moscovitch, D. A. (2012). Test-retest reliability of regional electroencephalogram (EEG) and cardiovascular measures in social anxiety disorder. *International Journal of Psychophysiology*, **84**, 65–73.
Schmidt, L. A., & Schulkin, J. (1999). *Extreme fear, shyness, and social phobia: origins, biological mechanisms, and clinical outcomes*. New York: Oxford University Press.
Schmidt, S., Mohr, A., Miltner, W. H., & Straube, T. (2010). Task-dependent neural correlates of the processing of verbal threat-related stimuli in social phobia. *Biological Psychology*, **84**, 304–12.
Schutter, D. J. L. G., & Knyazev, G. G. (2012). Cross-frequency coupling of brain oscillations in studying motivation and emotion. *Motivation and Emotion*, **36**, 46–54.
Schutter, D. J. L. G., Leitner, C., Kenemans, J., & van Honk, J. (2006). Electrophysiological correlates of cortico-subcortical interaction: a cross-frequency spectral EEG analysis. *Clinical Neurophysiology*, **117**, 381–7.
Schutter, D. J. L. G., & van Honk, J. (2004). Decoupling of midfrontal delta-beta oscillations after testosterone administration. *International Journal of Psychophysiology*, **53**, 71–3.

(2005). Salivary cortisol levels and the coupling of midfrontal delta-beta oscillations. *International Journal of Psychophysiology*, 55, 127–9.
Schwartz, C. E., Snidman, N., & Kagan, J. (1999). Adolescent social anxiety as an outcome of inhibited temperament in childhood. *Journal of the American Academy of Child and Adolescent Psychiatry*, 38(8), 1008–15.
Segalowitz, S. J., & Schmidt, L. A. (2008). Capturing the dynamic endophenotype: a developmental psychophysiological manifesto. In L. A. Schmidt & S. J. Segalowitz (Eds.), *Developmental psychophysiology: theory, systems, and methods*. New York: Cambridge University Press, 1–12.
Sewell, C., Palermo, R., Atkinson, C., & McArthur, G. (2008). Anxiety and the neural processing of threat in faces. *NeuroReport*, 19, 1339–43.
Shah, S. G., Klumpp, H., Angstadt, M., Nathan, P. J., & Phan, K. L. (2009). Amygdala and insula response to emotional images in patients with generalized social anxiety disorder. *Journal of Psychiatry and Neuroscience*, 34, 296–302.
Sotres-Bayon, F., & Quirk, G. J. (2010). Prefrontal control of fear: more than just extinction. *Current Opinion in Neurobiology*, 20, 231–5.
Staugaard, S. R. (2010). Threatening faces and social anxiety: a literature review. *Clinical Psychology Review*, 30, 669–90.
Stein, D. J., & Bouwer, C. (1997). Blushing and social phobia: a neuroethological speculation. *Medical Hypotheses*, 49, 101–8.
Stein, M. B., Goldin, P. R., Sareen, J., Zorrilla, L. T., & Brown, G. G. (2002). Increased amygdala activation to angry and contemptuous faces in generalized social phobia. *Archives of General Psychiatry*, 59, 1027–34.
Straube, T., Kolassa, I. T., Glauer, M., Mentzel, H. J., & Miltner, W. H. (2004). Effect of task conditions on brain responses to threatening faces in social phobics: an event related functional magnetic resonance imaging study. *Biological Psychiatry*, 56, 921–30.
Straube, T., Mentzel, H. J., & Miltner, W. H. (2005). Common and distinct brain activation to threat and safety signals in social phobia. *Neuropsychobiology*, 52, 163–8.
Theall-Honey, L. A., & Schmidt, L. A. (2006). Do temperamentally shy children process emotion differently than nonshy children? Behavioral, psychophysiological, and gender differences in reticent preschoolers. *Developmental Psychobiology*, 48, 187–96.
Tillfors, M., Furmark, T., Marteinsdottir, I., Fischer, H., Pissiota, A., Langstrom, B., & Fredrikson, M. (2001). Cerebral blood flow in subjects with social phobia during stressful speaking tasks: a PET study. *American Journal of Psychiatry*, 158, 1220–6.
Tillfors, M., Furmark, T., Marteinsdottir, I., & Fredrikson, M. (2002). Cerebral blood flow during anticipation of public speaking in social phobia: a PET study. *Biological Psychiatry*, 52, 1113–19.
Uhlhaas, P. J., & Singer, W. (2006). Neural synchrony in brain disorders: relevance for cognitive dysfunctions and pathophysiology. *Neuron*, 52, 155–68.
Van Ameringen, M., Mancini, C., Szechtman, H., Nahmias, O., Oakman, J. M., Hall, G. B., Pipe, B., & Farvolden, P. (2004). A PET provocation study of generalized social phobia. *Psychiatry Research*, 132, 13–18.

van Honk, J., Harmon-Jones, E., Morgan, B. E., & Schutter, D. J. L. G. (2010). Socially explosive minds: the triple imbalance hypothesis of reactive aggression. *Journal of Personality*, **78**, 67–94.

van Peer, J. M., Roelofs, K., & Spinhoven, P. (2008). Cortisol administration enhances the coupling of midfrontal delta and beta oscillations. *International Journal of Psychophysiology*, **67**, 144–50.

van Wingen, G., Mattern, C., Verkes, R. J., Buitelaar, J., & Fernandez, G. (2010). Testosterone reduces amygdala-orbitofrontal cortex coupling. *Psychoneuroendocrinology*, **35**, 105–13.

Wieser, M. J., McTeague, L. M., & Keil, A. (2011). Sustained preferential processing of social threat cues: bias without competition? *Journal of Cognitive Neuroscience*, **23**, 1973–86.

Yoon, K. L., Fitzgerald, D. A., Angstadt, M., McCarron, R. A., & Phan, K. L. (2007). Amygdala reactivity to emotional faces at high and low intensity in generalized social phobia: a 4-Tesla functional MRI study. *Psychiatry Research*, **154**, 93–8.

Zhang, D., & Raichle, M. E. (2010). Disease and the brain's dark energy. *Nature Reviews Neurology*, **6**, 15–28.

*Part III*

# The blush in social interaction

# 9 The interactive origins and outcomes of embarrassment

*Rowland S. Miller*

Let's consider a prototypical case of embarrassment: a hapless person suddenly realizes that he has misbehaved with others present, but his misdeed is not a grievous sin. Instead, his mistake is one of manners or deportment; he has spilled his soup or torn his trousers, and, had he been alone, his error may have been merely annoying. However, his misstep has occurred in public, and that aspect of his predicament is key. His witnesses may not have displayed any disapproval or disregard, and, indeed, they may not have given any sign that they have yet noticed his mistake. Nevertheless, it is enough that others *may* be aware of his misbehaviour. Our target becomes flustered and discombobulated as chagrin arises, and, as his cheeks redden in a blush, his embarrassment is plain. Two consequences ensue. First, our target is contrite and apologetic, and he is eager to redress any inconvenience he has caused. Second, and perhaps more importantly, his evident sheepishness has mollified his witnesses. Had he not become embarrassed, his misbehaviour might have made him seem a boor, a lout or a fool. But his chagrin has reassured his audience that he acknowledges his transgression and that he regrets it. By implication, his action is judged to be an aberration that is unlikely to recur. Placated, his audience may chuckle at his predicament, but their humour is good-natured, not malicious, and they remain tolerant and lenient despite his maladroit behaviour.

Actual embarrassments can be variously idiosyncratic, of course, but this prototype is probably familiar to you. All of its aspects – the public misstep, one's visible chagrin and conciliatory reactions, and the charitable, forbearing responses of others – are typical components of embarrassing circumstances (Miller, 1996). Indeed, this common pattern of events offers a template with which to make sense of the social effects of the singular physiological response that is 'the hallmark of embarrassment' (Buss, 1980, p. 129), blushing. The interactive origins and outcomes of embarrassment, in general, provide a framework for the usual operation of blushing, in particular. In this chapter, then, I will support the goals of this volume by surveying the social circumstances that cause embarrassment and by detailing the interactive consequences of embarrassing episodes. Important clues to the communicative and interactive effects of blushing may lie herein.

## Embarrassing circumstances

Back in the 1990s, I used two different procedures to compile a catalogue of the events that cause embarrassment (see Miller, 1996). In the first method, 350 high school or college students in Ithaca, New York, Winston-Salem, North Carolina, and Huntsville, Texas, described anonymously and in detail their most recent embarrassments, whether strong or weak. In the second procedure, which was undertaken in Texas, fifth-graders in elementary school and college students described their most recent embarrassments once a week for four and eight weeks, respectively; 753 accounts were obtained. Combined, the 1,103 reports delineated an impressive array of events that result in embarrassment in the United States.[1]

### Individual behaviour

Most embarrassments occur when people unintentionally violate consensual norms of deportment, civility, self-control or grace with an obvious lapse in their behaviour or judgment that may take several forms. The most common of these, as you can see in Table 9.1, is some sort of *clumsiness* or ungainliness – often slipping, tripping or spilling something – that makes the person seem momentarily inept or incompetent. People also frequently experience *losses of control* over (a) their possessions (such as stalled cars, overeager pets and unzipped clothes), (b) their bodies (via, for instance, inadvertent flatulence, belching and hiccupping), and, on occasion, (c) their emotions (usually with anger, fear or weepiness that seem excessive). A variety of *cognitive errors* is also commonplace. People make mistakes in judgment – an American journalist, Ann Landers, once carved a piece out of a doily believing it to be an 'unusual lacy coconut dessert' (Morley, 1983, p. 72) – and they can be forgetful, inattentive or temporarily stupid, forgetting the names of people to whom they have just been introduced. Other individual

---

[1] The scheme that follows may apply to some cultures better than others, and, because it is based on self-reports, it may be incomplete. Nevertheless, studies of embarrassment in other cultures (e.g., Cupach & Imahori, 1993; Edelmann & Iwawaki, 1987) suggest that embarrassment results from similar events all over the world, and the diverse (and sometimes subtle) nature of these accounts is reassuring: despite its possible imperfections, this scheme – based as it is on a very sizeable collection of embarrassing events – likely captures many of the circumstances that cause us to become embarrassed.

Table 9.1 *The sources of embarrassment in social life*

|  | Frequency of occurrence (%) |
|---|---|
| *Individual behaviour* | |
| (1) Normative public deficiencies | |
|     (a) Clumsiness and physical pratfalls | 17 |
|     (b) Losses of control | 16 |
|     (c) Cognitive errors | 15 |
|     (d) Harmdoing | 5 |
|     (e) Failures of privacy | 3 |
| (2) Undue sensitivity | 4 |
| (3) Departures from personal goals | 2 |
| (4) Conspicuousness | 2 |
| *Interactive behaviour* | |
| (5) Awkward interaction | |
|     (a) Loss of script | 4 |
|     (b) Guilty knowledge | 4 |
| (6) Partner sensitivity | 1 |
| *Audience provocation* | |
| (7) Others intend to embarrass | 7 |
| (8) Others do not intend to embarrass | 7 |
| *Bystander behaviour* | |
| (9) 'Team' transgressions | 10 |
| (10) Empathic embarrassment | 3 |

norm violations involve *harmdoing*, when one inconveniences, insults, embarrasses or otherwise does mild harm to others, and *failures of privacy*, in which private thoughts and actions (often involving bathrooms and bedrooms) become public. Altogether, most embarrassments (56 per cent in this sample) result from lapses like these in which all of us would agree that an individual's behaviour is unflattering or undesirable.

Other predicaments that result from individual behaviour are more subtle and/or idiosyncratic. People occasionally become embarrassed not because they have clearly misbehaved, but because they have done something in public that is personally disappointing or disconcerting (though not normatively incorrect). They are sometimes unduly *sensitive*, overreacting to situations that are only mildly awkward – as a young man might be, shopping with his girlfriend, when she buys a box of tampons. Alternatively, they may be chagrined by a *departure from a personal goal* in which they feel that their behaviour is deficient, but no one else does. Or, even more remarkably, they may be embarrassed by simple *conspicuousness*, becoming the object of others' attention even when they have done nothing wrong. Any action that makes one conspicuous can cause embarrassment, even when the action is entirely appropriate. Close inspection by others can be embarrassing all by itself; most embarrassments result from noticeable misbehaviour, but unwanted attention can be worrisome even when one is not at fault. This is an intriguing point to which I will return.

### Interactive behaviour

Other embarrassments result not from an individual's sole actions but from interactions of two or more people that go awry. Interestingly, interactions can become embarrassingly awkward or uncomfortable even when one is blameless, so these are other situations in which embarrassment does not depend on overt misbehaviour.

Awkward interactions occur for two reasons (Miller, 1996). The first is a *loss of script*: people can find themselves flustered and unsure of what to do or say as a result of an unanticipated event or revelation. *Guilty knowledge* of past events may also adversely affect current interactions; in these cases, one's private knowledge makes a present interaction problematic although, on the surface, nothing is amiss.

Another less frequent interactive circumstance causes embarrassment when a particular partner disapproves of one's behaviour when it is not normatively deficient. In such situations, it is the partner's (usually quite straitlaced or touchy) standards that are unusual, not one's behaviour, and the *partner's sensitivity* is the cause of one's discomfort. Once again, some embarrassments are not our fault.

### Audience provocation

Indeed, a remarkable number of embarrassments in young adults – one in every seven – are created by the actions of others. Most college students (75 per cent) have tried to embarrass someone at least once within the past six months (Sharkey, 1991), and they have often succeeded. Teasing, practical jokes and other manufactured predicaments can be deployed to intentionally embarrass an unfortunate target. In such cases, the targets are often entirely innocent of any real impropriety, and that's plain to all concerned; moreover, the audience's mischief is usually playful instead of malicious. Nevertheless, even playful mocking can cause people real chagrin (Sharkey *et al.*, 2001).

In addition, others can embarrass us even when they do not intend to do so. They make cognitive errors and suffer their own losses of control, and we are sometimes the unlucky victims of their mistakes. In one such instance, I once spilled a large soft drink on the head of a colleague's wife when I was being introduced to her at a campus eatery. I was gravely embarrassed, of course, but – what with cola dripping off her nose and pooling in her lap – I created a predicament for her, as well. She was not to blame, but she was quite soaked, and her public disarray embarrassed her, too.

A noteworthy audience provocation in which embarrassment is unplanned is *overpraise*, which can occur when public acclaim and compliments that are well intended nonetheless cause some discomfort. Episodes of overpraise that resulted in embarrassment were rather rare in my samples, comprising only 1 per cent of the embarrassments I collected. Still, it's impressive that, as was the case with simple conspicuousness, excessive attention from others can cause embarrassment – and what's intriguing here is that in episodes of overpraise the judgments of others are clearly favourable and the attention is admiring. Unwanted social attention evidently carries considerable power whether its valence is negative or positive, and this is a point that may be fundamental to an understanding of embarrassment and blushing.

### *Bystander behaviour*

In interactive predicaments, both we and others are active participants, and in audience provocations, we are the obvious targets of others' actions. Finally, people can become embarrassed when they are merely witnesses of others' predicaments and – yet again – haven't personally misbehaved at all. The most common events of this type occur when one's associates do something embarrassing and one is (perhaps rightly) concerned that, in the eyes of any third-party observers, their misbehaviour makes one look bad, too (e.g., Fortune & Newby-Clark, 2008). Parents who frequently spend time in public with their children are usually very familiar with these *'team' transgressions.*

Lastly, so potent is the power of embarrassment in social life that people can experience vicarious chagrin when they simply watch the embarrassments of complete strangers. Others' predicaments can certainly be amusing, but witnesses can also become embarrassed for and with hapless others when they are in a sympathetic frame of mind (Stocks *et al.*, 2011). The *empathic embarrassment* that results tends to be mild, but it is real embarrassment nonetheless (Miller, 1987).

## Why does embarrassment occur?

In their entirety, the diverse circumstances that can trigger embarrassment help to delineate *why* such situations can cause awkward, flustered sheepishness and chagrin. One possibility, a *dramaturgic model*, holds that embarrassment results from the disrupted scripts and disordered expectations that leave one at a loss of what to do or say next when predicaments arise. From this perspective, dramaturgic uncertainty and inadequacy cause the aversive arousal of embarrassment, and 'the only source of unpleasantness that *necessarily* accompanies embarrassment is flustering caused by the perception that there is no character that one can coherently perform' (Silver et al., 1987, p. 51). In fact, awkwardness and ungainliness characterize embarrassment, and maladroit interaction can elicit it. And one can reasonably argue that a rattled, befuddled loss of script occurs in most of the circumstances I described above.

Still, I think that there are several persuasive reasons to prefer a *social evaluation model* of the origins of embarrassment. According to this alternative perspective, embarrassment is fundamentally rooted in our concerns for what others are thinking of us: it is the acute threat of undesired evaluations from others that causes embarrassment to arise, and if we genuinely did not care what others thought of us, we would not become embarrassed (Miller, 2009). In my view, this approach more cleanly and parsimoniously fits the full range of events that cause embarrassment.

Consider, for instance, the physical pratfall that results when a fellow slips and falls in an icy car park. If he is completely certain that no one else is around, embarrassment is unlikely because it almost never occurs when people are alone (Tangney et al., 1996). When embarrassment *is* felt when no one else is actually present, it's either because discovery of some misbehaviour is imminent – there are headlights in the driveway or footsteps in the hall – or because one is vividly imagining what others would think if they knew what was happening (Miller, 2004). Embarrassment is quite clearly a *social* emotion that depends on the real or imagined presence of other people.

This fact is assumed by both the dramaturgic and social evaluation models, so as our protagonist gathers himself and cautiously stands up, both perspectives are faring well. But imagine that the only observer of his fall is a stranger driving by, 50 yards away; his pratfall is clearly witnessed, but his audience is gone before he gets up off the ice. In such a situation, there is little dramaturgic peril, but there is potential for an unwanted social evaluation (albeit one of little consequence). And because brief embarrassment could readily result from such a slip – pratfalls among strangers are common causes of embarrassment (Miller, 1992) – a causal process that involves unwanted attention from others seems more correct.

The greater utility of a social evaluation model is also evident in those various classes of embarrassing events in which unlucky targets haven't done anything wrong, aren't engaged in interaction with anyone, and/or are merely bystanders to others' misconduct. When simple conspicuousness is embarrassing, for instance, unwanted attention is clearly at work, but dramaturgic uncertainty need not be. An instructive example of the clout of conspicuousness is to pick someone at random in a large classroom and to ask everyone else in the room to gaze silently at him or her (Lewis, 1995). Unfortunate targets of such treatment usually smile and continue what they were doing (which is just sitting quietly), initially thinking the exercise to be a lark. However, the enormity of their conspicuousness gradually dawns on them, and, as it does, their discomfort grows. Thirty seconds of close inspection by others is reliably embarrassing, even when one's behaviour is impeccable and one is simply sitting there, following a leader's instructions. Similar sensitivity to unwanted attention from others is at work in team transgressions when one hasn't misbehaved, but one's associates have.

Nevertheless, a problem in assessing the relative merits of the social evaluation and dramaturgic models is that they are confounded in many embarrassments (e.g., Higuchi & Fukada, 2008). Young adults may be embarrassed by using condoms, for instance, *both* because of their concern about how they will be judged if they have condoms on hand, and because they feel ill-equipped to negotiate the use of the condoms with poise and skill (Higuchi & Nakamura, 2010). To address this complexity, I sought to disentangle the overlapping predictions of the two models in a scenario study in which an unwanted social evaluation occurred independently of the awkwardness of a present interaction (Miller, 2012). I asked college students to imagine a messenger bringing them news that they had been refused a date either for an innocuous, benign reason or for a reason that, because it was privately known to be false by the recipient, was a threatening rebuff. Further, the messenger was said to believe that the refusal was either inoffensive or a snub. Thus, the participants did or did not receive an unwanted social evaluation that was independent of the awkwardness of the interaction with the messenger, who did or did not think that they had been rejected.

Consistent with the dramaturgic model, an awkward interaction with a messenger who believed (correctly or not) that one had been snubbed was imagined to be more embarrassing than an interaction with someone who thought that nothing was amiss. However, an actual rebuff was even more embarrassing, whether or not that rebuff was apparent to one's present audience; a sudden encounter with an unwanted social evaluation was embarrassing even when an ongoing interaction was not maladroit and had not gone awry. Social evaluation was simply a more potent influence on the participants' expected embarrassment, explaining twice as much variance as the dramaturgic manipulation did.

Other research results also lend more support to the social evaluation perspective than to a dramaturgic approach. As I'll soon explain, embarrassed people are generally generous and charitable, and they tend to be helpful even in subsequent interactions with new audiences who are unaware of their prior predicaments (Apsler, 1975). They seem to be noticeably eager to gain continuing acceptance in new interactions in which nothing has gone wrong. These carryover effects of embarrassment are consistent with the social evaluation model, but they are problematic for a dramaturgic approach. Once a brand new, stable interaction with new partners begins, one's dramaturgic difficulties are past and prior embarrassments should be inert, but they're not.

Finally, individual differences in dispositional susceptibility to embarrassment – that is, variations from person to person in the trait of *embarrassability* – are more closely tied to social evaluative influences than to interactive ineptitude and a lack of social grace. Highly embarrassable people don't stumble into different types of public predicaments than the rest of us do; they just become embarrassed more easily and suffer stronger embarrassments when things go awry (Miller, 1992). And importantly, whereas embarrassability is unrelated to one's global level of social skill, it is highly correlated with fear of negative evaluation (Miller, 1995, 2009). Highly embarrassable people dread disregard from others, and they tend to believe that others' evaluations of them are more negative than they really are. Notably, they also receive higher scores on the attachment dimension of anxiety about abandonment than less embarrassable people do (Withers & Vernon, 2006). Social evaluation is very salient to them, and they compound their difficulties by also being high in *social sensitivity*, or attentiveness to the normative appropriateness of behaviour (Miller, 1995). They take heed of social rules, and presumably detect improprieties that go unnoticed by less embarrassable people. Thus, 'they (1) hold themselves to stricter, less forgiving codes of conduct; and (2) chronically worry about what others are thinking of them, more than the rest of us do' (Miller, 1996, p. 101).

Highly embarrassable people are thus situated squarely between a social evaluative rock and a hard place. They also tend to be less deft than others are at adjusting their behaviour to fit new situations (Miller, 1995). This is a specific component of social skill termed *social control*, and it, at least, is an aspect of embarrassability that is consistent with the dramaturgic model. Still, susceptibility to embarrassment has much more to do with alertness and concern about what others are thinking of us than it does with interactive skill and social adroitness. Awkward uncertainty is characteristic of embarrassment, but the situations that elicit it, the dispositions that invite it and (as we shall soon see) the responses that follow it all suggest that social evaluation is the wellspring of embarrassment (e.g., Robbins & Parlavecchio, 2006). Thus, embarrassment is most aptly defined as *'the acute state of flustered, awkward, abashed chagrin that follows events that increase the threat of unwanted evaluations from real or imagined audiences'* (Miller, 1996, p. 129).

Blushing is triggered by similar threats. People can be embarrassed without displaying a blush, and blushing sometimes occurs when people are not yet embarrassed (e.g., Hofmann et al., 2006). Nevertheless, blushing can rightly be considered 'the hallmark of embarrassment' (Buss, 1980, p. 129): it invariably involves social evaluation that threatens, or that has already engendered, disapproval from others (Miller, 1996). Thus, simple conspicuousness in the absence of any misbehaviour can cause people to blush (Drummond & Mirco, 2004)[2] – but blushing is even more likely, being commonplace, when one's behaviour is embarrassingly deficient (Leary & Meadows, 1991). At its core, blushing results from unwanted or threatening attention from others, and such attention is always at work when embarrassment occurs; thus, blushing and embarrassment routinely co-occur, and observers can reasonably assume that someone who is blushing is also, or may well soon be, embarrassed.

## Interactive consequences of embarrassment

Importantly, the social-evaluative concerns that elicit blushing and cause embarrassment direct and constrain social interaction both before and after embarrassment occurs. As I'll establish below, fears of embarrassment are largely misplaced. Most embarrassing incidents end positively because both the embarrassed parties and their audiences behave kindly and well. Nevertheless, people routinely fear embarrassing circumstances more than they should, and there are several likely reasons why (Miller, 2007). First, we generally think that our actions are more noticeable than they really are and that people care about our conduct more than they really do. This is a misperception known as the *spotlight effect* (Gilovich et al., 2000), and it unfairly intensifies the evaluative

---

[2] In fact, and remarkably, when someone is staring at them from off to one side, people blush more intensely on the side of the face that is visible to the observer than on the side that cannot be seen (Drummond & Mirco, 2004; see Drummond, Chapter 2, this volume).

implications of embarrassing circumstances. In fact, although we are usually painfully aware of our own clumsiness, cognitive errors and losses of control, we are less likely to notice the similar predicaments of others, and they, in turn, are less likely than we think to notice ours (Epley et al., 2002). We also incorrectly believe that others are bolder and less embarrassable than we are because we underestimate the reticence and dread with which they approach potentially embarrassing situations (Van Boven et al., 2005); thinking that we are more cowed than others are by the threat of embarrassment makes our own social qualms seem more serious. Finally, an *illusion of transparency* leads us to believe that any nervous fluster and disquiet we experience during a predicament is more obvious to observers than it really is (Savitsky & Gilovich, 2003). We overestimate how awkward and discombobulated we appear to be when embarrassment strikes, and that, too, needlessly exacerbates our evaluative peril.

Similar misperceptions are often at work among those who have strong fears of blushing. A person who blushes intensely in the absence of any (other) predicament is guilty of an embarrassing *loss of control*, and most people expect negative judgments from others in such circumstances (Dijk, Voncken et al., 2009). However, compared to the rest of us, people with undue fears of blushing believe that blushing does greater damage to our images in others' eyes (Glashouwer et al., 2011); they believe that blushing is costly and that others disapprove (Dijk et al., 2010; cf. Dijk & de Jong, 2009), but, as we will see, they are usually mistaken.

### Avoiding embarrassment

Thus, we tend to think that embarrassment is more fearsome than it really is, and our exaggerated dread of embarrassing circumstances can motivate behaviour that is intended to avoid potential predicaments, but that is nevertheless counterproductive. People go out of their way to avoid awkward situations that could engender embarrassment, and when they make small adjustments that protect their or others' poise, they are simply being polite. But people also do things that are unhelpful or perhaps even harmful to themselves or others in order to circumvent embarrassment, and those actions are often wasteful.

For instance, small kindnesses can go undone. A woman who drops a box of envelopes into the path of a man walking behind her can ordinarily expect to have them returned to her; when this event was staged by researchers, the men retrieved the envelopes three-quarters of the time (Foss & Crenshaw, 1978). In contrast, if she dropped a box of tampons, most men stepped over them and kept on walking; they picked up the tampons and returned them to the woman only a third of the time. Women were equally likely to retrieve the tampons and the envelopes, presumably because the tampons were less threatening to them. However, when a later study employed a similar procedure with a mitten or a box of condoms, both men and women were more helpful with the mitten than they were with the condoms (McDonald & McKelvie, 1992). People are less likely to help others (Zoccola et al., 2011), and they are less likely to ask for help themselves (Bohns & Flynn, 2010), when a threat of embarrassment exists.

More importantly, misplaced social evaluative concerns can keep people from doing things that they really ought to do (Consedine et al., 2007; Darby & Harris, Chapter 7, this volume). In order to avoid embarrassment, people may fail to obtain preventive medical checkups involving mammograms (Lerman et al., 1990), pelvic examinations (Kowalski & Brown, 1994), and prostate examinations, and they may understate their alcohol and drug use, smoking, and lack of exercise when they are asked (Leary & Kowalski, 1995). They may also fail to buy or use condoms, and this is true around the world (Bell, 2009; Moore et al., 2008). Then, once problems have arisen, they may actually fail to seek treatment for sexually transmitted infections (Lichtenstein et al., 2005), sexual dysfunction (Brown & Haaser, 2005), urinary incontinence (Horrocks et al., 2004), colorectal cancer (Hou, 2005), and mental illness (Outram et al., 2004) in order to avert the awkward interactions that (they fear that) such help may entail. In such instances, by behaving in an inhibited fashion, people are being situationally shy, rather than embarrassed. Nevertheless, by going to such lengths to keep embarrassment at bay, people treat embarrassment as if it were really quite awful. Is it such a calamitous event?

*Responses to embarrassment*

It's true that embarrassment is sometimes so mortifying and discombobulating that people simply abandon the situation and flee the scene, hastily departing in disarray. However, in the accounts of embarrassment I collected in Texas (see Miller, 1996), taking *flight* was not particularly common, and that's a good thing: abashed bolting is clumsy, and it compounds one's evaluative troubles by making a poor impression on one's audience (Levin & Arluke, 1982). It's fortunate, then, that people are generally more likely to behave in a variety of other, more adaptive, ways when they become embarrassed (as you can in see Table 9.2).

Table 9.2 *Actors' primary responses to their embarrassment*

| Response | Frequency of use (%) |
|---|---|
| Evasion | 28 |
| Remediation | 17 |
| Humour | 17 |
| Apology | 14 |
| Flight | 9 |
| Excuses | 8 |
| Aggression | 5 |
| Justification | 2 |

The most common response is simply to ignore one's predicament and to act as if nothing has happened. I term this response *evasion* because it evades most of the fluster that often accompanies an embarrassing event and forgoes a more elaborate response. Continuing an interaction without pausing to offer an account or an apology can actually be a graceful, poised response to trivial misbehaviour because 'belaboured apologies for minor social misdemeanors can create more commotion than they resolve' (Miller, 2007, p. 250). Moreover, the frequency with which evasion occurs suggests that many embarrassments are small matters, indeed.

The next most common responses are *remediation* and *humour*. When damage has been done or inconvenience caused to others, embarrassed people often take action to repair or redress the harm they've done. This is a conciliatory response that implies that one is apologetic even if nothing is said, and it makes a good impression on observers (Semin & Manstead, 1982). If no harm has occurred, people may poke fun at their predicament with a self-deprecating quip or some other light-hearted remark, and such attempts at humour help to define the situation as one that is silly rather than serious (Edelmann, 1982).

My survey of embarrassing events also found that an *apology* that expresses regret and remorse and that may offer restitution occurs in one of every seven embarrassments. Thus, with remediation, humour or apologies, people are explicitly contrite, conciliatory and/or agreeable in response to about half of the embarrassments they encounter. Another 10 per cent of the time they provide accounts for their behaviour, offering either *excuses* that reduce their responsibility for their untoward acts or *justifications* that downplay their negative ramifications. Overall, however, remediation and apologies that atone for one's behaviour are much more common than are explanations that excuse or justify one's actions.

In fact, only rarely are people actually antagonistic when they are embarrassed. *Aggression* occurs infrequently, and it is almost wholly limited to cases of audience provocation in which one's embarrassment results from others' (usually intentional) meddling or mockery. So, embarrassed people do indeed behave disadvantageously on occasion, sometimes being surly and sometimes being spooked by their predicaments. However, much of the time, they just carry on, barely acknowledging their missteps, and if their misbehaviour is admitted, it is usually addressed with conciliatory responses that – as it turns out – appease their audiences, defusing any disregard.

## The reactions of others

We have arrived at what may be the most compelling aspect of embarrassment in social life: notwithstanding our fears of embarrassment, and despite its aversive nature, embarrassment usually elicits supportive reactions from other people. Most of the time, others are helpful; they either collaborate with us in ignoring our miscues, or they respond to our predicaments with empathy and support or kindly humour (Lee, 2009; Metts & Cupach, 1989). On those occasions when others do react in ways that make our embarrassments worse, they are rarely critical or malicious; more often, their attempts at humour fall flat or they innocently draw more unwelcome attention to our plight. Audiences do sometimes single us out for rough treatment, jeering and ridiculing us for our pratfalls, but such derision is unusual among adults, and especially rare among strangers. It *was* commonplace in elementary school – my embarrassment diaries revealed that fifth-graders routinely respond with laughter and ridicule to slips and gaffes by their peers (Miller, 1996) – and that may be one reason why we dread embarrassment so much. But more often than not, adult embarrassments are met with understanding (e.g., 'I know how you feel; that happens to me all the time') or friendly, accepting jocularity.

Importantly, it appears that a key reason why others are usually agreeable in response to our predicaments is that appropriate embarrassment that is calibrated to its context *makes a good impression* on observers. When things go awry in social life, we are liked better when we do become embarrassed than we would be if we remained unruffled and unperturbed. In a clever demonstration of this point, research participants watched videos of a man who knocked over a stack of toilet paper rolls in a grocery store (Semin & Manstead, 1982). In different versions of the tape, the shopper reacted with evident embarrassment or cool aplomb and he either gathered up the rolls or left them spread across the floor. He received the kindest evaluations when he became embarrassed and cleaned up his mess (employing the response of *remediation*), but even the abashed actor who just fled the scene was preferred to the unflappable fellow who seemed unruffled as he picked up the rolls. Remarkably, becoming embarrassed in an embarrassing situation made a more favourable impression on others than staying cool and calm did.

Independently, blushing has similar effects. Whether or not they remain poised and calm, people who blush after a normative public deficiency (see Table 9.1) are evaluated more positively than are those who do not blush (Dijk, de Jong et al., 2009; see de Jong & Dijk, Chapter 12, this volume). Specifically, when social predicaments occur, people who blush seem more moral, trustworthy, likeable and sympathetic than those who do not blush (de Jong, 1999). Even those who have greedily exploited others receive more forbearance and forgiveness when they blush after their misdeeds than when they remain unabashed and implacable (Dijk et al., 2011). Evident embarrassment in general, and blushing in particular, apparently reassure any observers that one recognizes and regrets one's misbehaviour and that one will (try to) do better in the future. As a result, one may avert punishment or rejection by others that might otherwise have followed (Crozier, 2010).

Importantly, however, overwrought embarrassment that is disproportional to one's predicament does not elicit liking and support from an audience. Overreactions to small mishaps, such as fleeing the scene in disarray, merely add to one's woes, portraying one as bungling and overly sensitive (e.g., Levin & Arluke, 1982). In order for embarrassment to be beneficial, one's fluster and chagrin need to seem reasonable, being attuned to, and apt in, the circumstances in which they occur. This seems to be true of blushing, as well: blushing in the absence of any apparent provocation can arouse suspicion, leading observers to wonder if one has a guilty conscience (de Jong, Peters & De Cremer, 2003).

Nevertheless, when they are calibrated to their context, both embarrassment and blushing are *desirable* responses to unwanted events that arouse social-evaluative concerns. Given its role and functions in social life, embarrassment is clearly a blessing, not a curse (Miller, 2007).

## Conclusion

Things have gone wrong (or at least people think they have) when embarrassment occurs, and such events create acute concern about how one is being judged by others. But even in the midst of embarrassed disarray, people typically behave in conciliatory or amiable ways that elicit kindly judgments and reactions from others. These patterns jibe nicely with the analyses of the evolutionary origins and the communicative impact of blushing that appear in other chapters of this volume, and it is reasonable to conclude that, along with the singular physiological response of blushing that might be its hallmark, embarrassment has desirable functions in social life. It interrupts unwanted behaviour, generally engenders advantageous responses, and reassures others, and we would be less well off without it.

# REFERENCES

Apsler, R. (1975). Effects of embarrassment on behavior toward others. *Journal of Personality and Social Psychology*, 32, 145–53.

Bell, J. (2009). Why embarrassment inhibits the acquisition and use of condoms: a qualitative approach to understanding risky sexual behaviour. *Journal of Adolescence*, 32, 379–91.

Bohns, V. K., & Flynn, F. J. (2010). "Why didn't you just ask?" Underestimating the discomfort of help-seeking. *Journal of Experimental Social Psychology*, 46, 402–9.

Brown, G. R., & Haaser, R. C. (2005). Sexual disorders. In J. L. Levenson (Ed.), *The American Psychiatric Publishing textbook of psychosomatic medicine*. Arlington, VA: American Psychiatric Publishing, 359–86.

Buss, A. H. (1980). *Self-consciousness and social anxiety*. San Francisco: Freeman.

Consedine, N. S., Krivoshekova, Y. S., & Harris, C. R. (2007). Bodily embarrassment and judgment concern as separable factors in the measurement of medical embarrassment: psychometric development and links to treatment-seeking outcomes. *British Journal of Health Psychology*, 12, 439–62.

Crozier, W. R. (2010). The puzzle of blushing. *The Psychologist*, 23, 390–3.

Cupach, W. R., & Imahori, T. (1993). Managing social predicaments created by others: a comparison of Japanese and American facework. *Western Journal of Communication*, 57, 431–44.

de Jong, P. J. (1999). Communicative and remedial effects of social blushing. *Journal of Nonverbal Behavior*, 23, 197–217.

de Jong, P. J., Peters, M. L., & De Cremer, D. (2003). Blushing may signify guilt: revealing effects of blushing in ambiguous social situations. *Motivation and Emotion*, 27, 225–49.

Dijk, C., & de Jong, P. J. (2009). Fear of blushing: no overestimation of negative anticipated interpersonal effects, but a high-subjective probability of blushing. *Cognitive Therapy and Research*, 33, 59–74.

Dijk, C., de Jong, P. J., Müller, E., & Boersma, W. (2010). Blushing-fearful individuals' judgmental biases and conditional cognitions: an Internet inquiry. *Journal of Psychopathology and Behavioral Assessment*, 32, 264–70.

Dijk, C., de Jong, P. J., & Peters, M. L. (2009). The remedial value of blushing in the context of transgressions and mishaps. *Emotion*, 9, 287–91.

Dijk, C., Koenig, B., Ketelaar, T., & de Jong, P. J. (2011). Saved by the blush: being trusted despite defecting. *Emotion*, 11, 313–19.

Dijk, C., Voncken, M. J., & de Jong, P. J. (2009). I blush, therefore I will be judged negatively: influence of false blush feedback on anticipated others' judgments and facial coloration in high and low blushing-fearfuls. *Behaviour Research and Therapy*, **47**, 541–7.

Drummond, P. D., & Mirco, N. (2004). Staring at one side of the face increases blood flow on that side of the face. *Psychophysiology*, **41**, 281–7.

Edelmann, R. J. (1982). The effect of embarrassed reactions upon others. *Australian Journal of Psychology*, **34**, 359–67.

Edelmann, R. J., & Iwawaki, S. (1987). Self-reported expression and consequences of embarrassment in the United Kingdom and Japan. *Psychologia*, **30**, 205–16.

Epley, N., Savitsky, K., & Gilovich, T. (2002). Empathy neglect: reconciling the spotlight effect and the correspondence bias. *Journal of Personality and Social Psychology*, **83**, 300–12.

Fortune, J. L., & Newby-Clark, I. R. (2008). My friend is embarrassing me: exploring the guilty by association effect. *Journal of Personality and Social Psychology*, **95**, 1440–9.

Foss, R. D., & Crenshaw, N. C. (1978). Risk of embarrassment and helping. *Social Behavior and Personality*, **6**, 243–5.

Gilovich, T., Medvec, V., & Savitsky, K. (2000). The spotlight effect in social judgment: an egocentric bias in estimates of the salience of one's own actions and appearance. *Journal of Personality and Social Psychology*, **78**, 211–22.

Glashouwer, K. A., de Jong, P. J., Dijk, C., & Buwalda, F. M. (2011). Individuals with fear of blushing explicitly and automatically associate blushing with social costs. *Journal of Psychopathology and Behavioral Assessment*, **33**, 540–6.

Higuchi, M., & Fukada, H. (2008). Comparison of four factors related to embarrassment in nontypical situations. *Psychological Reports*, **102**, 328–34.

Higuchi, M., & Nakamura, N. (2010). The causes and effects of embarrassment on using or negotiating to use condoms. *The Japanese Journal of Social Psychology*, **26**, 151–7.

Hofmann, S. G., Moscovitch, D. A., & Kim, H. (2006). Autonomic correlates of social anxiety and embarrassment in shy and non-shy individuals. *International Journal of Psychophysiology*, **61**, 134–42.

Horrocks, S., Somerset, M., Stoddart, H., & Peters, T. J. (2004). What prevents older people from seeking treatment for urinary incontinence? A qualitative exploration of barriers to the use of community continence services. *Family Practice*, **21**, 689–96.

Hou, S. I. (2005). Factors associated with intentions for colorectal cancer screenings in a Chinese sample. *Psychological Reports*, **96**, 159–62.

Kowalski, R. M., & Brown, K. J. (1994). Psychosocial barriers to cervical cancer screening: concerns with self-presentation and social evaluation. *Journal of Applied Social Psychology*, **24**, 941–58.

Leary, M. R., & Kowalski, R. M. (1995). *Social anxiety*. New York: Guilford Press.

Leary, M. R., & Meadows, S. (1991). Predictors, elicitors, and concomitants of social blushing. *Journal of Personality and Social Psychology*, **60**, 254–62.

Lee, J. (2009). Escaping embarrassment: face-work in the rap cipher. *Social Psychology Quarterly*, **72**, 306–24.

Lerman, C., Rimer, B., Trock, B., Balshem, A., & Engstrom, P. F. (1990). Factors associated with repeat adherence to breast-cancer screening. *Preventive Medicine*, 19, 279–90.

Levin, J., & Arluke, A. (1982). Embarrassment and helping behavior. *Psychological Reports*, 51, 999–1002.

Lewis, M. (1995). Embarrassment: the emotion of self-exposure and evaluation. In J. Tangney & K. W. Fischer (Eds.), *Self-conscious emotions: the psychology of shame, guilt, embarrassment, and pride*. New York: Guilford Press, 198–218.

Lichtenstein, B., Hook, E., & Sharma, A. K. (2005). Public tolerance, private pain: stigma and sexually transmitted infections in the American deep South. *Culture, Health and Sexuality*, 7, 43–57.

McDonald, J., & McKelvie, S. J. (1992). Playing safe: helping rates for a dropped mitten and a box of condoms. *Psychological Reports*, 71, 113–14.

Metts, S., & Cupach, W. R. (1989). Situational influence on the use of remedial strategies in embarrassing predicaments. *Communication Monographs*, 56, 151–62.

Miller, R. S. (1987). Empathic embarrassment: situational and personal determinants of reactions to the embarrassment of another. *Journal of Personality and Social Psychology*, 53, 1061–9.

  (1992). The nature and severity of self-reported embarrassing circumstances. *Personality and Social Psychology Bulletin*, 18, 190–8.

  (1995). On the nature of embarrassability: shyness, social evaluation, and social skill. *Journal of Personality*, 63, 315–39.

  (1996). *Embarrassment: poise and peril in everyday life*. New York: Guilford Press.

  (2004). Emotion as adaptive interpersonal communication: the case of embarrassment. In L. Z. Tiedens & C. W. Leach (Eds.), *The social life of emotions*. New York: Cambridge University Press, 87–104.

  (2007). Is embarrassment a blessing or a curse? In J. L. Tracy, R. W. Robins & J. P. Tangney (Eds.), *The self-conscious emotions: theory and research*. New York: Guilford Press, 245–62.

  (2009). Social anxiousness, shyness, and embarrassability. In M. R. Leary & R. H. Hoyle (Eds.), *Handbook of individual differences in social behavior*. New York: Guilford Press, 176–91.

  (2012). *Delineating the causes of embarrassment*. Manuscript submitted for publication.

Moore, S. G., Dahl, D. W., Gorn, G. J., Weinberg, C. B., Park, J., & Jiang, Y. (2008). Condom embarrassment: coping and consequences for condom use in three countries. *AIDS Care*, 20, 553–9.

Morley, R. (1983). *Pardon me, but you're eating my doily*. New York: St Martin's Press.

Outram, S., Murphy, B., & Cockburn, J. (2004). Factors associated with accessing professional help for psychological distress in midlife Australian women. *Journal of Mental Health*, 13, 185–95.

Robbins, B., & Parlavecchio, H. (2006). The unwanted exposure of the self: a phenomenological study of embarrassment. *The Humanistic Psychologist*, 34, 321–45.

Savitsky, K., & Gilovich, T. (2003). The illusion of transparency and the alleviation of speech anxiety. *Journal of Experimental Social Psychology*, **39**, 618–25.

Semin, G. R., & Manstead, A. S. (1982). The social implications of embarrassment displays and restitution behaviour. *European Journal of Social Psychology*, **12**, 367–77.

Sharkey, W. F. (1991). Intentional embarrassment: goals, tactics, and consequences. In W. R. Cupach & S. Metts (Eds.), *Advances in interpersonal communication research – 1991*. Normal, IL: Personal Relationships Interest Group, 105–28.

Sharkey, W. F., Kim, M. S., & Diggs, R. (2001). Intentional embarrassment: a look at embarrassors' and targets' perspectives. *Personality and Individual Differences*, **31**, 1261–72.

Silver, M., Sabini, J., & Parrott, W. (1987). Embarrassment: a dramaturgic account. *Journal for the Theory of Social Behaviour*, **17**, 47–61.

Stocks, E. L., Lishner, D. A., Waits, B. L., & Downum, E. M. (2011). I'm embarrassed for you: the effect of valuing and perspective taking on empathic embarrassment and empathic concern. *Journal of Applied Social Psychology*, **41**, 1–26.

Tangney, J. P., Miller, R. S., Flicker, L., & Barlow, D. H. (1996). Are shame, guilt, and embarrassment distinct emotions? *Journal of Personality and Social Psychology*, **70**, 1256–69.

Van Boven, L., Loewenstein, G., & Dunning, D. (2005). The illusion of courage in social predictions: underestimating the impact of fear of embarrassment on other people. *Organizational Behavior and Human Decision Processes*, **96**, 130–41.

Withers, L. A., & Vernon, L. L. (2006). To err is human: embarrassment, attachment, and communication apprehension. *Personality and Individual Differences*, **40**, 99–110.

Zoccola, P. M., Green, M. C., Karoutsos, E., Katona, S. M., & Sabini, J. (2011). The embarrassed bystander: embarrassability and the inhibition of helping. *Personality and Individual Differences*, **51**, 925–9.

# 10 Performing the blush: a dramaturgical perspective

*Susie Scott*

The blush is not only a psychological phenomenon but also a sociological curiosity. Despite being experienced as something intensely personal that evokes individual distress, blushing also has evidently social causes, consequences and functions. As colleagues in this volume have noted, the blush has evolved as an adaptive response unique to humans, who have an awareness of other minds and external perspectives on the self, together with a sensitivity to the social norms and values of the groups to which they belong. It serves a communicative function, signalling regret, apology and appeasement for having transgressed these social rules, which may be triggered by a feeling of shame before the other (Castelfranchi & Poggi, 1990). Such a gesture of role distance, which separates the person from the acts they have committed, indicates his or her adherence to the group's shared values; the blush therefore has a restorative function in helping to repair situations of awkward or disrupted interaction (Dijk & de Jong, 2009; see Darby & Harris, Chapter 7, this volume). Moreover, this gesture cannot be faked or controlled, and so reads as an authentic sign of honesty and trustworthiness (Crozier, 2007). Paradoxically, therefore, despite its associations with deviance, shame and negative evaluation, blushing can be read as a prosocial, positive signifier of cooperativeness and commitment to maintaining interaction order (Goffman, 1983).

Central to the social meaning of the blush is the notion of self-presentation. Dramaturgical theory, a sociological approach developed by Erving Goffman (1959/1990), identifies this as a motive behind much human behaviour. Social life is compared metaphorically to a theatrical performance, wherein individual actors strive to create particular impressions to the audiences they meet in different situations, using artefactual props, settings and scenery. These performances are given publicly 'frontstage' but may be contradicted by actors' private thoughts, feelings and behaviours, which are displayed 'backstage' as they slip out of character and evaluate their success or otherwise. Actors also work in teams or casts, rehearsing their parts together and devising strategies to keep each other in face so that the show can go on. Not surprisingly, a key focus of interest is on what happens when this goes wrong: when actors fail to communicate the impression they had intended, or audiences remain unconvinced.

Dramaturgy has been applied to blushing by social psychologists to identify the features of some social situations that trigger the 'self-conscious emotions' of embarrassment, shyness, pride and shame (Crozier, 2006; Tangney & Fisher, 1995). Of key importance is the feeling of being the centre of unwanted social attention (Leary et al., 1992), which may be triggered by threats to an individual's public identity, such as norm violation; mere conspicuousness; praise and positive attention; and accusations of blushing (Leary et al., 1992). However, there seems to be an additional element of *exposure* involved: the blusher is concerned with the risk of communicating unwanted impressions of him- or herself to others, which may result in social disapproval. Crozier's (2004) exposure theory identifies the public revelation of private information that the individual would prefer to keep hidden, combined with a shift in perspective to that of the 'other': an internalized representation of the critical audience gaze. In what Cooley (1902/1983) called the 'looking glass self', we imagine how audiences might perceive our behaviour, anticipate their criticisms and judgments, and experience self-conscious emotions. While there are many aspects of the self that might be exposed in this way, such as secret information or guilty knowledge, a common trigger is the perceived exposure of one's incompetence at managing social encounters. This can induce shameful blushing, whereby the actor believes he or she has been seen as weak, inadequate or lacking self-control (Edelmann, 1990), as well as unable to interact effectively with others (Crozier, 2010). It is also a key element of the shy blush, which is the focus of this chapter, wherein actors are concerned with *anticipated* social reactions to interactional blunders that may not actually occur (Scott, 2007).

What remain unexplored, however, are the detailed social mechanisms through which these processes unfold, as constructed and experienced by actors themselves. This promises to locate the blush in a wider context of patterns of interaction that sustain over time to reproduce social order. Sociological dramaturgy is rooted in the theoretical tradition of Symbolic Interactionism, which considers how social actors collaboratively work to negotiate shared 'definitions of the situation' (Thomas & Thomas, 1928/1970) by interpreting the meaning of each other's symbolic gestures (Blumer, 1969). There is a shift in focus away from the individual mind to the interaction context in which *social* minds are shaped and understood (cf. Mead, 1934). Thus, rather than analysing the cognition of self-presentation or the skills of individual performers in isolation, the sociologist is interested in what these patterns reveal about the groups to which self-conscious behaviour is oriented, how meanings are imputed reciprocally between actors and audiences in a 'conversation of gestures' (Mead, 1934), and how social reactions to unexpected or deviant behaviour impact upon the actor's sense of self. Agency is also emphasized by this perspective: blush-inducing states, such as shyness, are not passively suffered but rather actively performed and managed, through the enactment of social roles (Scott, 2007).

We can also consider the longer-term effects of negative social evaluation upon self-identity. Symbolic Interactionists examine the social process of *becoming* deviant, as a career trajectory that unfolds through a sequence of contingent interaction episodes (Becker, 1963). Depending on the social reactions they encounter, actors may either become 'progressively committed' to their attributed role or status (Becker, 1963), or 'drift' out again through normalization into a more conformist social identity (Matza, 1964). This promises to explain why, if blushing is a universal human experience, only some people come to see themselves as 'chronic blushers' (de Jong & Dijk, Chapter 12, this volume) and deal with the social consequences of this as a stigma, or spoiled social identity (Goffman, 1963a). Finally, the perspective sheds more light upon the paradox that ostensibly deviant behaviour, such as blushing, might be prosocial in its intentionality and consequences. This is illustrated clearly in the case of shyness, insofar as the shy blush is elicited in actors who are highly concerned with their responsibility to cooperate in upholding interaction order (Goffman, 1983).

In the remainder of this chapter, I examine the social conditions and consequences of the shy blush, from this Symbolic Interactionist dramaturgical perspective. Drawing on Goffman (1963a), I suggest that the shy blush is experienced as doubly stigmatizing, insofar as it involves both the fear of a potentially discredit*able* attribute (one's perceived relative incompetence at managing social encounters) being revealed, and the resultant blush itself, as a visual signifier of shyness, being actually discredit*ing* in its effects upon the actor's social status. Although shy actors anticipate negative social evaluation to occur in response to their potential mistakes and blunders, what in fact evokes more indignation from others is the strategies they use to avoid this risk, by withdrawing from social encounters altogether and being seen as rude, aloof or misanthropic. Thus, it is not interactional incompetence that is regarded as deviant, but rather the embodied performance of the shy role. This is exemplified by accounts of how and why the shy blush is evoked and the social reactions that it generates.

The data I present come from an empirical study that I conducted with forty self-defined 'shy' people in the United Kingdom in 2003 (see also Scott, 2004a, 2004b, 2005, 2007). I conducted face to face semi-structured interviews with sixteen people who responded to advertisements placed locally; these were twelve women and four men, most of whom were white, middle class and relatively young. I also recruited twenty people (two of whom had also been interviewees) from internet-based self-help groups and forums about shyness to subscribe to an email list, through which they recounted personal narratives and engaged in group discussions. A further six individuals emailed me privately with their accounts of living with shyness. The online participants varied more in age, gender and social background, and came from a more geographically dispersed area, although still mainly Western countries (the United Kingdom, United States, Canada and Australia). Elsewhere (Scott, 2004a; Scott et al., in press), I have documented the methodological implications of conducting research with erstwhile 'shy' people, who, ironically, proved to be most forthcoming in accounting for their reticence. The rich body of qualitative data produced by the study is typical of the sociological approach, which allows for a more in-depth interpretive understanding of the meanings that social experiences hold for actors (Weber, 1904/1949). Thus, to complement the quantitative measures of blushing set out by other colleagues in this volume, I present some extracts from interviews, which serve to document my participants' accounts in their own words. To protect their anonymity, the names given are all pseudonyms.

### Evoking the shy blush: social incompetence as a discreditable stigma

When asked to describe the situations that made them blush, the 'shy' participants cited familiar themes of self-consciousness, concern about negative social evaluation, and feelings of exposure. Believing that they lacked certain social skills and competences that others took for granted, the shy worried about saying or doing the 'wrong' thing in a situation and being judged as ignorant, incompetent or inconsiderate at interaction: a poor team player. Central to the experience of shyness, then, was an imagined, prospective view of the self in the eyes of the other, as someone embarrassed, humiliated, shamed or rejected on the basis of a revealed flaw (Scott, 2007; cf. Crozier, 2001). For some participants, simply being the centre of attention was enough to evoke this feeling of conspicuousness (Leary et al., 1992) under the social spotlight:

So I suppose that was why I defined myself as shy, because I was always blushing. And it wasn't because I was embarrassed, although that was sometimes the reason, but it was just – a deep sense of self-consciousness. (Heather)

This was often associated with an awareness of the audience's expectation that one should make a defensible contribution to the encounter, together with a doubt about one's ability to do so (cf. Schlenker & Leary, 1982). Particularly daunting was the prospect of confronting situations in which there were no clearly defined roles or scripts to follow, and where actors had to improvise their performance: making small talk at a party, for example, was much more shyness-inducing than carrying out one's duties within a workplace role. When actors could not hide behind a pre-scripted persona but had to present their 'real' self, they felt much more exposed and vulnerable to scrutiny (Scott, 2005). Assuming that there were sets of unspoken rules that they did not understand, they sensed a much greater risk of saying or doing what might be judged by audience to be the 'wrong' thing:

If I start giving my opinion or say what I think or something, I just go red. So it doesn't have to be anything quite embarrassing, really, or confidential or anything ... I think it's sort of, um, not being sure of what you're saying. (Anna)

Elsewhere (Scott, 2004b, 2007) I have outlined a theory of the shy self, as a social object that is formed by the interplay between individual consciousness, other minds and wider cultural values. Drawing on Mead (1934), we can understand the shy self as an internal conversation, comprised of two distinct phases, which are mutually reinforcing. The Shy 'I' refers to the private feelings of inhibition, awkwardness and self-consciousness that arise when one confronts certain social situations, and which seem to be involuntary and uncontrollable. These instinctive reactions are translated into embodied, performative displays that render the actor socially visible, such as blushing, stammering and avoiding eye contact. The Shy 'Me', in turn, is an awareness of oneself as being viewed in this way, from the imagined perspective of others. It involves the anticipation of an audience making negative judgments about one's social competence and therefore one's right to belong to their performance team. Moreover, this generalized other (Mead, 1934) is imagined in quite a distinct way, as a *Competent Other*, who appears more poised, skilled and confident at managing interaction than the actor perceives him- or herself to be (Scott, 2004b). To the shy actor, it seems as if 'everyone else' understands what to do in a situation and it is only they who do not know the rules: to say or do anything is to risk exposing one's incompetence and subjecting oneself to ridicule and rejection. As Iz reflected,

> I think blushing may well be to do with the way we think we appear to others . . . for example, if someone asks me a question, expecting an answer (even if it's not the right one), and they sit there watching me until I say something, I go a deep shade of red.

In Goffman's (1963a) terms, the shy actor's perceived relative social incompetence is experienced as a discredit*able* stigma – one that could potentially be hidden but which threatens to reveal itself at any moment. This contrasts with the discredit*ing* stigma (in this case the blush), which is already socially visible and cannot be concealed. Discreditable stigmas are in some ways more dramaturgically stressful to manage in everyday life, insofar as the actor must work at keeping their attribute secret, and remain constantly vigilant about the threat of discovery. They may seek to pass as 'normal' or unblemished in the relevant attribute (as, for example, in Pilkonis's (1976) shy extrovert, who appears gregarious and confident), but know that their mask may slip at any moment to reveal their 'real' self. Goffman (1963a) defined stigma as a feeling of spoiled social identity, occurring when an actor's claims to be a certain type of person are undermined by the impressions they unwittingly give off: there is a discrepancy between their virtual and actual identities. For Heather, this centred on an awareness of herself as a shy extrovert, insofar as the gregarious character she was sometimes able to project belied what she saw as her true self – an incompetent fraud:

> I think my problem started in my teens when I was trying to come out of my shell and be more sociable . . . [blushing] happened in any situation – with family, friends and strangers; with individuals, groups, and performing in public – and was a generalized anxiety that my 'performance', my 'way of being in the world' was not satisfactory and I was being judged negatively . . . It's obvious to me now that there was a dissonance between my beliefs about myself (that I was insignificant, worthless, empty, inferior, etc) and my behaviour (an indiscriminate friendliness to anyone who showed any interest in me, a compulsive longing for friendship/company, an eagerness to leave home and meet new people, etc). My blushing reminded me that there was an inconsistency and made me feel uncomfortable.

Often this discrepancy is a situational state that emerges when an interaction context makes explicit performative demands upon the social actor. Whereas much behaviour in public places takes the form of unfocused encounters (Goffman, 1961), in which actors are co-present but not cooperating in a shared activity, other focused interactions (Goffman, 1961) or face engagements (Goffman, 1967) require all parties to take an active part. Many of the participants reported blushing in the context of a role performance, when they were expected to improvise a line or move in order to keep the situation flowing smoothly. They voiced a dread of their presumed social incompetence, a backstage flaw, being revealed through the inept performances they expected to give frontstage: as Toby put it, the blush seemed to convey the message to oneself, 'Oh dear, I've made a faux pas. I looked a fool.' Dijk and colleagues (2009) also found that people who blush tend to anticipate negative social reactions, which exacerbates their self-consciousness. This demonstrates the internal conversation between the Shy 'I' and Shy 'Me', as the actor reflects upon his or her behaviour and the impressions he or she may have unwittingly communicated. For example, Iz reported that she would blush when she was,

very self conscious of saying something silly which may be embarrassing, or just making a fool of myself! I'm always really worried about what others think about me.

This felt inadequacy was more salient because of its proximity to the success of the Competent Other, who never seemed to make any such mistakes. It was further exacerbated by an anticipated lack of dramaturgical loyalty (Goffman, 1959/1990): the shy believed that were they to make such a blunder, their fellow actors would not step in to repair the situation with protective facework (Goffman, 1967), but rather would leave them to flounder alone under the spotlight of centre stage. As Emma said, she 'worried about standing out as this red, shaking fool'. However, what subsequently emerged from the data was that dramaturgical team-mates proved to be more supportive than the shy expected: they were less concerned with these kinds of mistakes in performance – fluffing lines, losing one's place, showing inconsistent roles – which were reparable, than they were with actors opting out of the performance altogether and dodging their obligations to the team.

## Blushing as a discrediting stigma

The blush therefore emerges as an expression of dramaturgical stress, but that is not the end of the story. Blushing is not just a passive response to triggering stimuli, but rather a consciously enacted, embodied performance that sets off its own chain of consequential events, which are socially 'fateful' (Goffman, 1967) for individual status and identity. Thus, as well as grappling with private misgivings about their social incompetence, the actor must now also deal with the problems ensuing from blushing itself. That is, in the course of trying to disguise a potentially discreditable stigma, they find themselves displaying an actually discrediting one, the blush, which evokes further self-consciousness. Blushing was experienced by my participants as embarrassing because it exposed their shyness: it revealed to their audience the shameful (as they saw it) truth that they were ill-equipped to take part in the interaction and uncertain of how to behave. The Shy 'Me' persisted as blushers imagined themselves in the eyes of the Competent Other, and anticipated the negative judgments that might ensue:

> when I know I'm gonna blush, it gets worse... I just think, 'Oh no, I look really – they know I'm nervous now, because I've gone red'... they can tell that I'm either nervous or embarrassed or something. And I'd like it better if I didn't show that, you know, it'd be better if we could sort of keep people guessing. (Anna)

In this respect, blushing also discredits the actor's claims to a different virtual identity: the attempts they might otherwise have made to 'pass' as socially confident are undermined by this bold, stubborn, undeniable marker of incompetence. Almost independently of its original causes, therefore, blushing itself can evoke further feelings of shyness, embarrassment and shame, in a loop of self-conscious emotions (cf. Crozier, 2006). As Emma put it,

> I only seem to blush when I can see that the person I'm speaking to can see I'm shy. I think I get embarrassed about being shy.

Crozier (2010) points to the cruel irony that blushing occurs on the most visible, socially communicative areas of the body – face, neck and ears – just at those very moments when its victim most wants to disappear. This paradox, which I call the visibility of invisibility (Scott 2007), is also dramaturgically interesting, because it suggests that a slip out of character into one's backstage self puts the blundering actor further into the spotlight of centre stage, causing potential embarrassment for the whole cast. By trying to withdraw to the margins of a social situation, to hide from the penetrating social gaze, shy actors find that their embodied displays of awkward detachment actually make them more conspicuous than if they had tried to join in, and demand social attention. My participants voiced regretful concerns about the way in which blushing allowed their felt incompetence to leak out involuntarily; this made them feel helpless and lacking in agency, as they could not control the impressions they were giving off (Goffman, 1959/1990). There was a sense of betrayal of the private inner self by its outward expression, the body, which then became the object of critical reflection:

> I'm aware that when I'm with another person, however much I might try to hide my feelings, my body often reveals the truth about what I'm actually feeling. (Heather)

Feeling visibly different and conspicuous means that shy blushing engenders feelings of shame, as the actor imagines his or her discredited self, from the perspective of the Competent Other, as having posed a threat to the social bond (Scheff, 2000). Even though shyness is ubiquitous and we all experience it in some situations (Zimbardo, 1977), when consumed by self-consciousness, it is easy to assume that we are the only one suffering, and that everyone else is as poised as they appear. Consequently, my participants reported feeling ashamed about blushing, quite apart from their shame about their underlying incompetence, and experienced this as a deeply personal problem and a private source of humiliation. It increased the sense of there being a division between the more and less competent, or shy and non-shy, as if these were two distinct groups, and reinforced the actors' sense of themselves as outsiders: excluded and marginalized. As Heather reflected,

blushing does seem to be a problem that makes the sufferer feel very isolated. It almost feels as if there's some sort of taboo on talking about blushing – or perhaps an unspoken assumption between shy and non-shy people that blushing is something nobody ever talks about!

She went on to add,

... the awful thing is, when you're someone who suffers from blushing, is that you cannot talk to anyone about it. So you're trapped in this thing of, well, you can't talk about it because you'll blush, and so it's a terrible sort of private experience that we simply can't share with anybody.

Blushing was not necessarily perceived as an affliction to be passively endured. Some of the respondents described how they had devised self-presentational strategies for concealing their blushing, to reduce their social visibility. These were embodied symbolic gestures (Blumer, 1969) that communicated inaccessibility to interaction, and served as 'involvement shields' to discourage others from trying to engage the individual (Goffman, 1963b). For example, Urchin recollected that,

As a teenager, I was very aware of my ears turning red at awkward moments. I always made sure my hair was at least long enough to cover my ears, for precisely this reason. I also avoid eye contact ... I used to walk around looking at my feet.

In other cases, however, such gestures were experienced as beyond conscious control, almost as involuntary as the blush itself. Although they were effective in helping the actor to deflect social attention, they were subjectively experienced as further evidence of his or her powerlessness, helplessness and low self-efficacy. Sally's account illustrates this well:

During the bad days, like today for instance, just talking to certain people, whatever the subject, can cause me to blush. When it happens I am totally aware of it, and I have noticed that I instinctively put my hands up against my face, for example to scratch my forehead or rub my eye, or if I'm sitting I will lean on my hand to at least cover one cheek. I don't realise I'm doing it until I actually do it now! I tend to sit with as much of my face covered as possible during bad days, ready and prepared for if I blush. That's just my way of hiding it from others, although I know that it probably makes it worse as I draw attention to my face. When it's happening, I just think about how much I hate myself for letting it happen, although I have no control over it consciously.

Being aware of oneself as a blusher therefore reinforces shy actors' image of themselves as inadequate or 'failed' interaction partners, and so, as a discrediting stigma, spoils their social identities (Goffman, 1963a). Over time, repeated experiences of this interaction chain can make the actor progressively committed to their deviant status (Becker, 1963), both as a shy person and as a blusher. Some of the participants spoke about the iterative effects of blushing as a vicious circle, as the awareness of oneself as someone prone to this response created a fear and dread of it emerging in social situations; the fatalistic anticipation that this would occur led them to avoid some situations altogether. Although no one mentioned the psychiatric term erythrophobia (Bögels & Voncken, 2008), some who had been diagnosed with social phobia or social anxiety disorder spoke colloquially about their 'blushing phobia' and its detrimental effects upon their self-esteem. As Dijk *et al.* (2010) argue, blushing can be the source as well as the symptom of social anxiety, insofar as it involves the belief that it will lead to one's being judged less competent, self-assured, 'normal' and likeable than one would hope to be (Dijk *et al.*, 2010, p. 267). The resultant self-consciousness ironically may then lead to further blushing, as if through a self-fulfilling prophecy. The whole process was recounted by Heather:

> I got into a vicious circle of being nervous about blushing and then feeling self-conscious that I couldn't be in a group situation or in any public place. You know, even going to the hairdresser's, where I had to look at myself in the mirror, I thought, 'Oh dear, this is terrible, I might blush!' And the more you think about it, 'Oh and I might do that', the more likely you are to do it, and you also get very tense. You know, so it just got into a vicious circle: if I was anxious about blushing, it inhibited me from any kind of social interaction, because I was always fearful that I'd show how self-conscious I was.

## Social reactions to the blush

These thoughts and feelings about blushing, and perceptions of the blushing self, are not simply symptoms of individual psychopathology, but rather are firmly grounded in 'real' contexts of social interaction. Turning, then, to the actual social reactions that people received when they blushed, we can see how these were experienced by the actors as fateful for their self-identities. As outlined above, Symbolic Interactionist theories of deviance emphasize the ways in which the meaning of an actor's behaviour is defined and negotiated between different parties at various stages of an ongoing trajectory (Becker, 1963; Erikson, 1964; Kitsuse & Cicourel, 1963; Schur, 1971). They also encourage us to shift our attention to the social, interactional process of becoming, rather than simply being, deviant (Becker, 1963), through a dynamic sequence of events.

Social reactions to norm-breaking acts may define them either as deviant or conformist ('normal' and therefore socially acceptable), each definition having quite different consequences for the individual so labelled. Normalization occurs when audiences account for the norm-breaking act, making sense of it in relation to shared vocabularies of motive (Mills, 1959): the act is explained away as a rational, socially intelligible action that makes sense in context: for example, when understood as a response to situational demands. When an actor receives such a response, it allows him or her to 'drift' back out of the deviant pathway and return to a conformist identity (Matza, 1964). When audiences cannot make sense of the act in this way, because it breaks one of the fundamental assumptions or 'residual rules' (Scheff, 1966/1984) of interaction, it (or rather, the individual who committed it) is defined as deviant, shifting the focus of the alleged problem away from the social to the individual level.

Rule breakers who are labelled in this way then have to make sense of and come to terms with the label, which may have a profound effect upon their self-identities. Hughes's (1945) notion of the master status describes a social label that comes pervasively to define an individual's whole being in the eyes of the other, shaping the way in which these others relate to them and how they see themselves: it determines their social fate (cf. Goffman, 1967). Those regarded as deviant tend to become progressively committed to the status through a deviant career trajectory (Becker, 1963), and experience their future social relations in these terms. Consequently, as Lemert (1967) argued, the sociologist's role is to investigate not only primary deviance – why people commit norm-breaking acts in the first place, since everybody does – but rather secondary deviance, or how those who are caught and labelled adapt to the consequences of the social reactions to their primary deviance.

*Positive reactions*

Blushing is not necessarily regarded as deviant, and can indeed evoke some very positive social reactions. As Crozier (2007) notes, despite the distress and suffering it causes its victims, blushing can be viewed as an attractive attribute: whether physically, as an aesthetic signifier of youth, beauty, good health and sexual availability, or socially, as an indication of desirable qualities, such as modesty, coyness and a lack of egotistic self-regard. Similarly, we have seen how the evolutionary model of the blush explains it as an appeasement gesture, which evokes sympathetic reactions to an interactional faux pas, thus serving a remedial function to repair any potential damage to social relations (de Jong, 1999). I have also documented the positive connotations of shyness (Scott, 2007), which are often overlooked but which do emerge in some people's reactions to displays of the condition: shyness is associated with similar qualities to blushing, such as modesty, humility, caution, reserve and conscientiousness.

The participants in my study had encountered both positive and negative reactions to their shy blushing. In the first case, audiences were identified as sympathetic and understanding: dramaturgical team-mates who were prepared to step in and support the blusher with acts of protective facework (Goffman, 1967). For example, Emma said,

> people who notice that you are blushing react in two ways. They either treat you nicely and sort of help you, or laugh at you ... those who are nicer are normally a much more understanding person [sic] and someone who I would talk to again.

Other participants felt that their blushing sometimes evoked positive reactions, but only when the behaviour was normalized. Audiences were reported to be sympathetic if they could attribute the blush to a situation in which it was 'reasonable' to assume that 'anyone' would be shy, such as a job interview or a meeting with an authority figure. Similarly, shyness was explained away by reference to age- and gender-related norms: some who had blushed as children had been seen as endearingly 'cute' and 'good as gold' but found that, as adults, they were expected to have grown out of it. Female participants also encountered more tolerant reactions than males, perhaps because shyness, modesty and reserve were seen as compatible with stereotypical ideas about appropriately feminine deportment (McDaniel, 2003). For example, Georgia said that friends had fondly (if cynically) described her blushing as a 'damsel in distress act', which they felt engendered sympathetic responses from bystanders.

In other cases, reactions to the blush were experienced as harsh and critical at the time, but reinterpreted with hindsight as having been well intentioned. The perspective of the Competent Other could be re-imagined differently, with greater optimism, which then led the individual to view their Shy 'Me' more sympathetically. For example, Heather explained how she had been teased for blushing during her schooldays, which had exacerbated her self-consciousness about the attribute, but that she had re-evaluated this in adulthood and come to terms with – even positively valued – her shy identity. Subsequently, she described exploiting the cultural aesthetics that defined female blushing as physically attractive (Crozier, 2007) by wearing make-up, and enjoyed discovering this 'fun' side of being shy. This shift in attitude towards herself in turn helped her to empathize with other people who blushed in everyday life, whom she now encountered from the perspective of an audience member:

But interestingly, now, I really, really warm to people I see who blush – you know what I mean? I really feel, 'Oh, what a lovely person!' So I just think, well, perhaps people used to think that about me when I used to blush a lot, you know. I thought they were thinking, 'What a silly woman! What's the matter with her?, you know, or girls at school would say, 'Ooh, you're bright red, Heather!' or 'Cor, you're beetroot!', and I'd sort of think, 'Ooh – well, I can't do anything about it. I can't help it.' So girls were really cruel, I think. But I think when I grew up, I thought, 'Well, if I put make up on, it'll just look like blusher, and it'll look quite pretty!'

### Negative reactions

More salient in the participants' minds, however, were memories of their blushing evoking reactions that they perceived as annoyed, disapproving and excruciatingly embarrassing. This rarely, if ever, involved direct criticism for blushing, but rather took the form of teasing and joking, which was nevertheless experienced by the shy as highly unpleasant. Already feeling self-conscious about their presumed social incompetence leaking out through the blush, which they felt helpless to prevent, they now had to deal with being made the centre of attention for this very thing. This exacerbated the image of the Shy 'Me' as a deviant outsider with a spoiled identity. As Leary et al. (1992) point out, accusations of blushing may serve as a trigger of further blushing, albeit caused this time by embarrassment rather than shyness (cf. Edelmann, 2001; Miller, 1996). For example, Georgia recounted this story of a time when she had been working at a supermarket checkout and served an older man who noticed that she was smiling:

[He said,] 'Oh, you've got dimples!', and I could feel myself just cringing and blushing, and then, 'Oh, and you blush!' So I'm sitting there with my smiley dimples and blushing, and thinking 'I need the ground to open up', and – oh, I hated that. And of course, by him saying that, then other people were looking, and I was just thinking, 'Leave me alone!'

To these shy actors, it seemed a particularly cruel irony that, just when they most wanted to be inconspicuous, someone would point out their blushing and turn bystanders' attention to it, thrusting them into the social spotlight. Remarks such as those in the above example may, as Heather suggested, have been intended as humorous, good natured, even sympathetic, but were experienced by the shy blushers as unfair: they felt as if they were being singled out for ridicule for something they could not help. This only increased their feelings of frustration, fatalism and powerlessness to change. A glum comment from Megan demonstrated this:

That's the worst part of being shy, I thought. People always point it out to you and this makes you feel like crawling under a rock. People reacted to my shyness by pointing [it] out as if I didn't know.

Some who routinely encountered this kind of social reaction found it extremely distressing because they experienced it as bullying. Etta, for example, had been teased for her shyness and blushing throughout childhood by jocular family members, and seemed emotionally scarred by the memory. Her account conveys feelings of victimization, as wellmeant expressions of fondness appeared to her as a personal attack, which she found cruelly tormenting:

My parents always called me 'the shy one of the family' ... [My uncle] would always ask me, 'How's my shy girl?' He'd say it as if he took some enjoyment in watching me cringe. He knew I was shy and would pursue it to no end. My [other] uncle would also give me a certain look with a smile on his face. He would just stare at me until he could get me to put that shy look on my face. We all know the 'shy look', I think. I would turn beet red as I silently died inside ... The more I showed I was shy, the more they would taunt me.

What seemed to evoke actual social disapproval, however, was not blushing per se, but rather the strategies that individuals used to manage it, and the further actions this led to. Many actors felt so self-conscious about blushing, and fearful of the consequences of this discrediting attribute being visible, that they made further deviant moves: either retreating to the margins of social situations, concealing themselves from view, erecting involvement shields to make themselves invisible, or avoiding the situations altogether. It was these behavioural displays to which others objected, insofar as they indicated an unwillingness to take part and to pull one's weight in sustaining the interactional flow. In ethnomethodological terms (Garfinkel, 1967), such symbolic gestures challenge the unspoken rules and taken-for-granted assumptions on which others rely to keep situations flowing smoothly, and breach their normative expectations. As Garfinkel showed, there is a tacit moral order underlying much of the routine business of everyday life, and those who fail to observe it pose a threat to interactional harmony. As such, social withdrawal evokes reactions of indignation, as affronted audiences move in to defend their perceptual reality. Many of the participants reported being misperceived as rude, aloof and standoffish because of their reluctance to engage 'normally' in social encounters. This is another unfortunate irony, of course, as the shy are in fact highly committed, sociable, dramaturgically conscientious team players, who are frozen with fear precisely because they care so much about the risk of 'getting things wrong' (Scott, 2005). Thus, Etta recounted with shame an episode when her blush-induced shyness had got her into trouble:

By 'standoffishness' I mean that people have seen me as not wanting to chat to them, when in reality I have been feeling too inferior to think anyone would choose to talk to me, that they were doing so out of pity. For example, when I travelled by bus, I'd avoid sitting near anyone I knew might start a conversation and the whole bus could listen in. One particular lady with a loud voice shouted one day at me, down the length of the bus, 'Who do you think you are tossing your head at? You think you are too good to sit near me.' I was mortified, as all I'd done was scuttle past her, pretending not to see her!

From this it seems that what audiences object to, more than blushing per se, is the performance of the shy role more generally. This again points to an underlying morality to the interaction order (Goffman, 1983). Actors are expected to try their best and demonstrate dramaturgical loyalty (Goffman, 1959/1990) to their fellow cast members. Thus, if someone attempts to join in with a social encounter but blushes, blunders and gives an imperfect performance, they may be good-naturedly teased, but their efforts are nonetheless appreciated: it is reasoned that they 'at least *tried*' and are demonstrably committed to keeping the show running. If, however, blushing leads them to hide from, avoid or effectively snub their team-mates, then this does invite disapproval. It is perceived as unfair that someone should be benefiting from the work that everyone else is doing to maintain interactional flow, and so the shy actor may be resented as an ungenerous 'social loafer' (Latané *et al.*, 1979): a free rider and poor team player who is not pulling his or her weight. Titus encapsulated this sentiment when, taking the view of the Competent Other, he reflected that,

I think people don't like the idea [that] you are listening but not contributing because it's like stealing, like someone who uses your milk but never buys any. Does that make any sense? It must seem to these people that we are being aloof, like we won't talk to them because we think THEY aren't worth talking to. You can see why they'd get annoyed.

## Living with the blush: effects on self-identity

Being routinely seen as a shy blusher, and labelled as such, not surprisingly leads many people to view themselves in the same terms, and to think of themselves as inherently and inevitably this type of person. Shyness can become a powerful master status (Hughes, 1945) that defines an individual's social identity as an over-riding characteristic, and shapes the way that they see themselves. In the latter stages of the deviant career (Becker, 1963), therefore, we find people engaging in secondary deviance, as they come to terms with and adapt to the consequences of labelling (Lemert, 1967). For some, this means a fatalistic acceptance of the shy role, and the resolution to develop a thick skin in order to survive future encounters. Anna expressed this view:

> I think it's who I am now, cos after so many years of being like that, I think I am [shy]. And I think quite a few times, some people have said, 'Oh, Anna's the quiet one' ... it kind of stuck with me, I suppose.

For others, however, their fate was more anguished, as they found the shy role hard to play. As we have seen, there are many tragic ironies embedded in shy blushing: the way that the gesture attracts attention when we most want to hide; the sense of betrayal by one's own body; the misperception of shyness as rudeness or aloofness; and the assumption that a withdrawn actor is socially disengaged or disinterested, rather than riddled with frustrated sociability. While the shy may wish to avoid scrutiny and judgment, they do still care passionately about making defensible contributions to situations, and want to be 'where the action is' (Goffman, 1967), playing their part, albeit from the safety of the theatre wings. Blushing, and the social effects it generates, makes this difficult to achieve. Thus, in a final twist of irony, the shy find that their blushing renders them horrifyingly visible, yet simultaneously feeling rejected and ostracized. As Nook explained, negative social attention accumulates to undermine the actor's self-esteem:

> Labelling has been a painful experience for me. I've only ever wanted to be just someone in the background and barely seen ... it was just being constantly dragged into the spotlight for all the wrong reasons that made me shy. I associate being in the public eye with pain and it's not easy to shrug off when it's occurred so much over time.

## Conclusion

Sociological dramaturgy offers a different perspective on the blush by showing how social interaction affects its elicitation, performance and reception by audiences and its effects upon individual identity. My study revealed that those who self-identify as shy experience the shy blush as doubly stigmatizing: it involves both the fear of a discredit*able* stigma (one's perceived relative social incompetence) being revealed, and the display of an embodied signal (the blush) that is in itself discredit*ing* because it exposes their uncertainty and lack of poise. Actors anticipate that spectators of the blush will disapprove of any flaws in their role performance, and will refuse to provide protective facework should a humiliating blunder occur. Feelings of shame and embarrassment follow from this awareness of oneself as a shy blusher, creating a loop of self-conscious emotions. Shame about shyness, embarrassment about blushing, and an uncomfortable sense of conspicuousness do little to attenuate the feelings of difference and deviance that blushing entails.

However, reports of the actual social reactions that these individuals receive tell a slightly different story. Often the shy blush evokes sympathy and understanding: it may be normalized by reference to situational factors or status characteristics, such as age or gender, which allow onlookers to rationally account for the gesture within shared vocabularies of motive. Negative social reactions may be subjectively experienced by the shy blusher in the form of teasing and bullying, but these are likely to have been well-intended gestures of fondness. What audiences do tend to object to, however, are the strategies with which some actors manage their blushing as a felt stigma, by withdrawing to the margins or avoiding social interaction altogether. They are seen as poor team players who are uncommitted to the morality that underlies interaction order – a cruel irony, considering their frustrated sociability and concern with getting things 'right'. Those who routinely encounter such social reactions to their shyness may come to see themselves in these terms, drifting further into a deviant career that defines their social identity. Nevertheless, this chain of negotiated meanings and mutual (mis)perceptions suggests that shy actors and their audiences ultimately share the same goal of interactional harmony. The designation of some shy blushers as outsiders may just be a socially constructed definition of the situation, which remains open to constant reinterpretation and revision.

REFERENCES

Becker, H. S. (1963). *Outsiders: studies in the sociology of deviance.* New York: Free Press.

Blumer, H. (1969). *Symbolic interactionism: perspective and method.* Englewood Cliffs, NJ: Prentice-Hall.

Bögels, S. M., & Voncken, M. J. (2008). Social skills training versus cognitive therapy for social anxiety disorder characterized by fear of blushing, trembling or sweating. *International Journal of Cognitive Therapy,* **1**, 138–50.

Castelfranchi, C., & Poggi, I. (1990). Blushing as a discourse: was Darwin wrong? In W. R Crozier (Ed.), *Shyness and embarrassment: perspectives from social psychology.* Cambridge University Press, 230–51.

Cooley, C. H. (1902/1983). *Social organisation.* New Brunswick, NJ: Transaction.

Crozier, W. R. (2001). *Understanding shyness: psychological perspectives.* Basingstoke: Palgrave Macmillan.

  (2004). Self-consciousness, exposure, and the blush. *Journal for the Theory of Social Behaviour,* 34, 1–17.

  (2006). *Blushing and the social emotions: the self unmasked.* Basingstoke: Palgrave Macmillan.

  (2007.) In praise of blushing. *Journal of Cosmetic Dermatology,* 6, 68–71.

  (2010). The puzzle of blushing. *The Psychologist,* 23(5), 390–3.

de Jong, P. J. (1999). Communicative and remedial effects of social blushing. *Journal of Nonverbal Behavior,* 23, 197–217.

Dijk, C., & de Jong, P. J. (2009). Fear of blushing: no overestimation of negative anticipated interpersonal effects, but a high subjective probability of blushing. *Cognitive Therapy and Research,* 33, 59–74.

Dijk, C., de Jong, P. J., Müller, E., & Boersma, W. (2010). Blushing-fearful individuals' judgmental biases and conditional cognitions: an Internet inquiry. *Journal of Psychopathology and Behavioral Assessment,* 32, 264–70.

Dijk, C., Voncken, M., & de Jong, P. J. (2009). I blush, therefore I will be judged negatively: influence of false blush feedback on anticipated others' judgments and facial coloration in high and low blushing-fearfuls. *Behaviour Research and Therapy,* 47, 541–7.

Edelmann, R. J. (1990). Embarrassment and blushing: a component-process model, some initial descriptive and cross-cultural data. In W. R. Crozier (Ed.), *Shyness and embarrassment: perspectives from social psychology.* Cambridge University Press, 205–29.

  (2001). Blushing. In W. R. Crozier & L. E. Alden (Eds.), *International handbook of social anxiety.* Chichester: John Wiley & Sons, 301–23.

Erikson, K. T. (1964). Notes on the sociology of deviance. In H. S. Becker (Ed.), *The other side: perspectives on deviance.* London: Free Press/Collier-Macmillan, 9–21.

Garfinkel, H. (1967). *Studies in ethnomethodology.* Englewood Cliffs, NJ: Prentice-Hall.

Goffman, E. (1959/1990). *The presentation of self in everyday life.* Harmondsworth: Penguin.

  (1961). *Encounters: two studies in the sociology of interaction.* Indianapolis: Bobbs-Merrill.

  (1963a). *Stigma: notes on the management of spoiled identity.* Harmondsworth: Penguin.

  (1963b). *Behavior in public places.* New York: Free Press/Macmillan.

  (1967). *Interaction ritual.* New York: Pantheon.

  (1983). The interaction order. *American Sociological Review,* 48(1), 1–17.

Hughes, E. C. (1945). Dilemmas and contradictions of status. *American Journal of Sociology,* L (March), 353–9.

Kitsuse, J. I., & Cicourel, A. V. (1963). The use of official statistics. *Social Problems*, 11, 131–9.

Latané, B., Williams, K., & Harkins, S. (1979). Many hands make light the work: the causes and consequences of social loafing. *Journal of Personality and Social Psychology*, 37, 6, 822–32.

Leary, M. R., Britt, T. W., Cutlip, W. D., & Templeton, J. L. (1992). Social blushing. *Psychological Bulletin*, 107, 446–60.

Lemert, E. (1967). *Human deviance, social problems and social control*. Englewood Cliffs, NJ: Prentice-Hall.

McDaniel, P. A. (2003). *Shrinking violets and Caspar Milquetoasts: shyness, power and intimacy in the United States, 1950–1995*. New York University Press.

Matza, D. (1964). *Delinquency and drift*. New York: John Wiley & Sons.

Mead, G. H. (1934). *Mind, self and society from the standpoint of a social behaviorist*. University of Chicago Press.

Miller, R. S. (1996). *Embarrassment: poise and peril in everyday life*. London: Guilford Press.

Mills, C. W. (1959). *The sociological imagination*. New York: Oxford University Press.

Pilkonis, P. A. (1976). *Shyness: public behavior and private*. PhD thesis, Stanford University.

Scheff, T. J. (1966/1984). *Becoming mentally ill: a sociological theory*. New York: Aldine.

(2000). Shame and the social bond: a sociological theory. *Sociological Theory*, 18, 86–99.

Schlenker, B. R., and Leary, M. R. (1982). Social anxiety and self-presentation: a conceptualization and model. *Psychological Bulletin*, 92, 641–69.

Schur, E. (1971). *Labeling deviant behavior*. New York: Harper & Row.

Scott, S. (2004a). Researching shyness: a contradiction in terms? *Qualitative Research*, 4(1), 91–105.

(2004 b). The shell, the stranger and the competent other: towards a sociology of shyness. *Sociology*, 38(1), 121–37.

(2005). The red, shaking fool: dramaturgical dilemmas in shyness. *Symbolic Interaction*, 28(1), 91–110.

(2007). *Shyness and society*. Basingstoke: Palgrave Macmillan.

Scott, S., Hinton-Smith, T., Härmä, V., & Broome, K. (in press). The reluctant researcher: shyness in the field. *Qualitative Research*.

Tangney, J. P., & Fischer, K. W. (Eds.) (1995). *Self-conscious emotions*. New York: Guilford Press.

Thomas, W. I., & Thomas, D. S. (1928/1970). Situations defined as real are real in their consequences. In G. Stone & H. Farberman (Eds.), *Social psychology through interaction*. Waltham, MA: Ginn-Blaisdell, 154–5.

Weber, M. (1904/1949). *The methodology of the social sciences*. New York: Free Press.

Zimbardo, P. G. (1977). *Shyness: what it is and what to do about it*. London: Pan Books.

# 11 Blushing and the private self

*W. Ray Crozier*

## Introduction

Understanding more about the circumstances that give rise to a blush would yield valuable insight into its causes. Knowing when people do something (and when they don't) and detection of patterns in their behaviour can be informative about the reasons for their behaviour. Classifications of the circumstances of embarrassment have been influential (e.g., Gross & Stone, 1964; Miller, 1996) and have been used to distinguish alternative accounts: for example, the self-evaluation model and the dramaturgical model (see Miller, Chapter 9, this volume). In comparison, there has been little equivalent research into the circumstances of blushing. A number of factors may have contributed to the dearth of such studies: the general neglect of the blush as a research topic, the ready acceptance of Darwin's thesis that it is 'the thinking of what others think of us which excites the blush' (Darwin, 1872/1999, p. 324) and the assumption that blushing is the 'hallmark' of embarrassment (Buss, 1980) with the implication that the circumstances of blushing coincide with the circumstances of embarrassment and do not warrant separate investigation.

Yet the identification of blushing as specific to embarrassment is problematic (Keltner & Buswell, 1997). Of course, we blush when we are embarrassed and, for example, researchers typically aim to induce embarrassment in their participants in order to study the blush. Yet it has not been established that we invariably blush when we are embarrassed. The blush is not always mentioned in personal reports of embarrassment (Edelmann, 1990; Parrott & Smith, 1991), nor is it included in videotape analysis of embarrassed facial expressions (Keltner & Buswell, 1997). There is a need to identify which embarrassing circumstances trigger a blush and which do not. Moreover, blushing is said to accompany other emotions, notably shame, guilt and shyness (which Darwin (1872/1999, p. 343) described as 'the most powerful of the causes of blushing'). Is the blush associated with these emotions too, or are there certain elements shared by these emotions that are necessary for a blush?

In this chapter I set out and illustrate 'exposure theory', one account of what is common to situations that elicit a blush. I apply this conceptualization, together with an established content analysis scale for episodes of shame, to analysis of descriptions of blushing episodes in fictional sources and self-report questionnaire responses. I relate the exposure account of the blush to shame and embarrassment – what distinguishes these emotional experiences and what do they share?

## Exposure and the blush

### Assumptions

I begin by setting out some working assumptions. First, the blush is a response to something specific. It has rapid onset, is of brief duration (although this is variable since one blush can trigger another), and is restricted to (or only visible in) the 'blush region'. There may be another type of blush, labelled the 'creeping' blush by Leary, Britt, Cutlip and Templeton (1992), which has gradual onset, is of long duration (perhaps of several minutes) and extends over the face, neck and upper chest. The creeping blush has attracted little research attention and it is unclear whether it is a distinct form or an extended 'classic' blush. Observation suggests that it is induced when someone is exposed to prolonged public attention or evaluation: for example, when giving a public presentation or being interviewed. This leaves the question of what specific event triggers the classic blush.

The second assumption is that the blush is an emotional experience, and I suggest that it belongs to the domain of shame, embarrassment and shyness. There is dispute in the psychological literature whether these constitute distinct emotions (or even whether shyness is an emotion), but one strand of theorizing regards them as aspects of a common affect (Tomkins, 1963), or basic emotion (Izard, 1977) or as members of a family of related emotions (Tracy & Robins, 2004). I return to the relation of the blush to these emotions in a later section.

### Occasion to blush

My thesis is that the trigger of the blush is consciousness of being exposed. Specifically, an event X occurs for person B in context E. If X raises the prospect that Y will be exposed to observer O, and Y belongs to the class of things the exposure of which in context E will create difficulties for B: B will blush.

Exposure has long been a recurrent theme in accounts of shame and embarrassment and it figures in other definitions of blushing (Dennett, 2001; Tallis, 2008). A person feeling shame feels exposed (Taylor, 1985, p. 57); 'this exposure is accompanied by an urge to hide and disappear, to become invisible, to sink into the ground' (Zahavi, 2010, p. 220). Deigh (1983, pp. 242–3) has an alternative take on this, proposing that shame protects the self from exposure and is expressed by 'acts of concealment'. In an early contribution to the psychology of blushing MacCurdy (1930) argued that the causes of embarrassment are typically exposure of some kind. Finally, Lewis (1971) identified frequent references to exposure and vulnerability in psychiatric patients' accounts of shame experiences.

Being the object of social attention or public scrutiny can be a cause of blushing in its own right (Leary et al., 1992). However, exposure entails more than being revealed or open to view. It can mean being deprived of cover or protection, open to danger. Exposure is not only physical. Disclosure of *information* that we wish to keep private and unwanted revelation of our motives or our feelings for someone can create difficulties for us, difficulties that can encompass transient social awkwardness and intense, enduring shame. Dennett (2001) argued that we blush because we think someone knows some fact about us that we would rather that they didn't know. Tallis (2008, p. 117) suggested that 'blushing is associated with undesired social attention and heightened self-consciousness. We blush with embarrassment, with shyness, with uncertainty, with a sense of exposure, of undress.'

Consider the elements of the hypothesis: the event, the matter at risk of exposure, the observer and the blush. Often the event is something that is said or done by the person ('actor') who blushes or by others present, and the exposure is to these others. However, it is not necessary that some social event occurs: the actor might have a thought, a shift in consciousness that is sufficient to trigger the blush, and the 'observer' might not be present. Scheler (1913/1987, cited by Metcalf, 2006) introduced a vignette describing a woman who has been posing nude as an artist's model and who suddenly experiences shame when she becomes conscious that the artist is looking at her not as a model, but as a sexual object. This vignette has been analysed by Taylor (1985) and Williams (1993), who identify the cause of the model's shame as the shift in her awareness of her situation. It is not necessary that the artist is looking at her in a prurient way, only that she now believes that he is doing so. George Eliot's *The Mill on the Floss*, published in 1860, provides another example:

But they had reached the end of the conservatory, and were obliged to pause and turn. The change of movement brought a new consciousness to Maggie: she blushed deeply, turned away her head, and drew her arms from Stephen's. (Eliot, 1860/1976, p. 416)

In these examples, what is (might be) exposed and to whom? Taylor (1985) argued that the trigger of the model's shame is not the artist but the model's adoption of a higher-order observer-view, an awareness of how she could be seen from this viewpoint. She feels herself to be degraded in the state in which she has allowed herself to be seen. 'Maggie' blushes when she suddenly realizes that it is wrong to be alone with Stephen given their feelings for one another. It is wrong because of her obligations to particular others and the implications for her self-respect. Her adoption of a higher-order perspective on her position is surely crucial for her blush. 'Stephen' is not the 'observer' here even though he is the only other person present. The only change in the situation is this shift in her perspective. However, Williams (1993, pp. 200–1) disputed that another observer-perspective is required for shame, and conceived of the model's exposure in a different way. He argued that the change in the situation introduces a sense of unprotectedness or loss of power: 'this is itself constituted by an actual gaze, which is of a special, sexually interested, kind. She had previously been clothed in her role as a model; that has been taken from her, and she is left truly exposed, to a desiring eye.'

There are instances when people blush, suspecting that a topic might have significance even if they are unaware what this is; when they realize that they have inadvertently raised an issue even if the person who would be affected by this is not conscious of it; when they are accused of something but don't know what it is they are being accused of. In Philip Roth's (2001) *The Dying Animal* a florist compliments a woman customer on her hat and he blushes when her reply implies that she is wearing it for medical reasons. He realizes that he has inadvertently brought up a sensitive topic. In Elizabeth Bowen's (1964) *The Little Girls* a girl has hidden a chain under her skirt and when a boy asks what the clanking noise is, he blushes when she teases him that it is not the sort of question he should ask, and when another girl pretends to be shocked at his asking, he blushes more intensely. In my questionnaire study (see below) a woman reported blushing when an authority figure announced to her group that someone in the group had misbehaved; she blushed even though she was innocent, explaining that she feared that she might be suspected of the misconduct. In another questionnaire response, a woman reported blushing when someone mentioned the name of a man she was attracted to.

This thesis can have a strong form (blushing is always triggered by exposure) or a weak form (many occasions of blushing can be described in this way). Yet even if circumstances that trigger a blush take this form, there remains the question why this pattern elicits the specific reaction that constitutes a blush. Any answer to this question is speculative at our current stage in understanding the blush, and the notion of such a visible response as a blush being a reaction to exposure seems paradoxical. Yet the notion of exposure may have heuristic value, as I discuss below.

I have explored these patterns in literary sources and questionnaire data in previous publications (Crozier, 2000, 2001, 2006). In this chapter I analyse additional samples from literary sources and responses to self-report questionnaires in order to relate the notion of exposure to a theoretical framework drawing upon theories of shame produced by Lewis (1971) and Scheff and Retzinger (1991). Lewis's analysis of shame in patients' discourse identified references to feeling foolish, exposed, complimented and criticized as verbal markers of shame. These markers are represented in the Gottschalk–Gleser shame-anxiety Content Analysis Scale (Gottschalk *et al.*, 1969), which analyses the form and content of speech as a means of identifying emotional states. Shame is indexed by phrases that refer to deficiencies of the self, to feeling inadequate, embarrassed, humiliated and exposed, to being criticized or ridiculed by others, and to being complimented and praised.

## Shame, exposure and the blush: a content analysis

Six categories, four based on Scheff and Retzinger's (1991) application of the Gottschalk–Gleser scheme to text analysis and two additional ones, were applied to the fictional episodes and individual questionnaire protocols. One of the additional categories represents 'topic exposure', defined by specific references to the exposure of a topic; the other is defined by references to sexual matters. A single episode or protocol could represent more than one category. Table 11.1 displays the categories and markers.

### Sources of episodes

**Questionnaires.** A sample of 101 female students of education, nursing and social work was presented with a questionnaire that invited them to recall and describe in their own words an occasion when something was said to have made them blush. Participants were invited to say why they

Table 11.1 *Categories in content analysis*

| Category | Marked by mention of: |
| --- | --- |
| Public exposure | being out of place; conspicuous; looked at; in the presence of an audience |
| Being criticized | being accused; commented on; challenged; ridiculed; laughed at |
| Being complimented | being complimented or praised |
| Feelings of inadequacy | being embarrassed; feeling stupid; self-conscious; tongue-tied; uncomfortable; unsure how to respond |
| 'Topic' exposure | personal, private or taboo topics |
| Sexual references | sexual attraction, appearance, activities |

thought they had blushed and these reasons were also coded into the shame categories. A separate sample of 45 participants from the same population of students completed an alternative version of the questionnaire where 'you felt embarrassed' replaced 'you blushed' and participants rated the intensity of their embarrassment. This version made no reference to blushing.

**Fiction excerpts.** A selection of works of fiction written by seventeen novelists was exhaustively searched for references to blush, flush and redden and alternative forms of these key words (e.g., blush, blushed, blushes, blushing, etc.), omitting references to inanimate objects, nature (e.g., the blush of dawn) or conventional phrases such as 'at first blush'. The selection was opportunistic, related to my tastes in literary and detective fiction, but included a range of works produced by English-language authors from Britain, Ireland and the United States, writing from the end of the nineteenth century to the early years of this century. Episodes were transcribed and submitted to content analysis using the same categories as in the questionnaire study.

The search identified 119 blushing episodes in total, 99 describing an adult (65 women, 34 men) and 20 a child (14 boys, 6 girls). Nearly all the episodes (114) referred to a blush occurring in a social situation. The remaining five episodes were as follows. In two episodes the person was explicitly described as not blushing in the situation despite reacting to it. In two further episodes a male narrator, who was alone, said that he blushed to recall how he had behaved badly in the past – 'I blush to say', 'I blush to write it.' Finally, a character made a general comment about blushing, saying that 'showing-off was so bad it made you blush for those who did it'. In these last three episodes the reference to a blush seemed to serve as a figure of speech rather than a description of an actual blush.

### Findings

The outcomes of the coding analysis for the questionnaire responses and the fiction episodes, together with the percentages of blushing episodes that were coded for each category, are displayed in Table 11.2. Table 11.3 displays the proportion of individual questionnaire protocols and fiction episodes that were coded in zero or more categories for the four Gottschalk–Gleser categories and with the topic exposure category added.

Table 11.2 *Blushing episodes categorized as shame occasions*

| Category | Embarrassment questionnaire | Blush questionnaire | Fiction episodes (adults) | Fiction episodes (children) |
|---|---|---|---|---|
| Public exposure | 25 | 46 | 23 | 65 |
| Topic exposure | 26 | 24 | 71 | 40 |
| Criticism | 37 | 41 | 26 | 55 |
| Compliment | 7 | 26 | 11 | 5 |
| Feelings of inadequacy | 36 | 55 | 13 | 20 |
| Sexual references | 23 | 25 | 64 | 5 |
| *Number of coded episodes* | *44* | *100* | *94* | *20* |

Entries in the table refer to the percentage of questionnaire responses or fictional episodes in which an instance of each category was coded as present.

Table 11.3 *Distributions of numbers of categories coded within individual protocols (percentage data)*

| Number of categories in a protocol | Questionnaire: Gottschalk–Gleser categories | Questionnaire: topic exposure category added | Adult fiction: Gottschalk–Gleser categories | Adult fiction: topic exposure category added |
|---|---|---|---|---|
| 0 | 6 | 1 | 39 | 3 |
| 1 | 33 | 23 | 40 | 53 |
| 2 | 50 | 61 | 18 | 37 |
| 3 | 11 | 14 | 3 | 7 |
| 4 | n/a | 1 | n/a | 1 |
| Percentage coded as shame | 94 | 99 | 61 | 97 |

All four Gottschalk–Gleser categories are strongly represented in both sets of data – over 90 per cent of questionnaire protocols can be coded into at least one category and 61 per cent coded into two or more. Table 11.2 shows that accounts of blushing episodes in both sources were replete with references to being conspicuous, exposed, looked at, in front of an audience, embarrassed, praised, ridiculed and criticized.

Whereas the topic exposure category is well represented, its frequency varies between sets. It accounts for 71 per cent of the coded adult fiction episodes (see Table 11.2) and adding it to the distribution of categories data (see Table 11.3) raises the proportion of fiction episodes that are coded in at least one category to 97 per cent. This difference is associated with variation in the pattern of social situations: interactions between two individuals were much more frequent in fictional adult episodes (64 per cent) than in questionnaire responses (10 per cent). Fictional episodes were more likely to involve an encounter between members of the opposite sex (81 per cent of episodes) and there were significantly more sexual references in fiction (64 per cent of episodes) than in questionnaire responses (25 per cent). Within the sample of fiction episodes there was a statistically significant association between topic exposure and the presence of a sexual theme in the episode. Conversely, more people were present and there were more references to an audience in the questionnaire responses than in the fiction. Feelings of inadequacy were common in questionnaires (55 per cent) but rare in fiction (13 per cent). Embarrassment was explicitly mentioned in 35 per cent of questionnaires but in only 6 per cent of fiction episodes. When giving reasons for their blushing, 32 per cent of questionnaire respondents mentioned embarrassment and 21 per cent mentioned feelings of inadequacy other than embarrassment.

The blushing and embarrassment versions of the questionnaire attracted different patterns of responses. Embarrassment was twice as likely to be mentioned by participants in the blushing version (35 per cent) than blushing was mentioned in the embarrassment version (16 per cent). Public exposure and receiving a compliment were much more frequent and feelings of inadequacy somewhat more frequent in the blushing version. Compliments and praise also appeared in reasons given for blushing: 'I don't accept compliments easily'; 'Receiving praise makes me blush.' The paucity of compliments in spontaneous responses to the embarrassment version is consistent with previous findings that although people are frequently embarrassed by being praised, congratulated, thanked and so on, this is rarely represented in studies of participants' spontaneous accounts: for example, in Miller's (1996) analysis of recollections of embarrassing episodes.

In summary, accounts of blushing episodes, whether recalled by research participants or extracted from a sample of literary sources, can readily be coded in terms of shame categories, and the category of topic exposure is prominent in both sources, particularly the fictional source where it is the modal category. The analysis uncovers an extensive set of circumstances. A blush accompanies errors of all kinds, appearing foolish, and so on – occasions that Leary et al. (1992) classify as threats to public identity, such as violations of norms, inept performances, loss of control, behaving out of role. These are also common elicitors of embarrassment and have attracted the most research attention (see Miller, Chapter 9, this volume). Such incidents are common in the questionnaire study and are also found, albeit less frequently, in the fiction episodes. The actor reveals himself or herself to be foolish, inept, inattentive, out of touch, insensitive, immodest, selfish, socially awkward and so on. The actor discloses something that is revealing about the self that is inappropriate to the occasion or that he or she would not want others to know. Topics that ought to be kept hidden are diverse. They can be culturally shared or idiosyncratic and their significance depends on the immediate social context. People can blush when a sensitive or private matter is merely hinted at, is about to be raised, or there is anticipation that it might be raised. You can blush even though you are the only one present who is aware of the implications of the topic.

### Limitations

I acknowledge that the conception of shame that has guided the content analysis is a broad one that encompasses embarrassment as a 'marker' or sign of shame. Furthermore, it does not follow from the assumption that embarrassment is a marker of shame that embarrassment cannot be experienced without shame. The study has limitations. No rival scheme is applied to the content analysis to represent alternative theories of blushing. The occasions that are recalled or described in fiction may not be representative of situations of blushing more generally. Participants may recall embarrassing incidents when prompted by the word 'blush'. The use of literature as a data source can be criticized on the grounds that the episodes are invented. In defence of this, writers working within the realist tradition of the novel are constrained to provide convincing descriptions of situations, characters, emotions and motives, descriptions that have to withstand the test of time and survive close critical scrutiny. Hogan (2010) argues that literary material has a valuable place in the scientific study of emotion since authors do not simply experience emotion but also encode and represent experiences. Finally, it is important to go beyond descriptions of situations to test hypotheses in actual social situations.

## Blushing with embarrassment: blushing with shame

### *Embarrassment versus shame*

What is the relation of blushing to embarrassment and shame? Although the notion that blushing is the hallmark of embarrassment has achieved prominence, there are opposing views. Darwin (1872/1999) regarded the blush as an expression of shame, as have many philosophers (e.g. Taylor, 1985; Williams, 1993), anthropologists (Casimir & Schnegg, 2002; Strathern, 1977) and psychologists (Castelfranchi & Poggi, 1990; Lewis, 1971; see also van Hooff, Chapter 5, this volume). Nevertheless, there are cultural and historical dimensions to this question.

A substantial body of cross-cultural research has examined variation in the meanings of shame-related terms. For example, several studies have examined the emotion lexicon in the Indonesian archipelago, reporting on the use of *malu* (usually translated as 'shame' and referring to 'a defect, inferiority or misdeed by the self': Heider, 1991, p. 85) and comparing this with usage in Western societies including the United States (Fessler, 2004) and the Netherlands (Fontaine *et al.*, 2002). This research shows that patterns of connections among shame terms differ across cultures and between studies within cultures. Thus, Fessler's (2004) analysis of shame-eliciting events reported that there was no distinct term for embarrassment in Bengkulu Malay, concluding that embarrassing events were subsumed within shame events, making a separate term unnecessary. In the Californian sample, on the other hand, there were separate guilt and shame clusters; 'shamed-humiliated-embarrassed' formed one of these clusters, with a link between the terms embarrassment and 'red faced'.

Within the English language, shame has a much longer history than has embarrassment in its current meaning, and references to blushing with shame are prevalent in older texts. Samuel Johnson's *Dictionary of the English Language* of 1755 defined shame as 'the passion felt when reputation is supposed to be lost; the passion expressed sometimes by blushing'. Johnson also referred to instances of blushing in entries for shamefaced and shamelessness. Shakespeare's *Richard III* (Act I, Scene II) provides an example of calling upon someone to blush with shame after he has committed multiple murders (hardly cause for mere embarrassment): 'Blush, blush, thou lump of foul deformity.'

Embarrassment in its current meaning of being ill at ease in social encounters has a shorter history. The *Oxford Dictionary of Word Histories* (Chantrell, 2004) traces 'embarrass' to the early seventeenth century, meaning to hamper or impede, and to be embarrassed is to encounter difficulty: for example, in the context of financial problems. Johnson's *Dictionary* defined it in terms of perplexity and entanglement.

These observations on lexical changes are consistent with statistical data about trends in English documents since 1800 which show that references to blushing with shame have been much more frequent than references to blushing with embarrassment over this period. Inspection of the relative frequencies of two phrases, 'blush with shame' and 'blush with embarrassment', using Google Books Ngram Viewer (Michel et al., 2010) shows that 'blush with shame' has been consistently much more frequent since the period of measurement began in 1800, and that the frequency of 'blush with embarrassment' has only exceeded zero since about 1900. Within this overall pattern the phrase 'blush with shame' has been decreasing steadily since around 1940 whereas 'blush with embarrassment' has been steadily increasing since 1930. A similar pattern with only minor differences is found when 'reddening' and 'blushing' replace 'blush' in the analysis.

Current psychological positions range from arguing that shame and embarrassment are distinct emotions (e.g., Keltner & Buswell, 1997) to proposing that they differ only in intensity or seriousness (see also Darby & Harris, this volume, Chapter 7). According to the latter position, shame is more intense and persistent and involves lasting damage to social identity whereas embarrassment is a mild and less persistent form of shame. Shame involves a breach of a fundamental standard of conduct, a serious dereliction, a violation of moral rules and it affects the core self or character. Embarrassment involves minor breaches of standard or conventions; it concerns a flaw in the self being enacted or, as Sabini and Silver (1997) argue, an apparent rather than an actual flaw. Sabini and Silver propose that shame and embarrassment share a common state ('state x'), which is labelled according to whether a real or an apparent flaw in character is revealed. Their account resembles the exposure account of the blush: B experiences event E; B appraises that E discredits B's self or character in the eyes of O; this appraisal triggers state x; x is subsequently labelled either shame or embarrassment depending on how B perceives him- or herself to be discredited. Sabini and Silver (2005) acknowledge that their explanation covers episodes involving a faux pas on the person's part and that there are other circumstances of embarrassment to which it does not apply: namely, being the object of social attention and 'sticky' situations where someone's conduct threatens another person's 'face'. They do not discuss whether state x is accompanied by any particular expression or how a blush might relate to the assignment of a label to this state. Examples of the kinds of circumstances they describe as embarrassing (Sabini et al., 2000) – faux pas, being the object of attention, 'sticky' situations – all appear in the episodes analysed in the study reported here; all can elicit a blush. O'Farrell (1997, p. 111) relates the blush to both flaws in character and transient social difficulties, describing the blush as 'expressive of a deep personal truth (expressive of character, the self, of the body) ... and the appropriate local response to and inevitable product of the pressure of social circumstances – as a mechanism ... the workings of which forward the grander social work of legibility and manners'.

## Self-consciousness

Rather than focus on what differentiates shame and embarrassment it is useful to ask what it is that they have in common and how this might relate to the blush. Two recurrent themes in the literature are self-consciousness and exposure. Self-consciousness is a state of mind that brings together two perspectives on the self: the individual's own perspective and his or her imagination of how he or she appears to others or, as Taylor (1985) conceptualizes it, the adoption of a higher-order observer-view on the self. It is a distinct state that is brought about by something specific, and is distinguishable from self-consciousness in the sense of our ongoing concern with our self-presentation and reputation (Rochat, 2009). Harris (1990) defined this state as acute negative public self-attention (ANPS-A) and argued that 'blushing ... is the hallmark of ANPS-A' (p. 69).

In summary, one hypothesis is that the blush is not specific to either shame or embarrassment but accompanies a state of self-consciousness which is common to both of these and to shyness. As Rochat (2009) argues, the underlying concern is with reputation and ultimately with the fear of social rejection. Scheff (1988) construes shame – and embarrassment as a form of shame – as an emotion that exerts a powerful influence on our lives, and that forms part of what he termed the deference-emotion system. Like Darwin, Scheff relates shame to people's perception of how others view them; furthermore, like Darwin, he considers that blushing is caused by shame.

## Exposure and shame

A second recurrent theme in the literature on shame is exposure, as noted in the introduction to this chapter. I have examined the role of exposure in the blush and aimed to show that blushing often occurs when the self is exposed or threatened with exposure. The findings of the content analysis study are consistent with this position. They are also consistent with previous research findings. For example, factor analysis of a self-report measure of individual variation in tendency to blush (Leary & Meadows, 1991) identified two factors. One was interpreted in terms of unwanted social attention, and its items refer to being in the presence of an audience, being conspicuous and being the object of attention; all common themes in the study reported here and in Leary and colleagues' (1992) account of blushing (see Leary & Toner, Chapter 4, this volume). The second factor has proved less straightforward to interpret but its items refer to interactions between individuals and include talking about a personal matter or a sexual topic (Edelmann & Skov, 1993, labelled this factor 'personal exposure'). The items loading on this factor describe the kinds of social situations that recur in the fiction episodes analysed in this study.

While many of the occasions of blushing, particularly in the questionnaire sample, are consistent with the theory that the blush is a response to unwanted social attention, other occasions are more difficult to explain in these terms. A sudden shift in awareness can be sufficient to cause a blush. It may be triggered by an allusion to something that is known only to the blusher. The prospect of a sensitive topic being raised can be sufficient for a blush, in either the person about to raise it, the person who anticipates that he or she is about to hear it, or both. Unwanted attention can be elicited by the blush rather than be its cause.

While the findings from our study relate the blush to exposure, several questions remain. Can we go beyond the weak form of the theory and assert that all occasions of blushing can be analysed in terms of exposure? The person who is criticized or challenged or whose behaviour is the subject of comment is exposed to view. Being open to scrutiny means that everyone can potentially evaluate us, and we are at risk that people will think differently about us because of the new information they have about us or the insight they have gained into our motives. Being the recipient of praise, thanks and compliments is more problematic – why should these make us blush? These circumstances also pose a challenge to shame and embarrassment theorists. Being praised seems incongruous with the thesis that shame is a matter of concerns about being negatively evaluated by others. It may be shaming because it results in the individual appearing to be different from others. Or it may create awareness of a discrepancy between what is being publicly attributed to us and our private view of ourselves: 'even a "positive" global evaluation can be a trigger to a shame episode if the evaluation is incongruent with the individual's sense of self' (Poulson, 2000, p. 14).

Perhaps, too, there is something inherently shaming about being self-consciously conspicuous, about being open to evaluation by others. Finally, public praise can be a source of embarrassment by posing a challenge to the person to act appropriately in front of an audience, to display neither too much nor too little modesty, to play down the honour without appearing to criticize those who have bestowed it. More investigation needs to be undertaken; nevertheless, the findings serve as a caution about assuming that a violation of a social norm is necessary for shame, embarrassment or blushing.

The visible blush can contribute to a social encounter, noticed and perhaps acted upon by those present. It can make it difficult to sustain the identity that the individual has projected into the encounter. It has the potential to communicate to others something unwanted in what it says about the blusher or others who are present or who are known by those present, or in terms of its effect upon the encounter. What is exposed can alter an observer's view of the person who blushes; in particular it can discredit him or her in the eyes of the observer. It can create a predicament for the current encounter and have implications for future encounters. The difficulties that are created for the self can be of different kinds and degrees, and these differences might map onto distinctions between shame and embarrassment. How serious are the consequences for the individual in the short term and in the longer term? Some things cannot be unsaid or undone; other matters can be quickly forgiven or give rise to humour, if not immediately, at least in the future (see also Miller, Chapter 9, this volume).

### But why a blush?

Explanations of blushing come up against the question why our reaction to exposure or unwanted attention or our expression of shame, embarrassment or shyness takes this particular form at this specific site on the body. Darwin argued that the face is our most conspicuous body feature and attention that is paid to a region of the body causes vasodilatation of blood vessels in that region. Other writers have regarded the blush as a sign or 'badge' of shame: it visibly displays our shame, we are aware that it does so, and this, together with the fact that we cannot control our blushing and thus cannot hide it, acts as a constraint upon our behaviour. An alternative view is that the blush is a mask, an attempt to conceal our shame. Hart (2005, p. 4) provides an example from Pocaterra's *Due dialoghi della vergogna*, published in 1592: 'since shame threatens the soul revealed in the face, blood rushes to the face to cover it, with gestures of covering-up and concealment providing a second line of defence'. An English example from 1606 is: 'the minde finding that what is to be reprehended in us, cometh from abroade, it seeketh to hide the fault committed, and to avoid the reproach thereof, by setting that colour on our face as a maske to defend us withal' (Lodowick Bryskett, *A Discourse of Civil Life*, London, 1606, cited by Schoenfeldt, 2004, pp. 60–1).

Evolutionary explanations of shame regard its expression and associated action tendencies – gaze aversion, shrinking posture, hiding, fleeing – as appeasement displays that signal to dominant others the ashamed person's acceptance of a subordinate role (Fessler, 2004). From this perspective a blush is a component of a human appeasement display (van Hooff, Chapter 5, this volume).

This explanation of the blush is consistent with conceptions of shame in terms of deference to the group and fear of social rejection argued by Scheff (1994) and Rochat (2009). Castelfranchi and Poggi (1990) have explicitly conceived of the blush as a signal of apology and appeasement.

This implies that, whether or not the blusher has been guilty of some action that would bring about social disapproval or rejection, the fact that the action could be interpreted as such is sufficient to trigger a blush. De Jong and Dijk (Chapter 12, this volume) provide a thorough discussion of research into the signal properties of a blush. Nevertheless, a continuing problem with this explanation is the relatively poor visibility of the blush among people with dark skin pigmentation.

Thoughts on exposure encourage speculation on possible alternative explanations of the evolutionary origin of the blush. Being conspicuous or exposed is threatening for many species since it potentially brings them to the attention of predators. Organisms try to maintain cover and prefer to explore their environment from a safe base, often hurrying back there after forays for food, potential mates and so on. There may be something innately arousing about being exposed and unable to escape or hide. The evolutionary origins of the blush may lie in arousal that is triggered by being conspicuous and hence exposed and vulnerable; over time this has become associated with being socially conspicuous and at risk of social rejection.

An alternative view is that the blush represents a sudden shift in arousal that takes place when action is inhibited. Frijda (1986, p. 168) suggested that the blush is associated with a state of ambivalence: 'an action tendency that is stopped, blocked, or suppressed. Blushing thus could result from sudden inhibition of some tendency to act.' Salzen (2010) suggests why this inhibition would result in vasodilatation: he argues that the blush represents physiological rebound from the shift of blood to the musculature for immediate vigorous action and where that action fails to take place; blushing occurs when the desired escape from being the centre of social attention is thwarted. Certainly blushing, like embarrassment, is often accompanied by fluster: uncertainty what to do and difficulty in thinking clearly. But why does inhibition result in vasodilatation in the blush region? At our current state of knowledge these suggestions are speculative.

## Conclusion

We can gain insight into the circumstances of blushing by examining occasions of blushing, whether these are recalled by research participants or described in works of fiction. The content analysis reported in this chapter found that occasions can be categorized effectively using a scheme developed for the analysis of episodes of shame augmented by a category that codes protocols in terms of the exposure of something that ought not to be disclosed. This raises questions about the relation of the blush to shame and embarrassment. Cross-cultural and historical evidence shows that blushing is a sign of shame in different languages and that this usage has predominated in the English language, at least as represented in documentary material. The notion that blushing is the hallmark of embarrassment is consistent with a recent trend in English usage but not if a broader cultural or historical perspective is adopted. The kinds of occasions that trigger a blush can involve either shame or embarrassment; the examples provided in Darwin's chapter, such as undressing for a medical examination, might be labelled as embarrassing rather than shaming by a contemporary reader. It is useful to consider what experiences are common to shame and embarrassment. Self-consciousness and exposure are key elements in both experiences and in blushing.

In this chapter I have explored the relation between 'exposure theory' as a potential explanation of the circumstances of blushing and a theory of shame proffered by Lewis (1971) and Scheff (1988, 1994). This highlights the relation between the notion of 'what ought not to be exposed' and anxieties about social acceptance and social rejection. The notion of exposure does, I suggest, provide insight into occasions of blushing. The role of the blush in many of these occasions is subtle, sometimes scarcely noticed, and while this is identified in writers' descriptions of social encounters it may not be spontaneously mentioned when research participants are invited to nominate examples of blushing. The differences among sources in the content analysis study could be followed up in studies with larger sample sizes and perhaps experimental designs.

A frequent theme in questionnaires and fiction is reference to sexual matters including sexual attraction. The relation between these and the blush require more investigation. Darwin speculated on it in his *N notebook*, relating it to his thesis that blushing is triggered by imagining what others think of our appearance (Gruber, 1974). Psychoanalytical perspectives also tend to link the blush with sexual excitement: for example, Feldman (1962, cited by Karch, 1971, p. 44) argued that women (but apparently not men, where the picture is 'more complex') blush to 'prove their innocence and chastity, and ... to indicate sexual excitement and reveal their interest in sex'. Of course it might simply be that incidents with sexual implications are common merely because they are especially likely to produce embarrassment or unwanted attention among the young people who are typically recruited for psychological research (and who are often of most interest to novelists). Finally, literary perspectives (e.g., O'Farrell, 1997) draw attention to the sensual nature of the blush in literature. This is an issue that warrants further investigation.

Several questions about exposure theory remain to be addressed: can all instances of blushing be explained in these terms? Will this perspective prove fruitful in the analysis of actual occasions when people blush? Will it help explain why our response to certain circumstances triggers vasodilatation of blood vessels below the facial skin, resulting in the visible blush?

## REFERENCES

Bowen, E. (1964). *The little girls.* London: Panther Books.
Buss, A. H. (1980). *Self-consciousness and social anxiety.* San Francisco: Freeman.
Casimir, M. J., & Schnegg, M. (2002). Shame across cultures: the evolution, ontogeny and function of a moral emotion. In H. Keller, Y. H. Poortinga & A. Schölmerich (Eds.), *Between biology and culture: perspectives on ontogenetic development.* Cambridge University Press, 270–300.
Castelfranchi, C., & Poggi, I. (1990). Blushing as a discourse: was Darwin wrong? In W. R. Crozier (Ed.), *Shyness and embarrassment: perspectives from social psychology.* Cambridge University Press, 230–51.
Chantrell, G. (2004). *Oxford dictionary of word histories.* Oxford University Press.
Crozier, W. R. (2000). Blushing, social anxiety and exposure. In W. R. Crozier (Ed.), *Shyness: development, consolidation, and change.* London: Routledge, 154–70.
  (2001). Blushing and the exposed self: Darwin revisited. *Journal of the Theory of Social Behaviour,* **31**, 61–72.
  (2006). *Blushing and the social emotions.* Basingstoke: Palgrave Macmillan.
Darwin, C. (1872/1999). *The expression of the emotions in man and animals.* Corrected 3rd edn with an introduction, afterword and commentaries by Paul Ekman. London: HarperCollins.

Deigh, J. (1983). Shame and self-esteem: a critique. *Ethics*, **93**, 225–45.
Dennett, D. C. (2001). The computational perspective. *Edge* (17 November). Available at http://edge.org/conversation/the-computational-perspective. Accessed 26 May 2011.
Edelmann, R. J. (1990). Embarrassment and blushing: a component-process model, some initial descriptive and cross-cultural data. In W. R. Crozier (Ed.), *Shyness and embarrassment: perspectives from social psychology*. Cambridge University Press, 204–29.
Edelmann, R. J., & Skov, V. (1993). Blushing propensity, social anxiety, anxiety sensitivity and awareness of bodily sensations. *Personality and Individual Differences*, **14**, 495–8.
Eliot, G. (1806/1976). *The mill on the Floss*. London: Dent.
Feldman, S. (1962). Blushing, fear of blushing, and shame. *Journal of the American Psychoanalytic Association*, **10**, 368–85.
Fessler, D. M. T. (2004). Shame in two cultures: implications for evolutionary approaches. *Journal of Cognition and Culture*, **4**, 207–62.
Fontaine, R. J., Poortinga, Y. H., Setiadi, B., & Markam, S. S. (2002). Cognitive structure of emotion terms in Indonesia and the Netherlands. *Cognition and Emotion*, **16**, 61–86.
Frijda, N. J. (1986). *The emotions*. Cambridge University Press.
Gottschalk, L., Winget, C., & Gleser, G. (1969). *Manual for using the Gottschalk–Gleser Content Analysis Scales*. Berkeley: University of California Press.
Gross, E., & Stone, S. P. (1964). Embarrassment and the analysis of role requirements. *American Journal of Sociology*, **50**, 1–15.
Gruber, H. (1974). *Darwin on man: a psychological study of scientific creativity. Together with Darwin's early and unpublished notebooks*. Transcribed and annotated by Paul H. Barrett. London: Wildwood House.
Harris, P. R. (1990). Shyness and embarrassment in everyday life and in psychological theory. In W. R. Crozier (Ed.), *Shyness and embarrassment: perspectives from social psychology*. Cambridge University Press, 59–86.
Hart, P. (2005). The badge of shame: blushing in early modern English literature. *Ecloga Online Journal*, 4. Available at www.strath.ac.uk/media/faculties/hass/knowledgeexchange/ecloga/media_135062_en.pdf. Accessed 31 October 2011.
Heider, K. G. (1991). *Landscapes of emotion: mapping three cultures of emotion in Indonesia*. Cambridge University Press.
Hogan, P. C. (2010). Fictions and feelings: on the place of literature in the study of emotion. *Emotion Review*, **2**, 184–95.
Izard, C. E. (1977). *Human emotions*. New York: Plenum Press.
Karch, F. E. (1971). Blushing. *Psychoanalytical Review*, **58**, 37–50.
Keltner, D., & Buswell, B. N. (1997). Embarrassment: its distinct form and appeasement functions. *Psychological Bulletin*, **122**, 250–70.
Leary, M. R., Britt, T. W., Cutlip, W. D., & Templeton, J. L. (1992). Social blushing. *Psychological Bulletin*, **107**, 446–60.
Leary, M. R., & Meadows, S. (1991). Predictors, elicitors, and concomitants of social blushing. *Journal of Personality and Social Psychology*, **60**, 254–62.
Lewis, H. B. (1971). *Shame and guilt in neurosis*. New York: International Universities Press.

MacCurdy, J. T. (1930). The biological significance of blushing and shame. *British Journal of Psychology*, **21**, 174–82.
Metcalf, R. (2006). Unrequited narcissism: on the origin of shame. *Studies in the History of Ethics*, **8**. Available at www.historyofethics.org/092006/092006Metcalf.shtml. Accessed 8 November 2011.
Michel, J.-P., Shen, Y. K., Aiden, A. P., Veres, A., Gray, M. K., The Google Books Team, Pickett, J. P., Hoiberg, D., Clancy, D., Norvig, P., Orwant, J., Pinker, S., Nowak, M. A., & Aiden, E. L. (2010). Quantitative analysis of culture using millions of digitized books. *Science*, **331**(6014), 176–82.
Miller, R. S. (1996). *Embarrassment: poise and peril in everyday life*. New York: Guilford Press.
O'Farrell, M. (1997). *Telling complexions: the nineteenth-century novel and the blush*. Durham, NC: Duke University Press.
Parrott, W. G., & Smith, S. F. (1991). Embarrassment: actual vs typical cases, classical vs prototypical representations. *Cognition and Emotion*, **5**, 467–88.
Poulson, C. (2000). *Shame: the master emotion?* University of Tasmania School of Management, Working Paper Series, no. 20–3.
Rochat, P. (2009). *Others in mind: social origins of self-consciousness*. Cambridge University Press.
Roth, P. (2001). *The dying animal*. London: Vintage.
Sabini, J., Siepmann, M., Stein, J., & Meyerowitz, M. (2000). Who is embarrassed by what? *Cognition and Emotion*, **14**, 213–40.
Sabini, J., & Silver, M. (1997). In defense of shame: shame in the context of guilt and embarrassment. *Journal of the Theory of Social Behaviour*, **27**, 1–15.
(2005). Why emotion names and experiences don't neatly pair. *Psychological Inquiry*, **16**, 1–10.
Salzen, E. (2010). Letter: flushing and blushing. *The Psychologist*, **23**, 539.
Scheff, T. J. (1988). Shame and conformity: the deference-emotion system. *American Sociological Review*, **53**, 395–406.
(1994). *Microsociology: discourse, emotion, and social structure*. University of Chicago Press.
Scheff, T. J., & Retzinger, S. M. (1991). *Emotions and violence: shame and rage in destructive conflicts*. Lexington Press.
Scheler, M. (1913/1987). Shame and feelings of modesty, in *Person and self-value*, trans. M. Frings. Dordrecht: Martinus Nijhoff.
Schoenfeldt, M. (2004). 'Commotion strange': passion in *Paradise Lost*. In G. K. Paster, K. Rowe & M. Floyd-Wilson (Eds.), *Reading the early passions: essays in the critical history of emotion*. Philadelphia: University of Pennsylvania Press, 43–67.
Strathern, A. (1977). Why is shame on the skin? In J. Blacking (Ed.), *The anthropology of the body*. London: Academic Press, 99–110.
Tallis, R. (2008). *The kingdom of infinite space*. London: Atlantic Books.
Taylor, G. (1985). *Pride, shame and guilt: emotions of self-assessment*. Oxford: Clarendon.
Tomkins, S. S. (1963). *Affect, imagery, consciousness. Vol. 2: The negative affects*. New York: Springer.

Tracy, J. L., & Robins, R. W. (2004). Putting the self into self-conscious emotions: a theoretical model. *Psychological Inquiry*, **15**, 103–25.

Williams, B. (1993). *Shame and necessity*. Berkeley: University of California Press.

Zahavi, D. (2010). Shame and the exposed self. In J. Webber (Ed.), *Reading Sartre: on phenomenology and existentialism*. London: Routledge, 211–26.

# 12 Signal value and interpersonal implications of the blush

*Peter J. de Jong and Corine Dijk*

## Introduction

Blushing is a highly common response and most people blush at least occasionally (Edelmann, 1990). A remarkable feature of the blush is that it may occur in many different types of situations: when spilling coffee on someone's trousers, when making a stupid remark during a meeting, when construction workers start whistling at you as you're passing, when being praised by your boss, when getting caught as you are about to leave the shop without paying, when someone bluntly asks if you have had sex lately, when being stared at, or just when the neighbour says hello to you. One may wonder: what is the common factor? And if there is a common factor, what is the meaning of the blush? Does it convey any relevant information about the blushing actor, about his or her traits or state, or about the situation in which the blush occurred? And if so, is the blush consistently associated with a particular mental/motivational state or just loosely coupled? Is it sufficiently consistent (within a particular context) to be useful for observers to infer relevant information about the actor?

In an attempt to arrive at some answers to all of these questions, we will first evaluate to what extent the blush can be considered as a meaningful, reliable signal. Subsequently, we will address the issue of what might in fact be signalled by the sudden reddening of the face: what type of information may be provided by a blush, what mental/motivational state can be inferred? Then we will discuss the potential social implications of displaying a blush. In the final section we will critically evaluate the empirical support for the signalling properties of the blush.

### Is the blush a reliable signal?

Several theorists have hypothesized that blushing has signal value in interpersonal contexts (e.g., Burgess, 1839; de Waal, 1995). Some have even argued that the blush has distinct signalling properties and conveys particular information that would otherwise remain hidden from observing others (e.g., Castelfranchi & Poggi, 1990; Frank, 1988). Indeed, several aspects of the facial blush invite speculation about its properties as a signalling device. First, although the blush may be elicited in many different types of situations, all of these situations imply the presence of other people (Leary & Meadows, 1991). So the least one can say is that in a typical blush-eliciting situation there is not only a transmitter (actor) but also a potential receiver (observer).

Another remarkable feature of the blush is that it typically expresses itself on the face (e.g., Simon & Shields, 1996). In fact, the specific physiological make-up which enables the blush response (e.g., beta-adrenergic receptors in facial veins) is restricted to this specific area of the human body (Mellander et al., 1982; Wilkin, 1988): an area that is typically uncovered and at the centre of social attention (Darwin, 1872/1989). Since facial expressions play such a crucial role in human communication (e.g., Goffman, 1967), this feature of the blush provides further ammunition for the view that displaying a blush may have important social implications.

Moreover, there is evidence that humans are well equipped to perceive the blush. The visual system in humans has been found to be especially sensitive to colours in the frequencies reflecting the colour of oxygenated (i.e., arterial) and de-oxygenated (i.e., venous) blood (Changizi et al., 2006). Thus, people seem ready for detecting subtle changes in blood circulation of the skin, and to differentiate between a reddening of the skin because of vasodilatation of facial arterioles (e.g., in the context of thermoregulation) and reddening because of vasodilatation of facial veins in the context of social blushing, although it should be noted that thus far this has never been put to the test. To the extent that the sudden vasodilatation of facial veins strongly correlates with a particular state (just as the reddening of the external female sex organs of a baboon is associated with being in a fertile state), this may provide people with the opportunity to infer a particular physical or mental/motivational state on the basis of the blush.

Germane to this, the ethologist Tinbergen (1952) argued that for a signal to be reliable it should be strongly correlated with a particular physical or mental state; it should be difficult to fake; and its absence may be taken as signalling the absence of the associated physical or mental state. At the very least, it seems beyond doubt that the sudden reddening of the face is extremely difficult to fake, and we guess that most people would agree that the blush can neither be intentionally elicited (when it would be efficient to pretend to blush) nor be intentionally suppressed (when it would be efficient to pretend not to blush). The exact nature of the mental/motivational state that is associated with the blush might be more controversial. In the following section we will therefore explore whether this principle also applies to the blush response (see also Frank, 1988).

## Signal value of the blush

Several approaches may help us to gain insight into the 'blush-contingent' mental/motivational state. First, it would be helpful to see what state is implied by writings about the blush. As a more direct approach, it would also be highly informative to know what feelings or emotions the actors themselves tend to report during blush-eliciting events. Third, one could catalogue the blush-eliciting events and see whether there might be any commonalities in the blush-eliciting antecedents that might inform us about the mental/motivational state of the blusher. Finally, it seems important to consider the underlying physiological mechanisms of the blush, as these might also provide important clues that help us to infer what mental/motivational state might co-occur with the acute reddening of the face. In the following sections we will use these various approaches to explore the critical features of the blush-contingent mental/motivational state.

### *Concurrent emotional feelings*

**Shame.** In early religious texts such as the Bible, blushing is clearly linked to moral sentiments as reflected by the experience of shame. In line with the requirements of being a reliable signal, not only is the presence of a blush associated with the presence of moral sentiment (e.g., '... Oh, my God! I am ashamed, and blush to lift up my head to thee, my God.', Ezra, 9:6), but also the absence of the blush is interpreted as implying the absence of moral sentiment (e.g., '... Are they ashamed of these disgusting actions? Not at all – they don't even know how to blush!', Jeremiah, 8:12). In one of the first scientific essays on the blush, Burgess (1839) also maintained that the blush reflects a moral sentiment. He argued that 'blushing ... is a peculiar faculty of ... the internal emotions exhibiting themselves, for no individual blushes voluntarily; it would, therefore, appear to serve as a check on the conscience, and prevent the moral faculties from being infringed upon, or deviating from their allotted path' (p. 24). He further maintained that the probable intent of the Creator, in endowing man with this peculiar property, was that 'the soul might have the sovereign power of displaying in the cheek, that part of the human body which is uncovered by all nations, the various internal emotions of the moral feelings whenever they are infringed upon either by accident or design, and that this precaution had the salutary effect of enabling our fellow beings to know whenever we transgressed or violated those rules which should be held sacred, as being the bonds that unite man and man in the civilized state of social existence' (p. 49). Thus, Burgess's analysis seems to imply that the blush-contingent mental state is shame and/or the consciousness of guilt.

**Shame and embarrassment before others**. Darwin (1872/1989) also contended in his *The Expression of the Emotions in Man and Animals* that the blush is the signature expression of the self-conscious emotions such as shame and embarrassment. However, Darwin emphasized that the experience of a moral sentiment per se seems insufficient to elicit a blush. Accordingly, he noted, for example, that 'it is not the sense of guilt, but the thought that others think or know us to be guilty which crimsons the face ...' (p. 261). This important feature of the blush-contingent mental state is emphasized further in the work of Castelfranchi and Poggi (1990). They corroborate Darwin's view by pointing to the importance of differentiating between two types of shame: shame before others and shame before oneself. The critical difference between these types of shame is that only for shame before others is it critical that the actors assume that the observing others share the transgressed social rule. For example, only if the actor assumes that the observing others also find it very important to be exactly in time for a planned meeting will they feel shame before others when arriving a few minutes late. When they think that others are not very strict about this, they may still feel private shame upon arriving late, but not shame before others. Following Castelfranchi and Poggi (1990), the blush will only be evident in the former case as they assume that the blush will only occur if the actor experiences (also) shame before others.

They also noted two important prerequisites for arriving at this blush-eliciting state. First, they emphasized that shame before others will only arise before those whose esteem we seek. Thus, if a person is somehow indifferent about the judgment of the other persons who observe his or her violation of a particular rule, shame may be felt only before oneself but not before these others, and thus, in Castelfranchi and Poggi's (1990) view, blushing is not likely to occur. Second, they noted that it is critical that the actor assumes that the other person interprets the actor's behaviour as a transgression, even when in reality this may not be the case. Thus, even socially acceptable behaviour, such as comforting a colleague who has just heard very bad news by putting your arms around her, may still give rise to shame before others when the comforting actor assumes that a third person may misinterpret the situation as reflecting some kind of hidden love affair.

It seems relevant to note that in their analysis Castelfranchi and Poggi (1990) explicitly reserve the term 'shame' for the negative, painful mental state that is elicited when people regret or fear a loss of face following a transgression. Yet, others might argue that embarrassment, too, may be a blush-contingent state, depending on the type of social norm that has been violated (Keltner, 1995). Indeed there is evidence that people typically report feelings of embarrassment following less severe violations, or a breach of social conventions, whereas relatively severe flaws have been found to be more typically associated with feelings of shame (Tangney et al., 1996). In the light of this, one would predict that blushing might be correlated with both feelings of shame and embarrassment (see also see Miller, this volume, Chapter 9; Scott, Chapter 10).

Consistent with this, people report blushing in both embarrassing and shameful situations (e.g., Shields et al., 1990). In a similar vein, studies actually measuring the blush have shown that the blush can be elicited in embarrassing situations (e.g., being observed while singing a children's song; Shearn et al., 1992) as well as in shameful conditions (e.g., upon transgression of a moral value; de Jong et al., 2002). Interestingly, there is also evidence that it is not necessary to violate a rule oneself to reach a blush-contingent mental state; it has been shown that witnessing a significant other being involved in a self-presentational predicament may also give rise to an 'empathic' blush (Shearn et al., 1999). In this case the blush may not only signify that the actor feels shame/embarrassment before others, but also that he/she feels strongly associated with the actual actor.

### Antecedents

**Violation of shared rules.** In their analysis of conditions that may give rise to a blush, Castelfranchi and Poggi (1990) maintain that only violations of shared rules may give rise to the proper mental state that correlates with the blush. Thus far, it has not been directly tested whether a blush will indeed only occur following transgressions of *shared* social rules. There is, however, some indirect evidence from a vignette study which challenges this strong assumption (de Jong, 1999; experiment 3). In that study, we instructed participants to identify themselves with the actor, and used several scripts in which an observer saw the actor violate rules that are only complied with among restricted groups of the total population (e.g., 'One should not eat meat'). As the critical experimental manipulation, we systematically varied the actor's and observer's compliance with these rules and asked participants to estimate the probability that the actor (e.g., the one who ate the meat) would blush.

In line with the theoretical framework of Castelfranchi and Poggi (1990), the probability ratings of blushing were highest (i.e., 85 per cent) for the scenarios referring to violations of rules which were shared by the actors and the observers. Yet, in contrast to the idea that the blush response would only occur when the actor and the observer shared the violated rule, participants considered it also quite likely (approximately 50 per cent) that they would blush in the types of scenarios where only the observer or only the actor complied with the social rule. These results seem to suggest that the blush does not so much coincide with regret or fear because of having violated a shared rule, but rather with the more general regret or fear of making a negative social impression on the observer (e.g., as a result of violating one's own or the observer's rule) (cf. Leary *et al.*, 1992). Thus, it seems that the assumption of shared values is not a critical prerequisite for the blush to occur, and on the basis of the available evidence it seems most parsimonious to propose that the blush coincides with the more general feeling that one is thwarted in one's goals of esteem before others or that one is about to thwart them.

**Undesired social attention**. This seems also consistent with the conclusion of Leary and colleagues (1992; see also Leary & Toner, Chapter 4) that the various categories of situations in which people typically tend to blush all have in common that they are characterized by undesired social attention. Clearly, only if the actor is somehow subject to social attention can the other person become aware of the transgression. In the typical situation that one's goal of esteem before others is at stake this social attention will logically be undesired. Thus, it seems highly plausible that the blush often coincides with the experience of undesired social attention. Yet, there seems no perfect contingency between blushing and undesired social attention. First, one can think of situations involving undesired social attention which will probably *not* give rise to a blush. For example, consider a student who starts whistling at the distinguished professor when she enters the lecture hall, the famous television personality who is chased by paparazzi, the Olympic champion who is approached by pushy fans, or the girl who is playing the piano when her younger sister starts commenting on her skill, and so on. In such cases, undesired social attention is likely to result in irritation or even anger instead of blushing. Second, there also seem to be situations involving desired instead of undesired social attention that nevertheless can elicit a blush: for example, when a girl is asked out for a drink by the most handsome guy in the class, or when someone receives a deserved compliment from his or her superior. Of course in the latter cases the experienced social attention may become undesirable but not as an antecedent condition, rather as a consequence of their blushing, since people typically dislike being caught while displaying a blush (Shields et al., 1990). Thus, the strong view expressed by Leary et al. (1992) that undesired social attention is a necessary and sufficient feature of blush-eliciting situations is not beyond dispute.

**Submissiveness.** Meanwhile, both types of apparent exceptions seem helpful in specifying further the presumed blush-contingent mental/motivational state. First, the situations exemplifying 'no blush despite undesired social attention' seem to point to an important restricting condition: blushing seems not to occur if the actor is in a dominant/favourable position compared to the observing other (elder vs younger sister; professor vs student; champion vs fan). Thus, it seems that the actor not only needs to have a goal of esteem before the observing other and thus to care about his or her judgment, but also to be (experience being) in a subordinate position compared to the observer. This suggests that the blush co-occurs with a motivational orientation towards submissiveness (see also de Waal, 1995). The situations exemplifying 'a blush in the absence of undesired social attention' are also consistent with this suggestion. In both examples, the observing other seems to be in a dominant (supraordinate) position. Moreover, paying a compliment can perhaps even more generally be considered as an intrinsically dominant type of behaviour (apparently the sender has the authority to judge the actor's behaviour/accomplishment), which, therefore, may automatically place the receiver in a subordinate position.

*Physiological characteristics*

Finally, the specific physiological underpinning of the blush may also point to an important feature of the blush-contingent mental/motivational state. That is, the reddening of the face depends on a fast-acting neuronal system (see Drummond, Chapter 2). This may be taken to reflect that the blush relates to an acute awareness of an urgent threat that requires immediate action. In response to a typical external threat (e.g., an angry, barking dog) motivational systems are activated to sustain 'fight or flight' behaviours. Under these conditions the acute activation of the sympathetic branch of the autonomic nervous system can be explained as a functional reflex that sustains the metabolic requirements for these defensive responses. However, in the typical blush-eliciting situations, neither fight nor flight responses seem appropriate or helpful, and would probably even contribute further to loss of face (see also Miskovic & Schmidt, Chapter 8, this volume). Perhaps, then, the activation of the sympathetic nervous system is due to the paradoxical situation that, on the one hand, the actor experiences a strong urge to flee (disappear, become invisible), while, on the other hand, the actor needs to inhibit this initial tendency, as such a response would make things even worse (cf. Crozier, 2006; Frijda, 1986). Clearly, this remains highly speculative as it is still a matter of debate how exactly the blush response has evolved and what physiological purpose lies at the heart of the activation of the sympathetic nervous system in the blush-eliciting situations (see van Hooff, Chapter 5). It seems nevertheless safe to conclude that the acute activation of the sympathetic branch that causes the reddening of the face indicates that the actor is subject to an acute and salient concern. Moreover, because it is virtually impossible to bring these autonomic responses under intentional control, the physiological underpinnings of the blush bear witness to the 'sincerity' of the actor's response.

To conclude, facial blushing seems to share all the relevant properties of a reliable signalling device. It seems not only impossible to fake, it seems also to co-occur with a specific mental state: the acute awareness that one's goal of esteem before the other is at stake together with the impulse to take a subordinate position.

## Social implications of the blush

### Theoretical speculations

Since the blush seems to fulfil all criteria of being a reliable signal (cf. Tinbergen, 1952), it may have acquired important interpersonal signalling functions. Accordingly, people may use the blush to understand the actors' behaviours and to make inferences about the dispositional characteristics and/or emotional state of the actors. What exactly people might infer on the basis of the actor's blush will logically be dependent on the context and social setting in which the blush is observed (cf. Costa et al., 2001). For example, in the context of a self-presentational predicament (e.g., arriving apparently underdressed to a business meeting), the blush may be taken as a signal that the actor feels embarrassed, is aware of the fact that his or her behaviour is inappropriate or may be taken as inappropriate (violating the social standards), is sincerely bothered by the possibility that he/she has made a negative impression on the observer, and feels the urge to humbly apologize for this faux pas. In such a context the blush may well elicit sympathy and serve as a remedial gesture in accordance with other displays of embarrassment such as touching the face or suppressing a smile (e.g., Keltner et al., 1997).

Yet, in the context of a straightforward moral transgression people might make a slightly different type of inference, and the transgression may therefore also have different social consequences. When, for instance, people observe the actor blushing upon being caught attempting to leave the restaurant without paying, they may infer that the actor is aware that he or she has committed a serious transgression, does care about others' judgment, feels guilty, fears the social consequences of being caught (e.g., aggression), and feels the urge to express a submissive apology. The blush following a moral transgression may therefore inhibit aggression and elicit reconciliation-related behaviours (cf. Tangney et al., 1996). The fact that blushing cannot be voluntarily produced seems of particular relevance in these contexts, as it prevents blushing from being used instrumentally. One might even argue that were opportunistic people able to simulate blushing, the blush response would eventually lose its specific communicative properties.

The fact that the blush cannot be voluntarily *suppressed* seems of particular relevance in another class of social contexts: social settings that are ambiguous with regard to the actor's behaviour (Crozier, 2004; see also Crozier, Chapter 11, this volume). For example, consider situations that may reflect a transgression, but not necessarily so, such as a person who starts blushing when he cannot find his train ticket when asked for it by a train authority. In their causal interpretation of the transgressor's behaviour, the observers will tend to overemphasize the role of the actor's negative dispositions and to underemphasize the influence of situational factors (the fundamental attribution error; Ross, 1977). Due to the pervasive logical fallacy of 'affirmation of the consequent' (Evans et al., 1993) (e.g., 'if a person does something undesirable, then that person will blush; the person blushes, thus the person must have done something undesirable'), observers might interpret blushing in the absence of a clear-cut antecedent of the blush response as a further confirmation of the undesirable (immoral) motives behind the actor's behaviour. Thus, the blush may lead observers to interpret ambiguous behaviour as reflecting an intentional (and thus unfair) act. In such a case the observer may, therefore, infer from the blush that the actor intentionally did not buy a ticket. In other words, the observer may use the blush to disambiguate the situation and may use the heuristic 'true innocence doesn't need a blush'. Hence in these cases the blush may be taken to reveal guilt.

Thus, although we propose that the blush always coincides with the acute awareness that one's goal of esteem before the other is at stake together with the impulse to take a subordinate position, its concrete signal value and/or the concrete interpersonal consequences of signalling this state seem highly dependent on the *context* in which the blush is elicited. Moreover, the inferences and social implications may also depend on the *characteristics of the observer*. For example, the signalling properties of the blush in interdependent situations may vary as a function of the observer's social value orientation. That is, one might expect that blushing has a different meaning for people who value cooperation and a fair distribution of resources (i.e., prosocials) than for people who are more inclined to work alone and to keep resources to themselves (i.e., 'proselfs'). Proselfs may infer from others' blushing that these individuals are exploitable, whereas prosocial individuals may use the blush to infer the actors' (lack of) trustworthiness (cf. Liebrand *et al.*, 1986).

Clearly, the literature on blushing is heavily dominated by speculations and conjectures whereas empirical research on social blushing is very scarce. There are nevertheless some empirical studies that have tested some of the hypotheses that have been put forward in this chapter. In the next section of this chapter we will discuss these studies in the light of the alleged signal value and social implications of the blush.

### *Empirical evidence*

**Clear-cut mishaps and moral transgressions**. Because blushing cannot be voluntarily produced, it seems virtually impossible to specifically vary the actors' blush response as a function of experimental conditions under *in vivo* circumstances. Accordingly, the first studies that directly tested the alleged communicative properties of the blush used vignettes rather than real-time interactions. In a first attempt to empirically document the view that social blushing might serve a remedial function, participants were presented with a series of vignettes which described incidents that had taken place in a shop (e.g., a shopper pushes a vase from a shelf; cf. Semin & Manstead, 1982) and asked them to evaluate these situations as if they were shoppers observing the incident (de Jong, 1999). In the vignettes, the actor could show one of three types of responses: the actor just left the shop after the incident, the actor showed motoric signs of shame and left the shop, or the actor displayed a blush and left the shop. In line with the idea that blushing serves as a remedial gesture, participants rated the blushing actors as being more friendly as well as more reliable than their non-blushing counterparts (de Jong, 1999, experiments 1 and 2). Also the incident itself was rated as less serious in the blush condition. In line with the view that the involuntary nature of the blush might strengthen its signal value, the remedial effects of blushing were more pronounced than those of motoric signs of shame.

An important limitation of these first studies was that the vignettes did not isolate the blush from the other features of an appeasement display. It can, therefore, not be ruled out that the participants in these experiments did not just imagine a reddening of the face (in the blush condition), but a complete emotional display including a blush. Thus, it remained to be tested whether merely blushing does indeed have remedial properties. Moreover, the vignettes explicitly described the actor's response. Asking participants about their judgment of the blushing actor thus requires people's explicit appreciation of this response. It might well be that the blush exerts its influence at a more implicit level. Hence, it remained to be tested whether indeed the blush may also elicit its remedial effect when the observers are not explicitly informed about the actor's blushing.

Therefore, a subsequent study (Dijk *et al.*, 2009) presented the participants with *photographs* of the actors (on a computer screen) rather than with an explicit description of the actor's response. As an additional issue, this study investigated whether the effects of the blush are restricted to contexts reflecting a mild social transgression which are typically associated with embarrassment, or whether similar effects could also be traced in the context of more severe transgressions such as hurting others emotionally or shortcomings in moral worth: conditions that are usually associated with shame (Keltner *et al.*, 1997). Therefore, in this study we used both vignettes representing obvious mishaps (e.g., bumping into a rack full of wine glasses; upsetting a pile of cans in the supermarket) and vignettes representing obvious moral transgressions (e.g., missing a funeral because of a party; driving away after crashing a car), along with displaying the actors in a photograph on the screen (Dijk *et al.*, 2009). Again, participants were instructed to imagine that they were the observer of the situation. The colour photographs consisted of the head and upper chest of models displaying shame, embarrassment or a neutral face (see Keltner *et al.*, 1997). For each facial expression, half of the photographs were manipulated to show a lifelike blush.

This subsequent study (Dijk *et al.*, 2009) also found that blushing has remedial properties. Importantly, displaying a blush on a neutral face positively affected the observers' judgments not only in the context of obvious mishaps but also in the context of transgressions. Specifically in the context of moral transgressions, blushing also led to more positive observers' judgments when the blush was displayed on top of shame. This pattern of findings indicates that blushing indeed has signal value in addition to other facial expressions. For all displays a blush intensified the impression that the actor felt ashamed or embarrassed. Mediational analyses suggested that blushing might succeed in affecting the observer's judgment via the enhancement of the perceived intensity of the actor's shame or embarrassment. Thus, the blush seems to signal that one experiences the moral emotion relatively intensively, which subsequently might give rise to a more positive judgment. Because the available range of expressing shame/embarrassment via contraction of the relevant facial musculature is restricted, the blush might have useful complementary remedial value, especially when one has already reached a full-blown (muscular) expression of shame/embarrassment. Moreover, blushing might have complementary value by attesting to the apparent sincerity that one is ashamed or embarrassed, because it is impossible to control the blush intentionally.

To examine the differential signal value of the muscular facial expressions of the emotions versus the blush, we additionally examined the relative efficacy of a blush vis-à-vis the facial expressions of embarrassment or shame without a blush (Dijk et al., 2009). Following a clear-cut transgression, a neutral but blushing face was rated as less ashamed than a facial expression of shame without a blush. However, merely displaying a blush elicited similar remedial effects to showing the facial expression of shame without a blush. The sincerity of the signal may be an explanation for this remedial effect of blushing. A sincere acknowledgment that one is aware of the wrongdoing may decrease the expectancy that the blushing individual will defect again (Gold & Weiner, 2000). Clearly, future research is necessary to test the robustness of these findings and to reach firmer conclusions about the mechanisms that underlie this effect of the blush on the observer's judgment.

*Social implications in the context of ambiguous social situations*

The situations described thus far in this section have reflected straightforward transgressions and mishaps. It remains to be seen, therefore, what type of information people might infer from the blush in more ambiguous situations that could reflect a transgression but not necessarily so. As we argued above, in such situations observers might well use the blush to disambiguate the situation and might tend to infer that the person may have done something undesirable ('true innocence doesn't need a blush'). Thus, rather than having remedial properties, the blush would reveal 'guilt'.

As a first step to testing the validity of this hypothesis we again presented participants with a series of vignettes (de Jong et al., 2003). Yet, in this study we not only used scenarios that referred to apparently involuntary mishaps and more serious moral transgressions, but also scenarios reflecting ambiguous situations that could be interpreted either as a transgression or as an accident. Corroborating the studies described in the previous section, the results of this subsequent vignette study again showed that blushing has favourable effects in the context of both a seemingly involuntary mishap and more serious and apparently voluntary moral transgressions (de Jong et al., 2003). As hypothesized, similar remedial effects of blushing were completely absent in the context of more ambiguous social situations (de Jong et al., 2003; experiment 1), or violations of socio-moral rules that were ambiguous with respect to the actor's intentionality (de Jong et al., 2003; experiment 2). Thus, in the absence of clear-cut transgressions or straightforward information with respect to the intentionality of a transgression, blushing did not result in a more positive evaluation of the actor as was found in the context of a mishap or a voluntary moral transgression. Instead, in the absence of straightforward antecedent behaviour, blushing tended to further undermine rather than to sustain the actor's trustworthiness. Meanwhile, the incident itself was judged as being considerably more serious when the actor displayed a blush. All in all, it appears that in the ambiguous situations, displaying a blush may substantiate observers' lingering suspicions that the blusher has behaved in a socially inappropriate manner (cf. de Jong et al., 2002).

### Blushing in real-time interactions

The vignette studies described above clearly showed that blushing actors were judged differently than their non-blushing counterparts (de Jong, 1999; de Jong et al., 2003; Dijk et al., 2009). However, to demonstrate that blushing really influences social interactions, it would be critical to test the influence of the blush in concrete as well as in imagined interpersonal situations (e.g., Parkinson & Manstead, 1993). Testing the influence of blushing on interpersonal behaviours is notoriously difficult as it requires: (1) that the experimental manipulation reliably elicits a (visible) blush in the actors, (2) the presence of at least one other individual who may observe the blush and whose judgments and/or behaviour may be influenced by the blush, and (3) a (controllable) social interaction during which the potential influence of the actor's blush response on the observer's behaviour can be reliably assessed. After extensive pilot work we eventually arrived at a modified and morally framed prisoner's dilemma game (PDG; de Jong et al., 2002). A PDG[1] is characterized by the occurrence of two conflicting motives (cooperation vs defection) which individuals experience in interdependent situations. In such a context, moral concerns with respect to cooperation are likely to be strong (e.g., Kerr, 1995). Accordingly, it has been shown that prosocial individuals' response strategy is typically guided by the aim to maximize joint outcomes, and to restore equality in outcomes (van Lange, 1999). Thus, prosocials generally approach interdependent others in a cooperative manner and continue to do so until the interdependent other fails to exhibit cooperative behaviour (van Lange, 1999). When being cheated, prosocials typically turn to non-cooperation in a rather unforgiving manner (van Lange, 2000). Thus, after being cheated, prosocial individuals will tend to reciprocate by defecting themselves.

To test the impact of blushing on people's appreciation of defecting others as well as on their interpersonal behaviour we designed a ten-trial PDG and selected a homogeneous group of individuals sharing the important social goal of cooperation (i.e., prosocials; de Jong et al., 2002). These individuals participated as pairs. To elicit a shameful transgression, for each pair, one individual was instructed to select the (for them non-habitual) defect-option on a pre-defined target trial (and to cooperate on all other trials). Of course the interdependent other was not aware of this instruction. Within this particular context we tested whether the interdependent other would evaluate the defector less negatively as a function of the defector's blush intensity and if the prosocial victim's habitual tendency to reciprocate cheating behaviour (cheat him- or herself on the next trial) would be attenuated by the defector's blush response. As expected, defecting led to a significant blush response in the defecting participant. However, the perceived intensity of the blush response was not significantly associated with the interdependent other's actual choice behaviour on the 'post-being cheated' trial. Meanwhile,

---

[1] In a PDG, participants play several rounds of decision making (cooperate or defect) with an opponent. Participants make their decision without knowing the opponent's decision and money can be earned in each round. Payout depends upon the participant's decision and that of the opponent. Normally, when both cooperate the division of money is equal. When one person defects whereas the other cooperates, the defector earns more than is received in the case of a joint cooperation; the cooperator earns little or nothing. When both participants defect they both earn little, but usually more than the cooperator in the case of one participant cooperating and the other participant defecting. In a morally framed PDG the cooperation option is primed as the moral option.

there was a meaningful relationship between the perceived intensity of the cheater's blush and the observer's judgment. Yet, the intensity of the blush response was not associated with a more favourable judgment of the blushing 'cheater'. In contrast, results indicated that the more the defector blushed, the less positively she was judged by the interdependent other. One explanation for this could be that the present context was ambiguous with respect to the defector's motive. The opponent's defecting could reflect innocent playing around (e.g., to prevent the experiment from getting boring), but also an intentional – and thus unfair – act to maximize outcomes for the self at the expense of the other person in the game. Also, here the observer might reason that if the defector was really innocent, then why would she blush?

We therefore carried out a subsequent PDG study in which we disambiguated the actor's behaviour in half of the participants, via informing the interdependent other that it was not the choice of the actor to defect but that she was forced to cheat as part of the experimental manipulation (Smits, 2003). Sustaining the hypothesis that the absence of a remedial effect in the earlier study might be attributed to the ambiguity of the experimental context, a positive relationship between the perceived intensity of the blush and the rated trustworthiness of the actor did emerge in the group of informed observers but not in the group of uninformed observers (Smits, 2003).

Although we were thus successful in showing that in real-time interactions displaying a blush following a transgression was associated with a more positive judgment, there were at least two shortcomings in this design (Smits, 2003). First, the behavioural measure (i.e., choice behaviour on the trial after being cheated) might have been too insensitive to detect the positive effect of the blush at the behavioural level. Second, the blush was clearly not isolated from other concomitant behaviour that might co-occur with the blush and could also have influenced observers, such as looking away or stammering. Therefore, we designed a subsequent study in an attempt to remedy both shortcomings.

In this subsequent study participants played the PDG with a virtual opponent via the internet (Dijk et al., 2011). After each round of the PDG, a photograph of the virtual opponent was shown on the screen (cf. Dijk et al., 2009). During the PDG, the virtual opponent always defected in the second round. Following defection, the opponent displayed a neutral face, a neutral face with a blush, an embarrassed face, or an embarrassed face with a blush. Thus, in half of the cases the cheating opponents blushed afterwards. To test if blushing affects the observers' tendencies to (not) trust or forgive the opponent after this defection, participants' trust-related behaviour was measured in a subsequent trust task, which we hoped would be more sensitive than the original categorical measure (cooperation or defection). In a trust task, participants decided how much money (0–10 euros) they wanted to give to the virtual opponent. They were further informed that the amount of money that the opponent received would be tripled, and that the opponent could return to the participant any amount of the money that she had just earned. The amount of money a participant gives to the opponent can be seen as an index of how much he/she trusts the opponent (to give a fair amount of money back). Thus, this study employed a more sensitive (quantitative) behavioural index of sustained trust and used a virtual instead of a real interaction to allow tight experimental control of the facial expression of the opponent (blush or no blush), while also controlling for possible concomitant behaviours that might influence observers' judgments.

The results of this study supported further the alleged remedial function of blushing; blushing systematically improved judgments of the transgressing opponent. Most importantly, the findings indicated that the remedial effects were also evident in the observer's behaviour. Blushing positively affected trust-related behaviour towards the defector in an interpersonal context. When the virtual opponent blushed after she defected she was entrusted with more money in the subsequent trust task than when she did not blush. This sustains the view that blushing can function as a signal that recuperates trustworthiness after a social transgression.

The study also provided some results that may help explain how the blush succeeded in influencing the observer's behaviour. First, the study showed that blushing positively affected the expectations of the opponent's future behaviour. By showing a blush the opponent appeared to show that, although she cannot present herself as irreproachable on this occasion, she is at least disturbed by the transgression and may be cooperative at some other time (cf. Goffman, 1967). Second, participants' responses showed that they believed that the blushing opponent was more worried about the other's judgment than the non-blushing opponent. Finally, blushing led to the impression that the opponent sincerely regretted the defection and was not just pretending to regret the defection. Clearly, it requires further research to test whether the influence of the blush on the interdependent other indeed critically depends on modifying these types of judgments.

Of course the PDG represents a highly specific interpersonal context and it remains important to test the influence of the blush also in other social situations. Germane to this, Xueni Pan (2009) used a completely different approach to circumvent the inherent difficulty of studying the influence of the blush in real-time interactions. In her study, she manipulated the absence/presence of a blush in a virtual character (avatar) and tested the impact of avatar blushing on real persons' behavioural responses. She instructed participants that some information would be presented about the 2008 Olympic Games by an avatar who would present a video. However, this video repeatedly failed to load. The avatar then apologized and the participant was invited to try again to start the video. In one condition the avatar never blushed whereas in the critical condition the avatar showed a reddening of the cheeks. A similar 'error message' could occur a maximum of ten times. This design thus allowed testing of whether participants' willingness to (again) restart the programme would be affected by the blush of the avatar. Interestingly, the proportion of participants who continued to the end (ten restarts) was greatly affected by the absence/presence of a blush on the avatar's cheeks. More than half of the participants in the non-blushing condition appeared willing to restart ten times, whereas only a small minority (18 per cent) of the participants in the cheek-blush condition reached the final trial. Thus, participants tended to withdraw earlier and were less tolerant if the avatar was blushing following the failure of the video to load.

Thus, during interactions with a virtual character the blush affected the behaviour of the observer. Yet, in this context it did clearly not have a positive, desirable effect. One explanation for this might be that people may usually consider a computer failure as a random error that may be solved by restarting, and for which no one in particular can be blamed or held responsible. However, by displaying the blush, the avatar may have prompted observers to hold the avatar responsible for the failure to get the video loaded. One or two times displaying a blush after a failure to start up properly may then be acceptable, but at some stage it would require more than an apology. Participants may start 'thinking' along the lines that it would be preferable for the avatar to do a proper job instead of making another apology. Future research is needed to arrive at more solid conclusions in this respect.

## Conclusions and future research

The available evidence clearly corroborates the view that blushing has relevant signal value in interpersonal situations. Moreover, it has been found that blushing also has unique signal value over and above other signs of shame or embarrassment before others. Both the signal value and the social implications of the blush have been shown to be highly context-dependent. In situations that clearly imply some kind of misbehaviour such as a faux pas or an obvious transgression, the blush showed face-saving properties and seems to serve as a nonverbal submissive excuse. Yet, in many other situations that are more ambiguous with regard to the blushing actors' antecedent behaviours and/or their underlying intentions, the blush may have undesirable revealing effects.

There are also some preliminary findings that may help explain how the blush succeeds in affecting the observer's appreciation of the actor. Most importantly, the internet PDG study (Dijk *et al.*, 2011) showed that participants believed that the blushing opponent was more worried about the other's judgment than the non-blushing opponent was. In addition, the findings indicated that blushing led to the impression that the opponent sincerely regretted the defection and was not just pretending to regret the defection. Together, these findings sustain the view that the blush may have a special role within the submissive and placatory behavioural signalling system, as a valid signal of sincere concern about others' judgments.

To the extent that indeed the blush has unique signalling properties, one may wonder what the impact of skin complexion is on the efficacy of this signalling device. There is clear evidence from both self-reports (Simon & Shields, 1996) and physiological studies that the physiological blush response is independent of people's skin colour (Drummond & Lim, 2000). However, the visibility of the blush response seems nevertheless to vary as a function of people's skin complexion. It would therefore be interesting to actually test whether skin complexion is a critical factor here and whether people whose blushing cannot be accurately detected may have acquired other displays and/or strategies to signal the blush-contingent mental state. Germane to this, previous experimental research showed that after a clear-cut predicament, participants typically engaged in (alternative) self-presentational tactics to improve their damaged social image when they were led to believe that the experimenter *did not* notice their blushing (on a bogus apparatus) (Leary *et al.*, 1996). It would be interesting to see whether this represents a more general tactic that people also use in other contexts (e.g., following a moral transgression) and most of all whether the strength of such motivated expression of embarrassment and/or shame may also vary as a function of temporary (e.g., ambient light) or relatively stable (e.g., skin complexion) differences in the visibility of one's blushing.

Although in the studies reported in this chapter blushing was found to influence the behaviour as well as the judgments of the observing participants, during the post-experimental debriefings it became evident that these participants were often completely unaware of the fact that blushing was somehow involved in the studies (e.g., Dijk *et al.*, 2009;

Dijk *et al.*, 2011). This is consistent with the view that the signal value of the blush may operate quickly and at an implicit level (cf. Willis & Todorov, 2006; Glashouwer *et al.*, 2011). Knowing the neural basis of perceiving a blush might help in understanding the mechanisms involved in this complex interpersonal response. It has been shown that specific brain networks are involved in the implicit judgment of faces in terms of trustworthiness (e.g., Winston *et al.*, 2002; Singer *et al.*, 2004). It would be interesting to see whether similar brain patterns are evident when participants observe blushing actors. Furthermore, by comparing the neural response to shame (without a blush) with the response to a blushing person we might be able to test the hypothesis that blushing, in particular, elicits neural responses that are associated with trustworthiness. This would also be relevant for the question whether or not blushing signals something that otherwise could not be signalled in these contexts: namely, that one is sincerely ashamed or embarrassed before others and willing to take a subordinate position.

People do blush in many types of situations and the research discussed in this chapter clearly shows that the effect of blushing is context-dependent (e.g., de Jong *et al.*, 2003). The situations that have been tested thus far are nevertheless restricted to (apparent) mishaps and (apparent) transgressions of social/moral rules. In all of these situations a (nonverbal) apology from the actor may be expected. It would be interesting for future research to examine the signal value and social implications of the blush in social situations that seem not to require the actor's (nonverbal) excuse. For example, how would the blush affect the observer's judgment when the actor displays a blush while being the centre of attention or during the exposure of something personal, or in common situations in which people usually do not blush (cf. Dijk *et al.*, 2010)? Do people obtain a more favourable or less favourable judgment when they blush in these types of situations? And to the extent that the blush does influence the observer's judgment of the actor, what would be the most relevant dimensions? One could speculate that someone who blushes during the exposure of a secret might be considered to be weak or socially incompetent but might nevertheless be the preferred choice for a game that requires mutual cooperation because he or she might be considered easier to 'read' (Boone & Buck, 2003). Thus, a short-term effect of obtaining a negative judgment does not imply that the blush has no desirable consequences, since in the long run there can be an advantage in being known to be a blusher (Frank, 1988). Thus, besides examining the immediate interpersonal effects of blushing, it might be fruitful to examine the long-term interpersonal effects of the blush as well.

Finally, it might be relevant to extend the research on the social implications of the blush to the more general impact of phasic changes of people's skin colour on interpersonal behaviours. Since the human visual system seems equipped with an exceptional sensitivity to two dimensions of skin reflectance modulation – one associated with haemoglobin oxygen saturation and one associated with haemoglobin skin concentration – this seems to provide the opportunity to detect both the level of blood accumulation in the skin (e.g., because of blood pooling or increased circulation) and the type of blood (venous or arterial). So it would be interesting to see whether perhaps more subtle changes in skin colour may more generally affect interpersonal behaviours. In this respect it might be especially relevant to differentiate between the impact of the more reddish colour of arterial blood – which may be associated with a more dominant, aggressive mental state – and the impact of the more greenish colour of venous blood, which seems most relevant for social blushing. Moreover, it might be that the impact of the blush also depends on the level of blood accumulation. In some contexts, a subtle, mild reddening might have a positive influence, whereas under the same conditions a strong coloration might have detrimental social consequences. The same might be true for the social implications of other types of blood-related reddening of visible body parts, such as the blush that sometimes occurs in more prolonged social evaluative contexts and that seems to creep on your skin, especially around the neck. The (implicit) impact of such state-dependent facial coloration in interpersonal interactions might even open a completely new avenue of research on the (implicit) impact of signalling one's more subtle emotional and/or motivational states in interpersonal contexts.

REFERENCES

Boone, R. T., & Buck, R. (2003). Emotional expressivity and trustworthiness: the role of nonverbal behavior in the evolution of cooperation. *Journal of Nonverbal Behavior*, 27, 163–82.
Burgess, T. H. (1839). *The physiology or mechanism of blushing*. London: John Churchill.
Castelfranchi, C., & Poggi, I. (1990). Blushing as a discourse: was Darwin wrong? In W. R. Crozier (Ed.), *Shyness and embarrassment: perspectives from social psychology*. Cambridge University Press, 230-51.
Changizi, M. A., Zhang, Q., & Shimojo, S. (2006). Bare skin, blood and the evolution of primate colour vision. *Biology Letters*, 2, 217–21.
Costa, M., Dinsbach, W., Manstead, A. S. R., Ricci, B., & Pio, E. (2001). Social presence, embarrassment, and nonverbal behavior. *Journal of Nonverbal Behavior*, 25, 225–40.

Crozier, W. R. (2004). Self-consciousness, exposure, and the blush. *Journal for the Theory of Social Behaviour*, **34**, 1–17
(2006). *Blushing and the social emotions*. Basingstoke: Palgrave Macmillan.
Darwin, C. (1872/1989). *The expression of the emotions in man and animals*. New York University Press, 163–8.
de Jong, P. J. (1999). Communicative and remedial effects of social blushing. *Journal of Nonverbal Behavior*, **23**, 197–218.
de Jong, P. J., Peters, M. L., & De Cremer, D. (2003). Blushing may signify guilt: revealing effects of blushing in ambiguous social situations. *Motivation and Emotion*, **27**, 225–49.
de Jong, P. J., Peters, M. L., De Cremer, D., & Vranken, C. (2002). Blushing after a moral transgression in a prisoner's dilemma game: appeasing or revealing? *European Journal of Social Psychology*, **32**, 727–44.
de Waal, F. B. M. (1995). *Good natured: the origins of right and wrong in humans and other animals*. Cambridge, MA: Harvard University Press.
Dijk, C., de Jong, P. J., Müller, E., & Boersma, W. (2010). Blushing-fearful individuals' judgmental biases and conditional cognitions: an internet inquiry. *Journal of Psychopathology and Behavioral Assessment*, **32**, 264–70.
Dijk, C., & de Jong, P. J., & Peters, M. L. (2009). The remedial value of blushing in the context of transgressions and mishaps. *Emotion*, **9**, 287–91.
Dijk, C., Koenig, B., Ketelaar, T., & de Jong, P. J. (2011). Saved by the blush: being trusted despite defecting. *Emotion*, **11**, 313–19.
Drummond, P. D., & Lim, H. K. (2000). The significance of blushing for fair- and dark-skinned people. *Personality and Individual Differences*, **29**, 1123–32.
Edelmann, R. J. (1990). Chronic blushing, self-consciousness, and social anxiety. *Journal of Psychopathology and Behavioral Assessment*, **12**, 119–27.
Evans, J. St. B. T., Newstead, S. E., & Byrne, R. M. J. (1993). *Human reasoning: the psychology of deduction*. Hillsdale, NJ: Lawrence Erlbaum.
Frank, R. H. (1988). *Passions within reason: the strategic role of the emotions*. New York: Norton.
Frijda, N. H. (1986). *The emotions*. Cambridge University Press.
Glashouwer, K. A., de Jong, P. J., Dijk, C., & Buwalda, F. M. (2011). Individuals with fear of blushing explicitly and automatically associate blushing with social costs. *Journal of Psychopathology and Behavioral Assessment*, **33**, 540–6.
Goffman, E. (1967). *Interaction ritual: essays on face-to-face behavior*. Garden City, MI: Anchor.
Gold, G. J., & Weiner, B. (2000). Remorse, confession, group identity, and expectancies about repeating a transgression. *Basic and Applied Social Psychology*, **22**, 291–300.
Keltner, D. (1995). Signs of appeasement: evidence for the distinct displays of embarrassment, amusement, and shame. *Journal of Personality and Social Psychology*, **68**, 441–54.
Keltner, D., Young, R. C., & Buswell, B. N. (1997). Appeasement in human emotion, social practice, and personality. *Aggressive Behavior*, **23**, 359–74.
Kerr, N. L. (1995). Norms in social dilemmas. In D. Schroeder (Ed.), *Social dilemmas: perspectives on individuals and groups*. Westport, CT: Praeger, 31–47.

Leary, M. R., Britt, T. W., Cutlip, W. D., & Templeton, J. L. (1992). Social blushing. *Psychological Bulletin*, 112, 446–60.

Leary, M. R., Landel, J. L., & Patton, K. M. (1996). The motivated expression of embarrassment following a self-presentational predicament. *Journal of Personality*, 64, 619–36.

Leary, M. R., & Meadows, S. (1991). Predictors, elicitors, and concomitants of social blushing. *Journal of Personality and Social Psychology*, 60, 254–62.

Liebrand, W. B., Jansen, R. W., Rijken, V. M., & Suhre, C. J. (1986). Might over morality: social values and the perception of other players in experimental games. *Journal of Experimental Social Psychology*, 22, 203–15.

Mellander, S., Andersson, P., Afzelius, L., & Hellstrand, P. (1982). Neural beta-adrenergic dilation of the facial vein in man: possible mechanism in emotional blushing. *Acta Physiologica Scandinavia*, 114, 393–9.

Pan, X. (2009). *Experimental studies of the interaction between people and virtual humans with a focus on social anxiety.* Doctoral thesis, University College London.

Parkinson, B., & Manstead, A. S. R. (1993). Making sense of emotions in stories and social life. *Cognition and Emotion*, 7, 295–323.

Ross, L. D. (1977). The intuitive psychologist and his shortcomings: distortions in the attribution process. In L. Berkowitz (Ed.), *Advances in experimental social psychology.* Vol. 10. New York: Academic Press, 173–220.

Semin, G. R., & Manstead, A. S. R. (1982). The social implications of embarrassment displays and restitution behavior. *European Journal of Social Psychology*, 12, 367–77.

Shearn, D., Bergman, E., Hill, K., Abel, A., & Hinds, L. (1992). Blushing as a function of audience size. *Psychophysiology*, 29, 431–6.

Shearn, D., Spellman, L., Meirick, J., & Stryker, K. (1999). Empathic blushing in friends and strangers. *Motivation and Emotion*, 23, 307–16.

Shields, S. A., Mallory, M. E., & Simon, A. (1990). The experience and symptoms of blushing as a function of age and reported frequency of blushing. *Journal of Nonverbal Behavior*, 14, 171–87.

Simon, A., & Shields, S. A. (1996). Does complexion color affect the experience of blushing? *Journal of Social Behavior and Personality*, 11, 177–88.

Singer, T., Kiebel, S., Winston, J., Dolan, R., &. Frith, C. (2004). Brain responses to the acquired moral status of faces. *Neuron*, 41, 653–62.

Smits, A. (2003). *True innocence doesn't need a blush, or does it?* Unpublished Master's thesis, University of Maastricht.

Tangney, J. P., Miller, R. S., Flicker, L., & Barlow, D. H. (1996). Are shame, guilt, and embarrassment distinct emotions? *Journal of Personality and Social Psychology*, 70, 1256–69.

Tinbergen, N. (1952). Derived activities: their causation, biological significance, and emancipation during evolution. *Quarterly Review of Biology*, 27, 1–32.

van Lange, P. A. M. (1999). The pursuit of joint outcomes and equality in outcomes: an integrative model of social value orientation. *Journal of Personality and Social Psychology*, 77, 337–49.

(2000). Beyond self-interest: a set of propositions relevant to interpersonal orientations. *European Review of Social Psychology*, 11, 297–331.

Wilkin, J. K. (1988). Why is flushing limited to a mostly facial cutaneous distribution? *Journal of the American Academy of Dermatology*, **19**, 309–13.

Willis, J., & Todorov, A. (2006). First impressions: making up your mind after a 100-ms exposure to a face. *Psychological Science*, **17**, 592–8.

Winston, J. S., Strange, B. A., O'Doherty, J., & Dolan, R. J. (2002). Automatic and intentional brain responses during evaluation of trustworthiness of faces. *Nature Neuroscience*, **5**, 277–83.

*Part IV*

Blushing problems: processes and interventions

# 13 Red, hot and scared: mechanisms underlying fear of blushing

*Corine Dijk and Peter J. de Jong*

## Problems with blushing

While there is evidence that blushing is functional for interpersonal communication (e.g., de Jong, 1999; Dijk *et al.*, 2011; Leary *et al.*, 1996), people often experience their blushing as an undesirable response to the extent that they try to hide or prevent it (Shields *et al.*, 1990). Although people generally do not like to blush, most will not avoid going to social events because they might blush, nor do they use several layers of foundation to be sure that a possible blush will remain unseen. Yet, some people do. For these individuals fear of blushing elicits so much distress that they avoid situations where they fear they might blush, and if avoidance is not possible they endure these situations with intense fear (Mulkens *et al.*, 2001).

Fear of blushing is clearly a social fear. People with blushing-phobic concerns are typically afraid of displaying a blush in interpersonal contexts. Usually their core concern is the fear that other people will see them blushing and will therefore judge them as abnormal, weak or insecure (Dijk *et al.*, 2010). This indicates that fear of blushing is related to social phobia. Accordingly, several researchers have described fear of blushing as a marker or subtype of social phobia (e.g., Bögels & Reith, 1999; Fahlén, 1997; Pollentier, 1992; Scholing & Emmelkamp, 1993). In support of this notion, self-reported blushing and sweating distinguish best between social phobia and other anxiety disorders (Fahlén, 1997). Furthermore, the fear of showing bodily symptoms of anxiety, such as blushing, is the main complaint in about one third of the people who seek clinical help for their social fears (Bögels & Scholing, 1995; Essau *et al.*, 1999). Gerlach and Ultes (2003) examined the connection between fear of blushing and social phobia the other way around. They interviewed people who surfed on the internet searching for information about a

---

'Red, hot and scared' was also the title of Sandra Mulkens's doctoral dissertation; we thank her for giving permission to use this phrase in the title of our chapter.

surgical anti-blush treatment and asked them about their social fears. These authors found that more than half of the people who considered applying for this surgical treatment could be diagnosed with social phobia.

Just how many people suffer from fear of blushing is not exactly clear. Considering that the lifetime prevalence for social phobia is about 12 per cent (Kessler et al., 2005), and about one third of these people have fear of blushing as their main complaint (Essau et al., 1999), one would estimate that about 4 per cent of all people will suffer from fear of blushing at one point in their lives. Yet, unpublished results from questionnaire studies at the universities of Amsterdam and Groningen showed that this estimate might be too stringent. For several years, all first year students have been asked to fill out the 'blushing' subscale of the Blushing, Trembling and Sweating Questionnaire (Bögels & Reith, 1999) during the mass screening that takes place during the first month of the first semester. Results of several waves indicate that a substantial proportion (8–10 per cent) of the first year students score as high or higher than the mean scores that are usually reported for treatment-seeking groups (e.g., Mulkens et al., 2001). Thus, problems with blushing might be more prevalent than just in a small group of socially phobic individuals.

Once developed, fear of blushing can be a chronic condition (Dijk et al., 2010). Yet, although chronic, the level of experienced fear and related problems might vary over time. Similar to social phobia (cf. Wittchen & Fehn, 2003), fear of blushing can decrease and increase depending on life events and contextual factors. For example, when someone with fear of blushing has a familiar and friendly workplace, fear of blushing might become less of a problem, but can then increase again in a new work environment. Not only the pattern of symptoms but also the inadvertent social consequences resemble those of social phobia (Stein & Kean, 2000; Wittchen & Beloch, 1996). When people avoid social situations because of their fear of blushing, this can cause problems in many important social roles. Blushing-fearful individuals can experience difficulties in getting involved in friendships and romantic relationships. Furthermore, because they do not speak up, they might miss important promotions at work and hence also earn less money. The impaired quality of life can also give rise to other secondary psychological problems. For example, social fears are often followed by alcohol misuse, depression and suicidal ideation (Stein & Kean, 2000). All in all, blushing fear can be a very devastating condition.

In the following sections of this chapter we will focus on the mechanisms that may be involved in the development and maintenance of these symptoms. One prominent explanation that has been put forward is that fearful individuals may be characterized by a tendency to blush relatively easily and/or intensely (e.g., Bögels et al., 1996). Consistent with this, fearful individuals often attribute their problem to their physiological make-up; they claim that it is because of their physiological disposition that they blush more often and more intensely than others. However, it has been questioned whether they actually do so. Moreover, even if they are right that they blush relatively easily, this does not of course imply that their physiological wiring is the critical factor driving such heightened responsiveness. Before examining the validity of the explanations that have been put forward to suggest that blushing-fearful people blush more readily than others, we will first address the question as to whether they actually do blush more readily in the first place.

## Blushing-fearful individuals' propensity to blush

The first studies that aimed to examine whether people with social fears and fear of blushing are more inclined to blush than others used a questionnaire approach. In these studies the self-reported propensity to blush is often measured with the Blushing Propensity Scale (BPS; Leary & Meadows, 1991). The BPS asks respondents to indicate how frequently they feel themselves blushing in social situations, such as: 'when a teacher calls on me in class' or 'when I've looked stupid or incompetent in front of others'. These early studies consistently showed that self-reported chronic blushing was related to social anxiety and fear of blushing (Amies et al., 1983; Bögels et al., 1996; Crozier & Russell, 1992; Edelmann, 1990; Neto, 1996). Such studies have been used to support the view that people who fear blushing do blush more easily than people without this fear; however, in reality they only show that people who fear blushing *report* that they blush more easily than do those without such fear.

Since one may question whether people have insight into their actual blushing propensity, a series of subsequent studies investigated whether people who report blushing relatively easily also display a relatively strong physiological blush under controlled laboratory conditions (e.g., Drummond, 1997; Edelmann & Baker, 2002; Mauss et al., 2004; Mulkens et al., 1997; Mulkens et al., 1999). In these studies, participants who were high or low in self-reported blushing propensity or fear of blushing were asked to perform a stressful social task, such as watching a video of themselves while singing or giving a speech to an audience. During these tasks the physiological blush response was measured. After the task, participants were asked to provide an estimation of the intensity of their blush response. Typically, the results showed that high blushing-fearful (or high BPS) participants gave much higher subjective ratings of their blushing than low-fearful participants. The physiological measures, however, showed no systematic difference between high and low-fearful participants. This led the researchers to conclude that blushing-fearful individuals overestimate the intensity of their blush and actually do not blush more intensely or more often than people without fear of blushing.

However, there is reason to assume that the latter part of this conclusion might have been premature. All the tasks that were used in these studies (such as singing 'Old MacDonald had a farm' in front of an audience) were generally experienced as very embarrassing. This might have undermined the sensitivity of these studies to detect individual differences in the blush response. The tasks might have been so embarrassing that they elicited a full-blown blush even in people who normally do not blush that easily. In accordance with this suggestion, in one of the studies blushing-fearful participants did seem to blush more intensely when they were in the mere presence of the confederates of the study, thus before the embarrassing task actually started (Mulkens et al., 1997). Several subsequent studies provided similar evidence indicating that during relatively mild social events, such as a conversation with an unknown person, blushing-fearful individuals might blush more easily and/or more intensely than people without fear of blushing (Bögels et al., 2002; Dijk et al., 2009; Voncken & Bögels, 2009). There are also other pieces of evidence supporting the view that there might be differences between high- and low-fearful individuals' readiness to display a blush. For example, falsely telling people that they show a blush was found to have a relatively strong effect on blushing-fearful people (Drummond, 2001; Drummond et al., 2003). In addition, there is evidence for a prolonged response as indicated by the observation that it took longer for blushing-fearful individuals to recover from the blush and turn pale again (Drummond et al., 2007).

Clearly, then, there is some empirical support for blushing-fearfuls' claim that they blush more easily than others. There is growing evidence suggesting that especially in more common social situations such as having a conversation with unknown others, at least a subgroup of individuals with fear of blushing blush more easily and/or more intensely than non-fearful people (e.g., Bögels et al., 2002; Dijk et al., 2009; Drummond, 2001; Drummond et al., 2003; Gerlach et al., 2001; Hofmann et al., 2006; Voncken & Bögels, 2009). This evidence from controlled research accords well with our clinical impression that some blushing-phobic individuals tend to blush very easily in common social situations that usually do not tend to elicit a blush in other people. All in all, there seem sufficient grounds to tentatively conclude that (under some conditions) indeed (some) individuals with fear of blushing tend to blush more readily than non-fearful people, although it would require more rigorous research to arrive at more definite conclusions in this respect.

If indeed blushing-fearful individuals tend to blush relatively easily in common social situations, the next question is how to explain this enhanced tendency to blush. Insight into the factors that are responsible for a heightened tendency to blush may provide important clues for improving our understanding of the mechanisms involved in blushing phobia. One explanation could be that blushing-fearful individuals are the victims of a hyper-responsive physiological 'blush' system. Although such a somatic explanation is quite common among people with fear of blushing, it seems inconsistent with findings indicating that following successful treatment people not only report lower levels of fear but also a lower frequency of displaying a blush (e.g., Mulkens et al., 2001). This seems to suggest that more malleable psychological mechanisms rather than hard-wired physiological features may best explain blushing-fearfuls' liability to blush. This is explored further in the next section.

## Restricted standards

Perhaps people with fear of blushing do not blush more easily because of some physiological predisposition, but because they feel themselves more often confronted with blush-eliciting situations. They might have a biased need for social appeasement (e.g., Stein & Bouwer, 1997). As also argued in Chapter 12, this volume, blushing can be conceptualized as a submissive nonverbal apology that may mitigate a negative social impression and help to restore the actor's social identity (Keltner & Buswell, 1997). Accordingly, it has been argued that people typically blush when breaching a social rule (e.g., Castelfranchi & Poggi, 1990). Indeed, when people were experimentally forced to violate a normative rule, this elicited a blush in the 'violators' (e.g., de Jong et al., 2002). In such a context, the blush response is assumed to reflect the blusher's concerns about the negative social impression that may result from violating another's rules (cf. Leary et al., 1992).

This perspective points to two critical features that may jointly set people at risk of a heightened tendency to blush: a relatively high sensitivity to other people's judgment and a tendency to attribute relatively restrictive social standards to other people (e.g., about what is appropriate and what is not). There is ample evidence that people with fear of blushing are relatively sensitive to other people's judgments. For example, several studies showed a relationship between fear of negative evaluation and fear of blushing (e.g., Bögels et al., 1996; Neto, 1996). In a similar vein, treatment-seeking samples have been found to obtain heightened scores on the Fear of Negative Evaluation Scale compared to non-fearful controls (e.g., Mulkens et al., 2001; Dijk et al., 2011). Thus, their heightened sensitivity to other people's judgment may be one part of the story as to why people with fear of blushing may tend to blush relatively easily.

In a recent study in our laboratory we also explored the relevance of the second critical feature and tested whether blushing-fearful individuals indeed tend to attribute relatively restrictive social standards to other people (de Jong et al., 2011). Participants with varying levels of fear of blushing were presented with descriptions of common behaviours that may be considered as breaching social standards but not necessarily so. For example, they were asked to imagine that they ordered a dessert whereas no one else in their party did, or that they appeared in leisure wear at a formal party. Next, they were asked to rate to what extent they considered this behaviour as breaching the prevailing standards. Sustaining the line of reasoning, participants' level of blushing fear was indeed found to be associated with the tendency to attribute relatively restrictive social standards to others.

These findings thus support the view that a biased judgment about the need for social appeasement might be involved in blushing phobia. Thus, perhaps, people who fear blushing just blush more easily because they (think they) have more reasons to blush than low blushing-fearful people. A critical next step would be to test whether modifying blushing-fearfuls' conception of the prevailing social standards would indeed attenuate their tendency to blush.

## Self-focused attention and fear of blushing

Besides possibly blushing more easily, blushing-fearful individuals seem to overestimate the intensity of their blush response (e.g., Dijk et al., 2009; Mulkens et al., 1999). This judgmental bias logically acts in a way to confirm their fear. Several mechanisms might contribute to this threat-confirming judgmental bias. Perhaps most importantly, blushing-fearful individuals might focus too much attention on the self, which in turn might increase the awareness of internal bodily processes (see Scheier et al., 1983). This may enhance their sensitivity to detect even very small changes in facial temperature, which may be interpreted as evidence that they are displaying a blush.

In apparent contrast to this suggestion an early study failed to find a relationship between self-defined chronic blushing and self-reports of general bodily sensations (Edelmann, 1991). Similarly, a series of studies failed to find a convincing relationship between heightened self-awareness and enhanced blushing propensity (Crozier & Russell, 1992; Edelmann, 1990; Leary & Meadows, 1991). Yet, Bögels and colleagues (1996) noted that the Self-Consciousness Scale, which was most often used to measure self-awareness, does not specify the exact focus of attention. That is, the scale consists of items such as 'I am self-conscious about the way I look' and 'I am constantly examining my motives.' Yet, for blushing-fearful individuals, attention directed to bodily signs of anxiety, such as blushing and trembling, seems specifically of relevance. Therefore, they designed the Self-Focused Attention Scale, which does specify this direction of attentional focus. Attesting to the validity of this idea, their study showed that fear of blushing was clearly related to a tendency to focus on one's marks of arousal, such as the feeling of blushing, sweating or trembling (Bögels et al., 1996). Altogether, the available evidence suggests that the enhanced attentional focus is restricted to specific bodily sensations and/or that the enhanced attentional focus is typically elicited in people who experience fear of blushing rather than in people who are characterized by chronic blushing per se.

The tendency to focus on the bodily sensations and the self might have profound consequences. That is, enhanced self-focused attention might not only increase social anxiety (Bögels & Mansell, 2004) but might also trigger the actual blush response (e.g., Crozier, 2004). One study that was set up to test this idea, however, failed to support the alleged impact of enhanced self-focused attention on people's blushing (Bögels et al., 2002). In that study, participants were asked to engage in a conversation with two confederates. During this conversation the researchers tried to induce enhanced self-focused attention in half of the participants by showing them their reflection in three large mirrors. Although the manipulation worked in the sense that it successfully increased self-awareness, it did not result in more blushing. This negative finding might, however, have been due to the manipulation; perhaps the objective feedback about their facial coloration that could be derived from the mirrors might have counteracted the negative effects of the heightened self-focused attention. Future research using other experimental strategies to increase self-focused attention is necessary to examine whether enhanced self-awareness may indeed give rise to a blush response.

The evidence for the impact of self-focused attention on people's level of social anxiety seems more straightforward. In one study, high- and low-fearful participants were asked to read short scenarios describing social situations and were asked to imagine that they were the main character in these scenarios. The main character sometimes blushed and was always the centre of everybody's attention. Furthermore, in the stories the direction of attention was manipulated: thus, the main character either was focused on the self or was focused on the social task. In line with expectations, self-focused attention led to more social anxiety than task-focused attention in both high- and low-fearful participants (Bögels & Lamers, 2002). Zou and colleagues (2007) found similar findings in a more naturalistic setting. They asked high and low blushing-fearful participants to engage in a 5-minute conversation with an unknown person. Before this conversation, the participants received an instruction that was meant to either induce self-focused attention or task-focused attention. The self-focused attention instruction, for example, informed participants that they needed to fill out a questionnaire concerning certain aspects of themselves during those 5 minutes. The instruction further asked them to focus attention inwards by concentrating on breathing, heart rate, voice or any signs of blushing. The task-focus instruction was similar but then participants were informed that they would receive a questionnaire about the conversation and they were asked to direct their attention outward. Results showed that self-focused attention increased anxiety, but only in the high anxious group. This pattern of findings suggests that self-focused attention might be especially detrimental for vulnerable individuals.

It has been argued that, besides enhancing fear, too much attention towards the self might also cause people to perform poorly in social situations (Bögels et al., 1997; Clark, 2001). This seems a plausible suggestion; directing attention to the self will logically reduce attention to the social task, which in turn might well result in a decline in these people's social performance. Yet, studies that were specifically designed to more directly examine the relationship between self-focused attention and social performance deficits did not find evidence for a causal relationship (e.g., Bögels et al., 2002; Woody & Rodriguez, 2000). Other studies did show that a relationship between self-focused attention and performance deficits did not rule out other explanations of poor social performance, such as the use of safety behaviours and/or an increase in anxiety (Alden et al., 1992; McManus et al., 2008).

Moreover, a recent study by Voncken and colleagues (2010) showed that self-focused attention did not mediate the relationship between blushing-fearfuls' social anxiety and the judgment they received from others. In that study, high and low blushing-fearful participants were asked to engage in a conversation with two confederates, and half of the participants were falsely led to believe that they blushed intensely (see also Dijk *et al.*, 2009). After the conversation participants were asked about their beliefs regarding the confederate's judgments. The confederates were asked to evaluate the participants and to indicate the extent to which they wished to have future interactions with these participants. Results showed that the blush feedback gave rise to heightened anxiety and self-focused attention in all participants. Furthermore, the confederates indicated that they wished to have less future contact with these participants. The researchers then used structural equation modelling to examine whether the self-focused attention mediated the relationship between social anxiety and social rejection (i.e., the wish not to interact in the future). As an alternative explanation they also included negative beliefs of the participants as a mediator between social anxiety and social rejection. That is, social anxiety can strengthen beliefs such as 'Others don't like me' or 'Others think I am not competent.' Earlier studies had already shown that the conviction that someone dislikes you can make people behave in such a way that these beliefs become true (e.g., Curtis & Miller, 1986). The results of the structural equation modelling clearly showed that these negative beliefs, and not self-focused attention, mediated the relationship between social anxiety and poor social performance.

Together, the available findings thus indicate that in addition to self-focused attention, negative beliefs about others' judgments might play an important role in fear of blushing. The following section will explore further the potential importance of negative beliefs in fear of blushing.

## Negative beliefs about the consequences of blushing

In a recent study we asked a group of blushing-fearful individuals, recruited from a German internet forum, about their fear of blushing as well as about their beliefs regarding the social consequences of their blushing (Dijk *et al.*, 2010). Several types of beliefs were examined: about others' evaluations (e.g., 'When I blush others will think I am weak'); about self-evaluations (e.g., 'When I blush, I will think I am socially insecure'); and, because blushing is an uncontrollable autonomic response, beliefs about the loss of control when blushing (e.g., 'When I blush people will find out things about me that I want to keep private'). For each type of belief, blushing-fearful individuals were clearly characterized by relatively negative ideas about the consequences of displaying a blush. This finding is in line with the results of an earlier study by Bögels and Reith (1999), who also showed that socially phobic individuals (with and without fear of blushing) were marked by more negative and less positive beliefs about blushing.

Thus, blushing-fearful individuals have negative beliefs about the social consequences of displaying a blush. Accordingly, it has been suggested that blushing-fearful individuals may overestimate the undesirable social consequences of displaying a blush (de Jong & Peters, 2005). That is, compared to people without fear of blushing, blushing-fearful individuals might hold the belief that others will judge them relatively negatively when they blush. Furthermore, blushing-fearful individuals might have biased judgments about the probability of blushing and hold the belief that they will blush relatively easily and intensely. Such overestimations of the costs and probability of an event have been referred to as judgmental biases, where the term 'bias' refers to the difference between the beliefs of high and low-fearful individuals (e.g., Foa et al., 1996; Voncken et al., 2003).

A series of studies was set up to test whether blushing-fearful individuals indeed show these types of judgmental biases for displaying a blush in several types of situations: after a social transgression, while being the centre of attention, or during the exposure of something personal (de Jong & Peters, 2005; de Jong et al., 2006; Dijk & de Jong, 2009). In these studies, participants were asked to read short scenarios in which social situations were described. Participants were always prompted in the perspective of the (blushing) actor and were asked to indicate their beliefs about the impressions they conveyed to hypothetical others. These studies showed that high-fearful individuals reported a relatively high subjective probability of blushing when being the centre of attention or during the exposure of something personal. Yet, the results did not show that high-fearful individuals were marked by an enhanced anticipation of social costs of blushing in these situations.

A more recent study focused on the anticipated influence of displaying a blush in common social situations in which people tend not to blush; ordinary situations such as: 'Your neighbour asks if you have already heard about the increase in the rent' (Dijk et al., 2010). Interestingly, individuals with fear of blushing did show a judgmental bias regarding the social costs of blushing in these types of situations. Thus, this pattern of findings seems to indicate that people with fear of blushing do overestimate the social costs of blushing but only within particular types of contexts. However, it should be noted that there were several methodological differences between the study that did find and the studies that did not find heightened cost estimates related to displaying a blush. Most importantly, the only study that did find a difference between high- and low-fearful individuals relied on high-fearful individuals from an internet forum about fear of blushing (Dijk *et al.*, 2010), whereas the other studies relied on high blushing-fearful students. Perhaps, then, the difference in findings might be attributable to sample differences rather than to a context-dependent influence of the blush. It seems reasonable to assume that for the forum visitors, their fear interfered more strongly with their daily life than was the case for the high blushing-fearful students. Perhaps only people for whom their fear of blushing is a real burden tend to overestimate the social costs of displaying a blush, and for these people this judgmental bias may not be restricted to particular contexts.

To test this possibility, we recently conducted a follow-up study among treatment-seeking individuals (Dijk & de Jong, 2012). In this study we included several types of situations that had also been used in previous research. The results of this study replicated the previous findings obtained with the forum visitors and meanwhile showed that the overestimation of the social costs of blushing was not restricted to a particular context but proved to be a more general tendency of treatment-seeking individuals. Thus, whereas both analogue and clinical samples report a similar tendency to overestimate the probability of displaying a blush, the judgmental bias regarding the social costs of blushing seems restricted to individuals with clinical levels of blushing fears.

To test more specifically whether high-fearful individuals overestimate the costs of their blushing and/or low-fearfuls underestimate the social costs of displaying a blush, a subsequent experiment was designed to examine the effects of blushing in the same contexts on the judgment of observers (Dijk & de Jong, 2012). Thus, rather than being prompted as the blushing actor, participants in this subsequent scenario study were prompted in the observer's perspective and asked to judge the blushing actor. This study showed that the observers' judgments were very similar to the judgments anticipated by the low-fear control participants in the previous study. Thus, the judgmental bias that was evident in the treatment-seeking individuals can be best interpreted as an overestimation of the social costs of displaying a blush. This pattern of findings not only supports the view that an overestimation of the social costs may contribute to blushing phobia, it also points to the clinical implication that it might be worthwhile to challenge blushing-fearfuls' costs expectancies (Nelson *et al.*, 2010).

## Implicit associations

Thus far, the focus has been on explicit self-reported beliefs. Recent dual-process models, however, emphasize the need to distinguish between these explicit, consciously accessible, beliefs and more implicit, automatic associations in memory. These models assume that behaviour is not only guided by cognitions of which people are consciously aware, but also by processes that occur more automatically and often outside awareness (e.g., Gawronski & Bodenhausen, 2006). People who fear blushing often describe their fear symptoms as dysfunctional, but at the same time as difficult to control or to ignore. This points to the potential relevance of automatic associations in blushing phobia. Yet, thus far, research into fear of blushing has predominantly focused on the more explicit, consciously accessible blushing cognitions. To fill this gap in the literature, a recent study examined whether fear of blushing is also characterized by more automatic associations between blushing and negative social outcomes (Glashouwer et al., 2011). Interestingly, this study showed that indeed high-fearful individuals not only reported enhanced explicit expectancies of social costs but also showed relatively strong automatic associations between blushing and social costs.

Although the pattern of results in that study was in the same direction for automatic as well as explicit blushing associations, both types of associations appeared highly independent as their correlation was close to zero. This pattern of findings fits well with the view that explicit and automatic associations should be considered as distinct cognitive processes that influence different kinds of behaviours (e.g., Gawronski & Bodenhausen, 2006; Ouimet et al., 2009). In individuals with fear of blushing, automatic associations between blushing and social costs might trigger relatively uncontrollable fearful thoughts and behavioural responses (cf. Strack & Deutsch, 2004). Even when individuals with a fear of blushing have sufficient time and cognitive resources, they will probably not correct these initial dysfunctional associations on a more explicit level, because their explicit beliefs about blushing are similarly negative and dysfunctional. In this way, automatic and explicit cognitions about blushing may both act to sustain or even enhance the preoccupation with blushing in individuals with fear of blushing (cf. Gawronski & Bodenhausen, 2006).

## Some directions for future research

There are no compelling reasons to assume that some physiological aberration is at the heart of blushing phobia, whereas the research reviewed in this chapter provides ample evidence that all kinds of biased judgments and negative beliefs might fuel people's fear of blushing. As already noted in the previous section, current cognitive models of anxiety disorders emphasize the importance of differentiating between more deliberate and more automatic cognitive processes in the origin and maintenance of irrational fears. Several leads have already been discussed in the previous sections of this chapter for future research to improve further our insight into the exact role of the more deliberate processes in the generation and maintenance of fear of blushing. Here we would like to highlight the relevance of complementing these research efforts, with studies on the more implicit processes that might also be involved in fear of blushing. The previous section reported tentative evidence for the potential importance of more automatic associations in fear of blushing. For a more proper appreciation of the actual relevance of automatic associations, it would be important to test the alleged differential predictive validity of these associations for more spontaneous fear behaviours (cf. Huijding & de Jong, 2006). For testing further the causal influence of this type of association in the maintenance of symptoms it would be critical to test whether specifically modifying these automatic associations would have a favourable influence on the strength of symptoms (cf. Clerkin & Teachman, 2010).

Apart from investigating further the role of more automatic associations, it seems relevant to explore more broadly the potential role of information-processing biases that might contribute to blushing-fearfuls' dysfunctional preoccupation with their blushing, such as attentional bias and interpretation bias (e.g., Koster et al., 2009). There is a growing body of evidence that this type of cognitive bias plays a critical role in the origin and maintenance of anxiety disorders including social phobia (e.g., Amir et al., 2008). Therefore, it seems reasonable to assume that this type of bias might also be at work in fear of blushing. As a first step to exploring the relevance of such a cognitive approach, we recently set up a pilot study in which we let high and low blushing-fearful participants read several short ambiguous stories that could be interpreted negatively, but not necessarily so, such as: 'You walk into a room and start blushing; everybody falls silent.' Then, after some time had passed, participants were asked to recall the situations they had read about. We presented them with several interpretations and asked them to choose the one that matched most closely with that story. Some descriptions were clearly positive ('People in the room felt silent because I looked great') and others negative ('People in the room felt silent because I looked terrible'). Of course, interpretation can clearly be made consciously but by presenting it as a memory test we tried to test the interpretations more implicitly. Whereas people without fear of blushing clearly preferred positive interpretations, people with fear of blushing did not, indicating that they might lack a positivity bias that might protect people from developing fear of blushing. These preliminary findings seem to suggest that it is a promising direction for future research to test further the impact of implicit cognitive mechanisms in the generation of blushing fears.

Improving insight into these biases may not only have theoretical importance but may also have direct clinical implications. As a relatively new development, several authors have designed so-called cognitive bias modification (CBM) procedures (for a clinical comment see March, 2010). A rapidly growing number of studies has shown that CBM focusing on attentional and interpretation bias has the potential to result in clinically significant and prolonged reductions in anxiety symptoms (e.g., Amir *et al.*, 2008). If indeed cognitive biases appear also to be involved in fear of blushing, similar CBM procedures may be tailored to reduce symptoms of blushing phobia as well.

## Conclusion

In this chapter we have discussed several mechanisms that seem to be involved in fear of blushing: one's conviction that one is blushing (which can be biased or correct); negative automatic associations as well as more deliberate negative beliefs about the social costs of blushing; relatively restricted social standards together with enhanced concerns about others' evaluations; and the tendency to focus attention on bodily sensation and the self. Interventions for fear of blushing are addressed in Chapter 14, but the mechanisms described in the current chapter clearly suggest several possible entrees. For example, dysfunctional beliefs about blushing or about other people's social standards seem a logical target for cognitive behavioural techniques (Scholing & Emmelkamp, 1993), whereas enhanced self-focused attention may be addressed via attentional training in which blushing-fearful people learn to cope with the distracting influence of their blushing and to remain focused on the social task (Bögels, 2006).

As already implied throughout the chapter, the mechanisms we have described are probably not independent but interrelated, and may well act in concert to fuel people's fear of blushing (see, e.g., Dijk *et al.*, 2009). For example, the conviction that one is beginning to blush may trigger dysfunctional cognitions and beliefs about the consequences of the blush. If people believe that blushing is charming, they will not experience fear when they think they blush. Yet, if the same people believe that the blush causes others to judge them as weak and incompetent, the conviction that they are blushing can clearly elicit fearful concerns. Thus, negative beliefs about the costs of blushing may mediate the relationship between one's conviction to blush and fear of blushing.

In the same interrelated manner, fear of blushing will probably enhance people's vigilance towards threatening information (e.g., a bodily sensation that may reflect a blush: Wegner & Giuliano, 1980), which logically will lower the threshold for perceiving minor (and perhaps also blush-irrelevant) changes in blood circulation in the cheek, thereby reinforcing the conviction that one is displaying a blush. In its turn this may enhance their fearful preoccupation with the blush, and eventually people with fear of blushing may end up in a threat-confirming downward spiral. Clearly future research is necessary to critically test the proposed causal influence for each of the proposed mechanisms.

## REFERENCES

Alden, L. E., Teschuk, M., & Tee, K. (1992). Public self-awareness and withdrawal from social interactions. *Cognitive Therapy and Research*, **16**, 249–67.

Amies, P. L., Gelder, M. G., & Shaw, P. M. (1983). Social phobia: a comparative clinical study. *British Journal of Psychiatry*, **142**, 174–9.

Amir, N., Weber, G., Beard, C., Bomyea, J., & Taylor, C. T. (2008). The effect of a single-session attention modification program on response to a public-speaking challenge in socially anxious individuals. *Journal of Abnormal Psychology*, **117**, 860–8.

Bögels, S. M. (2006). Task concentration training versus applied relaxation, in combination with cognitive therapy, for social phobia patients with fear of blushing, trembling, and sweating. *Behaviour Research and Therapy*, **44**, 1190–210.

Bögels, S. M., Alberts, M., & de Jong, P. J. (1996). Self-consciousness, self-focused attention, blushing propensity and fear of blushing. *Personality and Individual Differences*, **21**, 573–81.

Bögels, S. M., & Lamers, C. T. J. (2002). The causal role of self-awareness in blushing-anxious, socially-anxious and social phobics individuals. *Behaviour Research and Therapy*, **40**, 1367–84.

Bögels, S. M., & Mansell, W. (2004). Attention processes in the maintenance and treatment of social phobia: hypervigilance, avoidance and self-focused attention. *Clinical Psychology Review*, **24**, 827–56.

Bögels, S. M., Mulkens, S., & de Jong, P. J. (1997). Task concentration training and fear of blushing. *Journal of Clinical Psychology and Psychotherapy*, **4**, 251–8.

Bögels, S. M., & Reith, W. (1999). Validity of two questionnaires to assess social fears: the Dutch Social Phobia and Anxiety Inventory and the Fear of Blushing, Trembling, and Sweating Questionnaire. *Journal of Psychopathology and Behavioural Assessment*, **21**, 51–66.

Bögels, S. M., Rijsemus, W., & de Jong, P. J. (2002). Self-focused attention and social anxiety: the effects of experimentally heightened self-awareness on fear, blushing, cognitions, and social skills. *Cognitive Therapy and Research*, **26**, 461–72.

Bögels, S. M., & Scholing, A. (1995). Behandeling van angst om te blozen, trillen of zweten. *Tijdschrift voor Psychotherapie*, **21**, 248–67.
Castelfranchi, C., & Poggi, I. (1990). Blushing as a discourse: was Darwin wrong? In W. R. Crozier (Ed.), *Shyness and embarrassment: perspectives from social psychology*. Cambridge University Press, 230–51.
Clark, D. M. (2001). A cognitive perspective on social phobia. In W. R. Crozier & L. E. Alden (Eds.), *International handbook of social anxiety: concepts, research and interventions relating to the self and shyness*. New York: John Wiley & Sons, 405–30.
Clerkin, E. M., & Teachman, B. A. (2010). Training implicit social anxiety associations: an experimental intervention. *Journal of Anxiety Disorders*, **24**, 300–8.
Crozier, W. R. (2004). Self-consciousness, exposure, and the blush. *Journal for the Theory of Social Behaviour*, **34**, 1–17.
Crozier, W. R., & Russell, D. (1992). Blushing, embarrassability and self-consciousness. *British Journal of Social Psychology*, **31**, 343–9.
Curtis, R. C., & Miller, K. (1986). Believing another likes or dislikes you: behaviors making the beliefs come true. *Journal of Personality and Social Psychology*, **51**, 284–90.
de Jong, P. J. (1999). Communicative and remedial effects of social blushing. *Journal of Nonverbal Behavior*, **23**, 197–218.
de Jong, P. J., & Peters, M. L. (2005). Do blushing phobics overestimate the undesirable effects of their blushing? *Behaviour Research and Therapy*, **43**, 747–58.
de Jong, P. J., Peters, M. L., De Cremer, D., & Vranken, C. (2002). Blushing after a moral transgression in a prisoner's dilemma game: appeasing or revealing? *European Journal of Social Psychology*, **32**, 627–44.
de Jong, P. J., Peters, M. L., & Dijk, C. (2011). *Fear of blushing: the role of attributing relatively restrictive standards to others*. Manuscript submitted for publication.
de Jong, P. J., Peters, M. L., Dijk, C., Nieuwenhuis, E., Kempe, H., & Oelerink, J. (2006). Fear of blushing: the role of the expected influence of displaying a blush on others' judgments. *Cognitive Therapy and Research*, **30**, 623–34.
Dijk, C., Buwalda, F. M., & de Jong, P. J. (2011). Dealing with fear of blushing: a psychoeducational group intervention for fear of blushing. *Clinical Psychology and Psychotherapy*. Advance online publication. doi: 10.1002/cpp.764.
Dijk, C., & de Jong, P. J. (2009). Fear of blushing: no overestimation of negative anticipated interpersonal effects, but a high subjective probability of blushing. *Cognitive Therapy and Research*, **33**, 59–74.
(2012). Blushing fearful individuals overestimate the costs and probability of their blushing. *Behaviour Research and Therapy*, **50**, 158–62.
Dijk, C., de Jong, P. J, Müller, E., & Boersma, W. (2010). Blushing-fearful individuals' judgmental biases and conditional beliefs: an internet inquiry. *Journal of Psychopathology and Behavioral Assessment*, **32**, 264–70.

Dijk, C., Koenig, B., Ketelaar, T. & de Jong, P. J. (2011). Saved by the blush: being trusted despite defecting. *Emotion*, 11, 313–19.
Dijk, C., Voncken, M., & de Jong, P. J. (2009). I blush, therefore I will be judged negatively: influence of false blush feedback on anticipated others' judgments and facial coloration in high and low blushing-fearfuls. *Behaviour Research and Therapy*, 47, 541–7.
Drummond, P. D. (1997). The effects of adrenergic blockade on blushing and facial flushing. *Psychophysiology*, 34, 163–8.
  (2001). The effect of true and false feedback on blushing in women. *Personality and Individual Differences*, 30, 413–25.
Drummond, P. D., Back, K., Harrison, J., Helgadottir, F. D., Lange, B., Lee, C., Leavy, K., Novatscou, C., Orner, A., Pham, H., Prance, J., Radford, D., & Wheatley, L. (2007). Blushing during social interactions in people with a fear of blushing. *Behaviour Research and Therapy*, 45, 1601–8.
Drummond, P. D., Camacho, L., Formentin, N., Heffernan, T. D., Williams, F., & Zekas, T. E. (2003). The impact of verbal feedback about blushing on social discomfort and facial blood flow during embarrassing tasks. *Behaviour Research and Therapy*, 41, 413–25.
Edelmann, R. J. (1990). Chronic blushing, self-consciousness, and social anxiety. *Journal of Psychopathology and Behavioral Assessment*, 12, 119–27.
  (1991). Correlates of chronic blushing. *British Journal of Clinical Psychology*, 30, 177–8.
Edelmann, R. J., & Baker, S. R. (2002). Self-report and actual physiological responses in social phobia. *British Journal of Clinical Psychology*, 41, 1–14.
Essau, C. A., Conradt, J., & Petermann, F. (1999). Frequency and comorbidity of social phobia and social fears in adolescents. *Behaviour Research and Therapy*, 37, 831–43.
Fahlén, T. (1997). Core symptom pattern of social phobia. *Depression and Anxiety*, 4, 223–32.
Foa, E. B., Franklin, M. E., Perry, K. J., & Herbert, J. D. (1996). Cognitive biases in generalized social phobia. *Journal of Abnormal Psychology*, 105, 433–9.
Gawronski, B., & Bodenhausen, G. V. (2006). Associative and propositional processes in evaluation: an integrative review of implicit and explicit attitude change. *Psychological Bulletin*, 132, 692–731.
Gerlach, A. L., & Ultes, M. (2003). Überschneidung von sozialer Phobie und übermäßigem Schwitzen und Eröten – eine internetbasierte Studie. In R. Ott & C. Eichenberg (Eds.), *Klinische Psychologie im Internet*. Göttingen: Hogrefe Verlag, 327–41.
Gerlach, A. L., Wilhelm, F. H., Gruber, K., & Roth, W. T. (2001). Blushing and physiological arousability in social phobia. *Journal of Abnormal Psychology*, 110, 247–58.
Glashouwer, K. A., de Jong, P. J., Dijk, C., & Buwalda, F. M. (2011). Individuals with fear of blushing explicitly and automatically associate blushing with social costs. *Journal of Psychopathology and Behavioral Assessment*, 33, 540–6.
Hofmann, S. G., Moscovitch, D. A., & Kim, H. (2006). Autonomic correlates of social anxiety and embarrassment in shy and non-shy individuals. *International Journal of Psychophysiology*, 61, 134–42.

Huijding, J., & de Jong, P. J. (2006). Specific predictive power of automatic spider-related affective associations for controllable and uncontrollable fear responses toward spiders. *Behaviour Research and Therapy*, **44**, 161–76.

Keltner, D., & Buswell, B. N. (1997). Embarrassment: its distinct form and appeasement functions. *Psychological Bulletin*, **122**, 250–70.

Kessler, R. C., Chiu, W. T., Demler, O., & Walters, E. E. (2005). Prevalence, severity, and comorbidity of 12-month DSM-IV disorders in the national comorbidity survey replication. *Archives of General Psychiatry*, **62**, 617–27.

Koster, E. H. W., Fox, E., & MacLeod, C. (2009). Introduction to the special section on cognitive bias modification. *Journal of Abnormal Psychology*, **118**, 1–4.

Leary, M. R., Britt, T. W., Cutlip, W. D., & Templeton, J. L. (1992). Social blushing. *Psychological Bulletin*, **112**, 446–60.

Leary, M. R., Landel, J. L., & Patton, K. M. (1996). The motivated expression of embarrassment following a self-presentational predicament. *Journal of Personality*, **64**, 619–36.

Leary, M. R., & Meadows, S. (1991). Predictors, elicitors, and concomitants of social blushing. *Journal of Personality and Social Psychology*, **60**, 254–62.

McManus, F., Sacadura C., & Clark, D. M. (2008). Why social anxiety persists: an experimental investigation of the role of safety behaviours as a maintaining factor. *Journal of Behavior Therapy and Experimental Psychiatry*, **39**, 147–61.

March, J. S. (2010). Attention bias modification training and the new interventions research. *Biological Psychiatry*, **68**, 978–9.

Mauss, I. B., Wilhelm, F. H., & Gross, J. J. (2004). Is there less social anxiety than meets the eye? Emotion experience, expression, and bodily responding. *Cognition and Emotion*, **18**, 631–62.

Mulkens, S., Bögels, S. M., de Jong, P. J., & Louwers, J. (2001). Fear of blushing: effects of task concentration training versus exposure in vivo on fear and physiology. *Journal of Anxiety Disorders*, **15**, 413–32.

Mulkens, S., de Jong, P. J., & Bögels, S. M. (1997). High blushing propensity: fearful preoccupation or facial coloration? *Personality and Individual Differences*, **22**, 817–24.

Mulkens, S., de Jong, P. J., Dobbelaar, A., & Bögels, S. M. (1999). Fear of blushing: fearful preoccupation irrespective of facial correlation. *Behaviour Research and Therapy*, **37**, 1119–28.

Nelson, E. A., Deacon, B. J., Lickel, J. J., & Sy, J. T. (2010). Targeting the probability versus cost of feared outcomes in public speaking anxiety. *Behaviour Research and Therapy*, **48**, 282–9.

Neto, F. (1996). Correlates of social blushing. *Personality and Individual Differences*, **20**, 365–73.

Ouimet, A. J., Gawronski, B., & Dozois, D. J. A. (2009). Cognitive vulnerability to anxiety: a review and an integrative model. *Clinical Psychology Review*, **29**, 459–70.

Pollentier, S. (1992). Wie aus der Erythropobie eine soziale Phobie wurde: eine Übersicht der klinisch-diagnostischen Problematic. *Nervenarzt*, **63**, 28–33.

Scheier, M. F., Carver, C. S., & Matthews, K. A. (1983). Attentional factors in the perception of bodily states. In J. T. Cacioppo & R. E. Petty (Eds.), *Social psychophysiology: a sourcebook*. New York: Guilford Press, 510–42.

Scholing, A., & Emmelkamp, P. M. (1993). Cognitive and behavioural treatments of fear of blushing, sweating, or trembling. *Behaviour Research and Therapy*, **31**, 155–70.

Shields, S. A., Mallory, M. E., & Simon, A. (1990). The experience and symptoms of blushing as a function of age and reported frequency of blushing. *Journal of Nonverbal Behavior*, **14**, 171–87.

Stein, D. J., & Bouwer, C. (1997). Blushing and social phobia: a neurological speculation. *Medical Hypotheses*, **49**, 101–8.

Stein, M. B., & Kean, Y. M. (2000). Disability and quality of life in social phobia: epidemiologic findings. *American Journal of Psychiatry*, **157**, 1606–13.

Strack, F., & Deutsch, R. (2004). Reflective and impulsive determinants of social behavior. *Personality and Social Psychology Review*, **8**, 220–47.

Voncken, M. J., & Bögels, S. M. (2009). Physiological blushing in social anxiety disorder patients with and without blushing complaints: two subtypes? *Biological Psychology*, **81**, 86–94.

Voncken, M. J., Bögels, S. M., & de Vries, K. (2003). Interpretation and judgmental biases in social phobia. *Behaviour Research and Therapy*, **412**, 1481–8.

Voncken, M. J., Dijk, C., de Jong, P. J., & Roelofs, J. (2010). Not self-focused attention but negative beliefs affect poor social performance in social anxiety: an investigation of pathways in the social anxiety–social rejection relationship. *Behaviour Research and Therapy*, **48**, 984–91.

Wegner, D. M., & Giuliano, T. (1980). Arousal-induced attention to self. *Journal of Personality and Social Psychology*, **38**, 719–26.

Wittchen, H. U., & Beloch, E. (1996). The impact of social phobia on quality of life. *International Clinical Psychopharmacology*, **11**, 15–23.

Wittchen, H. U., & Fehn, L. (2003). Epidemiology and natural course of social fears and social phobia. *Acta Psychiatrica Scandinavica*, **108**, 4–19.

Woody, S. R., & Rodriguez, B. F. (2000). Self-focused attention and social anxiety in social phobics and normal controls. *Cognitive Therapy and Research*, **24**, 473–88.

Zou, J. B., Hudson, J. L., & Rapee, R. M. (2007). The effect of attentional focus on social anxiety. *Behaviour Research and Therapy*, **45**, 2326–33.

## 14 Psychological interventions for fear of blushing

*Michelle C. Capozzoli, Imke J. J. Vonk, Susan M. Bögels and Stefan G. Hofmann*

Fear of blushing (erythrophobia) is a severe and persistent condition (Edelmann, 1990) and is generally considered to be difficult to treat (Bögels, 1994; Scholing & Emmelkamp, 1993). Along with fear of showing other physiological symptoms in social situations, such as trembling, sweating or freezing (going 'blank' or being unable to speak because of physiological symptoms), fear of blushing may be difficult to treat because of the persistent desire not to blush, although such a physiological symptom cannot be voluntarily controlled. In this persistence, and their resultant search for surgical treatment, patients with fear of blushing may resemble those with body dysmorphic disorder (Bögels *et al.*, 2010; Kelly *et al.*, 2010; Veale, 2004). Despite such features, only a handful of treatments have been developed specifically for fear of blushing and preliminary results support their efficacy (Bögels, 2006; Bögels & Voncken, 2008; Chaker *et al.*, 2010; Mulkens *et al.*, 2001; Scholing & Emmelkamp, 1993).

Blushing appears to be an important psychophysiological marker of shyness and social anxiety (Hofmann *et al.*, 2006), supporting the notion that fear of blushing is closely associated with social anxiety disorder (SAD). Concerns about blushing, trembling and sweating are commonly considered to be symptoms of SAD, but no diagnosis or specifier in the DSM-IV (American Psychiatric Association, 2000) captures fear of blushing or other physiological symptoms. To address this, some authors have suggested the addition of a specifier of SAD that reflects these fears (Bögels *et al.*, 2010; Bögels *et al.*, 1997). In fact, such a specifier already exists in Japan's indigenous diagnostic classification system. Within taijin-kyofusho, a disorder similar to SAD but commonly considered to be specific to Asian cultures, the subtype sekimen-kyofu, a phobia of blushing, is included (Hofmann, Asnaani *et al.*, 2010; Takahashi, 1989).

In support of such a diagnosis, there is evidence that patients with SAD and a fear of blushing are distinct from those who have SAD without this fear. Among patients who had completed semi-structured clinical interviews containing additional questions about fear of blushing, trembling and sweating, SAD patients with fears of blushing, trembling or sweating could be reliably differentiated from SAD patients without these fears by a self-report questionnaire on fear and avoidance of blushing, trembling or sweating (Bögels & Reith, 1999). Furthermore, in a recent evaluation of a sizeable sample of participants, individuals with fear of blushing (n = 142) were found to significantly differ in a number of ways from individuals with SAD and fear of blushing and also from those with SAD alone (Pelissolo et al., 2012). In comparison to the other two groups, individuals with fear of blushing alone had later age of onset, less comorbidity, lower behavioural and temperamental inhibition, and higher self-esteem. Despite these seeming indications of reduced severity in those with fear of blushing, levels of social anxiety (as measured by the Liebowitz Social Anxiety Scale and the Fear Questionnaire 'social phobia' subscale; Heimberg et al., 1999; Marks & Mathews, 1982) and functional impairment remained relatively high in these individuals. Physiological responses in those with SAD and fear of blushing also appear to differ from those with SAD alone, as SAD patients with fear of blushing have been found to blush more than those with SAD alone while watching an embarrassing video (Gerlach et al., 2001) and while completing a social task (Voncken & Bögels, 2009; but see Mulkens et al., 1999, for conflicting results). However, because physiological symptoms in social situations are common among those with SAD (Amies et al., 1983), for treatment reasons it is important to distinguish such patients from the minority of patients with SAD who present with these symptoms as their primary complaint.

In this chapter, we summarize the findings on treatments for fear of blushing, which is a relatively new area of study (see Table 14.1 for a comparison of treatment findings). Because it is a recent focus of research, only one novel treatment has been developed specifically for fear of blushing: task concentration training (Bögels et al., 1997). The remainder of treatments for fear of blushing described in this chapter are adaptations of existing treatments for SAD that have been evaluated among individuals with fear of blushing. It should be noted that some studies described include individuals with fear of blushing only, whereas others also include those with a fear of trembling, sweating or freezing. Throughout the chapter, however, we will consider the implications of such findings on individuals with fear of blushing, but these findings likely also apply to those with fear of other physiological symptoms. Where the data are sparse, we will supplement findings with studies on the treatment of SAD in order to guide clinicians and researchers seeking effective treatments for patients with fear of blushing.

Table 14.1 Summary of treatment studies for fear of blushing

| Study | Design | N | Treatments | Outcome measures | p-value[1] | Effect size (Cohen's $d$)[2] |
|---|---|---|---|---|---|---|
| Scholing & Emmelkamp (1993) | RCT | 35 | – EXP followed by CT (EXP-CT)<br>– CT followed by EXP (CT-EXP)<br>– CBT (integration of CT, EXP) | (a) Target situations – 'avoidance behaviour' subscale<br>(b) SCL-90 somatic complaints | (a) n.s.<br>(b) n.s. | (a) EXP-CT: 1.01 (block 1); 1.63 (block 2); 1.86 (FU)<br>CT-EXP: 0.68 (block 1); 1.14 (block 2); 0.99 (FU)<br>CBT: 1.10 (block 1); 1.82 (block 2); 1.88 (FU)<br>(b) EXP-CT: 0.43 (block 1); 0.95 (block 2); 1.02 (FU)<br>CT-EXP: 0.44 (block 1); 0.45 (block 2); 0.44 (FU)<br>CBT: 0.21 (block 1); 0.72 (block 2); 0.50 (FU) |
| Mulkens et al. (2001) | RCT | 31 | – TCT<br>– EXP | (a) BTS-Q – fear of blushing<br>(b) BTS-Q – negative cognitions<br>(c) Blushing responsiveness and consequences[3]<br>(d) CCM | (a) $p = .06$ (post; TCT > EXP); n.s. (FU-1; FU-2)<br>(b) n.s. (post); $p < .05$ (FU-1; TCT > EXP); n.s. (FU-2)<br>(c) n.s.<br>(d) n.s. | (a) TCT: 1.03 (post); 1.36 (FU-1); 1.53 (FU-2)<br>EXP: 0.45 (post); 1.17 (FU-1); 1.28 (FU-2)<br>(b) TCT: 1.09 (post); 1.42 (FU-1); 1.84 (FU-2)<br>EXP: 0.57 (post); 0.56 (FU-1); 0.73 (FU-2)<br>(c) TCT: 0.56 (post); 0.95 (FU-1); 0.97 (FU-2)<br>EXP: 0.88 (post); 0.88 (FU-1); 1.32 (FU-2)<br>(d) TCT: 1.11 (post); 1.68 (FU-1); 1.82 (FU-2)<br>EXP: 1.72 (post); 2.01 (FU-1); 1.37 (FU-2) |

| Study | Design | N | Treatment | Measures | Results | Effect sizes |
|---|---|---|---|---|---|---|
| Bögels (2006) | RCT | 65 | – TCT followed by CT (TCT-CT)<br>– AR followed by CT (AR-CT) | (a) BTS-Q<br>(b) CCM | (a) n.s. (post, FU-1); n.s. (post; FU-1); $p < .05$ (FU-2; TCT-CT > AR-CT)<br>(b) n.s. | (a) TCT-CT: 1.98 (post); 1.98 (FU-1); 2.64 (FU-2) AR-CT: 1.63 (post); 1.69 (FU-1); 1.47 (FU-2)<br>(b) TCT-CT: 2.54 (post); 2.49 (FU-1); 3.14 (FU-2) AR-CT: 2.01 (post); 2.12 (FU-1); 2.16 (FU-2) |
| Bögels & Voncken (2008) | RCT | 55 | – CT<br>– SST | (a) FQ Main Phobia<br>(b) TFBTS | (a) n.s.<br>(b) n.s. | (a) CT: 0.79 (post); 0.67 (FU-1); 1.0 (FU-2) SST: 0.81 (post); 0.75 (FU-1); 1.10 (FU-2)<br>(b) CT: 1.06 (post); 1.28 (FU-1); 1.42 (FU-2) SST: 1.41 (post); 1.52 (FU-1); 2.14 (FU-2) |
| Chaker et al. (2010) | Open trial | 31 | – Group treatment primarily consisting of TCT | BTS-Q – 'blushing' subscale:<br>(a) Positive cognitions<br>(b) Negative cognitions<br>(c) Behavioural problems<br>(d) Avoidance<br>(e) Physiological reactions | (a–e) $p < .001$ (post; FU) | (a) 0.68 (post); 0.69 (FU)<br>(b) 1.27 (post); 0.99 (FU)<br>(c) 1.76 (post); 1.34 (FU)<br>(d) 1.24 (post); 0.87 (FU)<br>(e) 1.15 (post); 1.24 (FU) |

Table 14.1 (*cont.*)

| Study | Design | N | Treatments | Outcome measures | p-value[1] | Effect size (Cohen's $d$)[2] |
|---|---|---|---|---|---|---|
| Dijk *et al.* (2011) | Open trial | 47 | – Cognitive behavioural group intervention in a course setting | (a) BTS-Q – 'blushing' subscale | (a) $p < .05$ (post; FU-1; FU-2) | (a) 1.13 (post); 1.55 (FU-1); 2.07 (FU-2) |

AR = applied relaxation; BTS-Q = Blushing, Trembling and Sweating Questionnaire; CCM = causal catastrophic misinterpretations; CT = cognitive therapy; EXP = exposure *in vivo*; FQ = Fear Questionnaire; RCT = randomized clinical trial; SST = social skills training; TCT = task concentration training; TFBTS = trouble and frequency of blushing, trembling and sweating

[1] The p-values listed are for differential effects of treatments, except for uncontrolled studies (open trials), for which there was no comparison treatment and therefore data listed are for overall treatment effects; n.s. = not significant ($p > .05$) at all time points.

[2] Effect sizes were initially calculated as if they concern between-groups effects and were subsequently corrected to indicate within-effects following the approach advocated by Garssen and Hornsveld (1992).

[3] Composite scores of Blushing Propensity Scale and BTS-Q subscales: 'bodily reactions while blushing', 'blushing consequences', and 'avoidance of blushing'.

## Social skills training

A great deal of research on social skills training (SST) has been carried out in patients with SAD. Investigators initially considered SAD to result from poor social skills, since those with SAD have been found to have deficits in social skills (Alden & Bieling, 1998; Baker & Edelmann, 2002; Beidel et al., 2010; Meleshko & Alden, 1993; Stopa & Clark, 1993; Voncken & Bögels, 2008). By explicitly teaching patients social skills, the experience of anxiety in social situations was expected to improve. Although several researchers have suggested that individuals with SAD may in fact possess social skills but are unable to utilize them due to their excessive self-focus (e.g., Clark & Arkowitz, 1975; Bellack, 1983; Clark & Wells, 1995), SST training has nevertheless been found to be an effective treatment for those with SAD. As in SAD, SST has served as a treatment comparison in treatment outcome studies for fear of blushing, despite some of the problems with the underlying rationale for such treatment, as noted above.

Regardless of the cause of social skills deficits, training that aims to improve social skills has been shown to decrease symptoms of SAD, including fear of blushing. SST, a multicomponent approach consisting of coaching, modelling, roleplaying, completion of homework assignments (which include exposure to feared situations and behavioural rehearsal) and providing corrective feedback and social reinforcement, teaches patients new behaviours or appropriate modifications of existing behaviours, which is expected to lead to improvements in social relationships and quality of life (Mersch et al., 1989; Van Dam-Baggen & Kraaimaat, 2000).

Preliminary evidence suggests that interventions that focus on improvement of social skills effectively treat fear of blushing. Bögels and Voncken (2008) randomly assigned patients with SAD and fear of blushing, trembling or sweating as the primary complaint to twelve weekly group sessions of SST or cognitive therapy (CT; discussed further in section 'Cognitive therapy'). CT focused on identifying, analysing and challenging dysfunctional beliefs, performing behavioural experiments to test these beliefs and identifying assumptions regarding fear of bodily symptoms. Both treatments reduced the fear of blushing, sweating or trembling, as well as general complaints and no differences were found in treatment efficacy of SST or CT (Bögels & Voncken, 2008).

Most of the research on SST has been carried out with patients with SAD and has shown that while effective for some patients (perhaps in part because of the inherent exposure to feared situations), it is unclear whether this is an essential treatment for all patients with SAD

(Rodebaugh et al., 2004). To our knowledge, only one study has examined SST as a treatment for patients with fear of blushing, trembling or sweating. Taking into account the different studies that have tested the effectiveness of SST, it appears to be an effective treatment method for patients with SAD and a promising treatment for patients with fear of blushing as their primary complaint, although more research on SST in this population is needed in order to confirm this finding.

## Applied relaxation

The aim of applied relaxation (AR) is to reduce bodily tension and induce relaxation rapidly in feared situations (Öst, 1987). AR may be considered a skill and coping technique that may be employed whenever anxiety and related physiological reactions arise. The rationale is that the more this skill is employed, the faster the relaxation response will occur (Öst, 1987). When using AR in the treatment of anxiety disorders, the goals are to help patients recognize early signs of anxiety and to teach them how to cope effectively with anxiety. AR is practised in stages throughout treatment, beginning with tensing and relaxing different muscles (progressive relaxation) and then relaxing the muscles directly (release-only relaxation). Once these and other relaxation skills are mastered, patients practise relaxation in non-stressful situations in order to reduce the time it takes to become relaxed (rapid relaxation) and, finally, to apply relaxation during stressful situations (applied training) (Öst, 1987).

A number of studies have examined AR in the treatment of SAD. Öst, Jerremalm and Johansson (1981) found that in patients with SAD, both AR and SST led to significant improvement in symptoms. Furthermore, patients were classified as 'behavioural reactors' or 'physiological reactors' (based on their behavioural and physiological responses to a social interaction test) and the authors found that behavioural reactors benefited more from SST, while physiological reactors improved more with AR. These results suggest that therapeutic methods that are tailored to the patient's response pattern achieve the best results. Because patients with fear of blushing may be classified as 'physiological reactors', such patients may be more likely to benefit from AR, which addresses physiological reactions, in comparison to treatments addressing behavioural or cognitive components of anxiety. In a later study by Jerremalm, Jansson and Öst (1986), SAD patients who were divided into 'cognitive reactors' and 'physiological reactors', based on cognitive and physiological responses to a social interaction task, received cognitive training or AR. Both treatments produced significant improvements in social anxiety.

However, in contrast to findings of the previous study, reactor type (i.e., cognitive or physiological) did not predict different outcomes by treatment.

AR is also commonly combined with exposure treatments. Although CT has been found to be superior to combined exposure therapy and AR in those with SAD (Clark et al., 2006), to date, only one study has examined the efficacy of AR in SAD patients with a fear of blushing. In this study, Bögels (2006) randomly assigned patients with a principal diagnosis of SAD and a main fear of blushing, trembling, sweating or freezing to eight weekly sessions of AR or task concentration training (TCT; a treatment that teaches patients to redirect attention away from bodily symptoms to the task at hand, further described in section 'Task concentration training'). Both treatments were followed by eight weekly sessions of CT. Although patients assigned to TCT reported greater reductions in fear of bodily sensations and dysfunctional beliefs immediately after treatment, both treatments were highly effective in reducing symptoms of SAD and fear of blushing. Differential treatment effects disappeared after both groups received CT and remained absent at three months post-treatment, although patients who received TCT-CT reported greater reductions in fear of bodily sensations than patients who received AR-CT at one year post-treatment.

No studies have examined AR as a stand-alone treatment for fear of blushing and, given its application as an addition to treatments for other anxiety disorders, AR is perhaps most likely to be utilized as an adjunct to treatment. Furthermore, in treatments for SAD that combined AR with exposure therapy or CT, the AR combination treatments did not outperform comparison treatments and in fact Bögels (2006) found a combination treatment of TCT and CT to be superior to AR and TCT in reducing fear among these patients. However, AR is often well accepted by patients and may help to increase retention (Clark et al., 1994), which is crucial for achieving response to exposure treatments.

## Task concentration training

SAD has been found to be effectively treated by addressing the attentional processes that serve to exacerbate the disorder and this strategy appears promising for fear of blushing as well. Patients with SAD tend to focus their attention inward in social situations (e.g., Bögels & Mansell, 2004; Clark & Wells, 1995; Daly et al., 1989; Hope et al., 1989) and salient physiological arousal has been found to increase self-focused attention (see Scheier & Carver, 1983, for a review), findings that are especially significant for fear of blushing. In turn, heightened inward attention increases awareness of physiological reactions, intensifies such reactions and may cause one to overestimate the intensity of such arousal (Mandler et al., 1958). It has been suggested that blushing is a particularly salient cue, as one senses warm cheeks when blushing (Bögels et al., 1997) and increased self-focus decreases outward attention to the social task at hand, which is likely to result in poor social performance (Bögels et al., 1997; Clark & Wells, 1995).

To modify self-focused attention in those with fear of blushing, Bögels, Mulkens and de Jong (1997) developed the attention-retraining strategy task concentration training (TCT). The aim of TCT is to redirect attention away from bodily symptoms and towards the social task, which may help patients to re-evaluate their thoughts about feared situations. Furthermore, because task focus appears to be incompatible with self-focused attention, TCT may serve as a coping mechanism for self-focused attention. Bögels, Mulkens and de Jong (1997) outline instructions for practising TCT with patients with fear of blushing: first, therapists provide patients with a rationale for treatment by explaining how blushing and self-focused attention reinforce each other and result in anxiety, negative thoughts about the self, difficulty concentrating and unskilled behaviour. Patients are told that they may intervene in this destructive cycle by redirecting their attention outward. Patients keep daily self-monitoring logs of situations in which blushing has occurred, level of anxiety in these situations, and percentage of concentration directed towards the self, social task and environment in such situations. TCT is then practised in sessions by engaging in listening and speaking exercises of increasing difficulty, in which the goal is to employ task concentration and redirect attention when distracted by worrying about blushing. Finally, patients practise TCT in non-threatening situations (e.g., walking through the woods) and subsequently in threatening situations (e.g., speaking with a supervisor).

When examined in randomized controlled trials, TCT has demonstrated some superiority over other treatments for fear of blushing and other physiological concerns. Mulkens, Bögels, de Jong and Louwers (2001) compared TCT to *in vivo* exposure in patients with SAD and a primary fear of blushing in social situations. At post-treatment, greater reduction in fear of blushing was reported by patients who had received TCT, although this effect had disappeared at a six-week follow-up. Notably, at six months post-treatment, patients who had received TCT reported a greater reduction in negative beliefs about blushing. Although this effect had once again disappeared at twelve months post-treatment, the finding is nevertheless significant since the treatment did not address cognitions or employ cognitive restructuring, suggesting that TCT may promote cognitive change by presenting disconfirming information and increasing awareness of the objective environment.

TCT has also been found to be effective when provided in an intensive format. Chaker, Hofmann and Hoyer (2010) studied participants with a primary fear of blushing who received thirteen hours of treatment in a three-day treatment that included psycho-education, a description of the cognitive model of SAD (Clark & Wells, 1995), elimination of safety behaviours and TCT. Participants practised TCT while listening to short stories, created fear and avoidance hierarchies and performed role plays with instructions to reduce safety behaviours and redirect attention to the task. For six weeks following treatment, participants were instructed to keep homework diaries to practise focusing and redirecting attention in non-threatening situations and then to start engaging in social situations listed on their fear and avoidance hierarchies. At six weeks post-treatment, 63 per cent of participants reported clinically significant reductions in fear of blushing. Although the design of the study did not allow for the separation of TCT and CBT and relied on self-reported measures, the results of this trial provide preliminary support for adapting TCT for use in an intensive group treatment format for patients with a fear of blushing (Chaker, Hofmann & Hoyer, 2010). Finally, TCT has been successfully combined with CT for fear of blushing (Bögels, 2006) and has shown to be slightly superior to AR and CT (results are further described in the 'Applied relaxation' section).

TCT may also be an effective addition to treatments for SAD. In a pilot study, a nine-session group treatment that combined TCT with an adaptation of Segal, Williams and Teasdale's (2002) mindfulness-based cognitive therapy was found to be well accepted by patients and highly effective in reducing SAD, and results were maintained at two months post-treatment (Bögels, Sijbers & Voncken, 2006). This study provides initial support for utilizing TCT beyond fear of blushing, for the treatment of SAD. For patients who seek treatment for both fear of blushing and SAD, TCT may a therefore be an efficient treatment choice.

### Exposure therapy

Exposure therapy is considered a highly effective psychological treatment for SAD. Although cognitive change is considered necessary to effectively treat SAD, changes in cognition have been demonstrated to occur in behavioural treatments that do not include cognitive restructuring (Feske & Chambless, 1995; Gould *et al.*, 1997; Hope *et al.*, 1995; Newman *et al.*, 1994; Taylor, 1996). For example, meta-analyses comparing cognitive behavioural therapy (CBT) to exposure therapy for SAD have found both treatments equally effective. Compared to exposure therapy, CBT did not lead to greater improvement on self-report measures of social anxiety and cognition (Feske & Chambless, 1995; Taylor, 1996). In the context of fear of blushing, it has been found that cognitive changes occurred after interventions (e.g., TCT) that did not include cognitive restructuring (Mulkens et al., 2001). In contrast, a few studies have found treatments incorporating cognitive elements to be superior to exposure therapy alone for SAD (Hofmann, 2004; Mattick & Peters, 1988).

The exposure therapy treatment package for SAD generally includes repeated in-session *in vivo* exposure to social performance situations, didactic training and weekly homework assignments to practise *in vivo* exposure exercises and decrease safety behaviours (e.g., Hofmann & Otto, 2008). For patients with fear of blushing, exposure exercises could include maintaining eye contact during silences or while talking about embarrassing topics, drinking coffee and alcohol if that increases blushing, drawing attention to themselves, breaking social rules and discussing with others their fear of blushing. During the completion of exposure exercises, it is also important to prevent the use of safety behaviours that are typically employed by patients with fear of blushing (e.g., wearing thick make-up to reduce visibility of blushing, avoiding artificial light, year-round sun-tanning, wearing blouses with closed necks and shawls, escaping to the bathroom while blushing).

To our knowledge, only two controlled studies have examined exposure therapy alone for fear of blushing. For patients with SAD and fear of blushing, sweating or trembling as their primary complaint, Scholing and Emmelkamp (1993) compared three treatment packages, each consisting of two treatment blocks, separated by four weeks without treatment sessions: (1) exposure *in vivo* followed by CT; (2) CT followed by exposure *in vivo*; and (3) cognitive behavioural treatment. No differences were found between the treatment packages. Significant time effects after both treatment blocks and at follow-up assessments indicated that patients in all three treatment packages improved and results were maintained at eighteen months post-treatment (Scholing & Emmelkamp, 1996). The results of this study also suggest that when combining cognitive and behavioural techniques, the order in which these techniques are provided does not make a difference. A second study examining stand-alone exposure for fear of blushing was described previously in the 'Task concentration training' section (Mulkens et al., 2001). Both treatments were highly effective in reducing fear of blushing symptoms. Although TCT outperformed exposure at certain time points, this differential treatment effect ultimately disappeared at the twelve-month post-treatment assessment.

## Cognitive therapy

According to Clark and Wells's (1995) model of SAD, patients with SAD hold distorted beliefs about themselves (e.g., 'I am stupid'). These distorted thoughts, along with negative assumptions about themselves and others (e.g., 'If people see my anxiety they will think I am stupid') and rigid rules about behaviour in social situations (e.g., 'I should never show signs of anxiety'), create a higher likelihood that a person will experience high levels of anxiety in social situations. Perhaps particularly applicable to those with fear of blushing is the finding that socially anxious patients overestimate the visibility (McEwan & Devins, 1983) and consequences (Bögels & Reith, 1999) of behavioural signs of anxiety such as blushing. These dysfunctional beliefs are considered to be central to the maintenance of SAD and a logical extension is that patients with fear of blushing also maintain their symptoms through such cognitive distortions. By directly challenging such beliefs, CT aims to change the cognitions that contribute to psychopathology.

Cognitive restructuring for patients with fear of blushing is employed as it is with other disorders; it is only the cognitive distortions that will differ. Commonly held dysfunctional beliefs regarding blushing include: '(1) being the center of attention; (2) viewing others as criticizing and evaluating; (3) mind reading: *I know what they think*, and *they know what I think*; (4) thinking that physical symptoms can be controlled; and (5) having a one-dimensional evaluation, for example, *My ability as a manager is exclusively dependent on a secure appearance*' (Bögels & Voncken, 2008, p. 143). Patients may identify, analyse and challenge such dysfunctional thoughts through the use of daily self-monitoring and cognitive restructuring forms and by conducting behavioural experiments to test the validity of particular beliefs.

Despite the cogent rationale of CT for psychopathology, the employment of cognitive strategies has been demonstrated to be unnecessary to produce cognitive change in patients with SAD, as cognitive change occurred with behavioural intervention strategies (e.g., Newman *et al.*, 1994) including those for fear of blushing (Mulkens *et al.*, 2001). Nevertheless, it has been suggested that because fear of bodily symptoms is severe and persistent (Edelmann, 1990), cognitive intervention may help to ensure long-term change and that coping strategies such as AR and TCT alone may be insufficient to treat enduring symptoms of fear of blushing (Bögels, 2006). More research is needed to examine whether CT does in fact lead to long-term change in those with fear of blushing, since the results of the sole study that has examined this hypothesis did not support this theory (Bögels & Voncken, 2008); that is, SST appeared as effective as CT. Regardless, cognitive therapy is useful for helping patients to modify the dysfunctional thoughts and core beliefs that serve to maintain fear of blushing.

## Cognitive behaviour therapy

Many of the previous studies have enlisted separate cognitive or behaviour therapy, often in order to test the differential effects of these treatments. These studies are helpful for illuminating which treatment techniques may be most effective for fear of blushing. However, in practice, clinicians are more likely to employ all tools at their disposal, including both cognitive and behavioural techniques. Dijk, Buwalda and de Jong (2011) describe the clinical impression that patients with fear of blushing do not easily seek psychological help for their complaints. To address this, they designed a low threshold psycho-educational group intervention based on CBT which appeared to be effective in reducing fear of blushing as well as symptoms of social anxiety (Dijk *et al.*, 2011). Because this study employed an uncontrolled design, it is necessary for future studies to evaluate the intervention in a controlled study. This intervention could be a useful approach for patients with fear of blushing who have difficulty seeking psychological help.

## Fear of blushing interventions for children

For children, somatic symptoms such as blushing are common features of SAD (Ginsburg *et al.*, 2006) and blushing is also frequently reported in children with other anxiety disorders. With a prevalence of 51 per cent, blushing is one of the most common somatic symptoms in children with SAD, separation anxiety disorder and generalized anxiety disorder. Furthermore, Ginsburg, Riddle and Davies (2006) found that somatic symptoms were significantly and positively correlated with anxiety severity, impairment and global functioning. A study by Colonnesi, Engelhard and Bögels (2010) showed that children aged 4–7 years self-reported blushing frequently and reliably. Despite the high prevalence of self-reported blushing symptoms in children, it is unclear whether they actually demonstrate increased frequency of blushing that is noticeable to others; perhaps they only *perceive* that their blushing is visible to and noticed by others. To our knowledge, this question has not been addressed in the literature and no studies have evaluated treatments specifically for fear of blushing in children. However, a number of treatments have been found to be effective for children with SAD and these treatments may also be beneficial when adapted for children with fear of blushing.

As in adults, children with SAD have been found to have social skill deficits (Beidel et al., 1999) and methods paralleling SST for adults have been developed to improve social skills in children. Social effectiveness therapy for children (SET-C; Beidel et al., 1998) is a behavioural treatment for children with SAD and has been used to reduce social anxiety, improve social skills and interpersonal functioning and increase participation in social activities. The programme consists of parent and child education, SST, *in vivo* exposure and homework assignments and peer generalization programming, in which children are paired with outgoing peer volunteers to practise newly learned social skills. Compared to children with SAD who received a nonspecific intervention targeting test anxiety and test-taking skills, children treated with SET-C demonstrated significantly greater improvement in social skills and social anxiety levels and engaged more in social interactions (Beidel et al., 2000). Furthermore, 67 per cent of participants in the SET-C group no longer met diagnostic criteria for SAD at post-treatment, as compared to 5 per cent in the test-anxiety treatment group, and most gains in the SET-C group were maintained long term (Beidel et al., 2006; Beidel et al., 2005).

Support has also been found for individual or group CBT as an effective treatment method for children and adolescents with SAD (Hayward et al., 2000; Herbert et al., 2009; Melfsen et al., 2011; Spence et al., 2000). In comparison to a waiting-list condition, children with SAD assigned to an integrated programme of intensive SST and group CBT interventions with or without parental involvement reported significant reductions in social and general anxiety and demonstrated increased social skills (Spence et al., 2000).

If SAD presents similarly in children and adolescents as it does in adults, then treatment methods for adults with SAD and fear of blushing could potentially be effective for children and adolescents. In an attempt to determine whether the cognitive model of SAD in adults (Clark & Wells, 1995; Hofmann, 2007) also applies to children, Hodson, McManus, Clark and Doll (2008) compared social anxiety in adults and children/adolescents and found that high socially anxious children scored significantly higher than low socially anxious children on negative social cognitions, safety behaviours, self-focused attention and pre- and post-event processing. Thus, treatments developed for adults for SAD (e.g., TCT) with fear of blushing may also translate to younger patients.

## Measures for fear of blushing

A number of self-report measures have been developed for fear of blushing, such as the Blushing, Trembling and Sweating Questionnaire that consists of the subscales 'fear of blushing', 'bodily reactions', 'positive and negative consequences about blushing', 'blushing consequences', 'blushing avoidance' and 'blushing frequency' (Bögels & Reith, 1999). In addition, Bögels (2006) had patients formulate five main idiosyncratic beliefs about their bodily symptoms, termed central causal misinterpretations (CCM; e.g., 'If I blush, everybody will find me weak') and patients rated their conviction of these beliefs on visual analogue scales before and after each therapy session. Finally, the Blushing Propensity Scale (Leary & Meadows, 1991; Bögels et al., 1996) measures how often people blush in different social situations. Psychometric properties of these measures have generally been found to be good to excellent (see Chapter 3, this volume, for a more detailed analysis of measures for fear of blushing).

## Conclusion

Although the body of literature on treatments for fear of blushing has grown substantially since about 1990, randomized controlled trials on treatments for this condition are relatively few and the most effective treatment package has yet to be solidly established. Nevertheless, some important findings have been reported in this area, including the development of TCT as a treatment and coping mechanism for fear of blushing and other physiological symptoms (Bögels et al., 1997), as well as the finding that cognitive intervention may not be necessary to change cognitions in those with fear of blushing (Mulkens et al., 2001; Bögels et al., 2006).

Regardless of the course of treatment selected, some factors appear common to effective treatments for fear of blushing: administration of self-reports specific to fear of blushing, completion of self-monitoring forms throughout treatment and completion of exposure exercises addressing feared and avoided situations. Self-monitoring forms, which are common to a number of effective treatments for anxiety and mood disorders, may also be completed by patients each week to monitor blushing and, depending on the treatment utilized, the practising of various therapeutic techniques. For example, if patients receive CT for fear of blushing, they may record automatic thoughts about blushing, cognitive distortions and rational responses for each situation, whereas with TCT, patients would record the amount of attention they devoted to the social task at hand versus thinking about blushing. Finally, *in vivo* exposures or other types of opportunities to practise these techniques in everyday life should be employed.

We advocate treatments designed specifically for fear of blushing because patients with this specific fear appear to differ from patients with SAD (e.g., Gerlach *et al.*, 2001; Voncken & Bögels, 2009). However, we recognize that, because fear of blushing resembles and overlaps with SAD symptoms and is not a separate diagnosis in the DSM-IV (American Psychiatric Association, 2000), it will be common practice for patients with this fear to be treated with interventions for SAD. In order to examine whether patients with fear of blushing respond differently to psychological treatments that have proven effective for SAD patients in general and to further demonstrate the necessity of a specific treatment for fear of blushing future research should focus on the comparative effects of psychological treatments that were originally designed for SAD versus interventions that have been specifically tailored to reduce fear of blushing.

Also, research is needed on the effects of psychological treatments for patients with SAD in general, specifically on the reduction of (fear of) blushing. Such research would give further insight into how effective the treatments we have are for that particular complaint. Furthermore, it would be interesting to investigate preventive approaches to fear of blushing. For example, can universal prevention programmes in the beginning of adolescence (a period in which self-focused attention and blushing peaks) that explain the function and normality of blushing, as well as the self-fulfilling prophecy of forbidding oneself to blush, prevent excessive fear of blushing?

Recent therapeutic developments have demonstrated promise for other anxiety disorders, but have not yet been explored for fear of blushing. One such therapeutic development is computerized attention-retraining programmes, which have demonstrated promise for the treatment of anxiety disorders (Hakamata *et al.*, 2010) and SAD in particular (e.g., Amir *et al.*, 2009; Schmidt *et al.*, 2009). Such programmes target subconscious attentional biases (e.g., to negative facial expressions in SAD) and retrain attention by redirecting it to other stimuli (e.g., to positive or neutral facial expressions in SAD). That is, by manipulating this biased attention towards threat, anxiety may be decreased (e.g., Mohlman, 2004). This treatment modality may also be beneficial for fear of blushing, if individuals with fear of blushing also demonstrate an attentional bias towards certain negative stimuli.

Other potentially promising treatments for fear of blushing that have not yet been explored are treatments focusing on or incorporating aspects of mindfulness. Mindfulness refers to the purposeful non-judgmental attention to the present moment experience (Kabat-Zinn, 2003). The cultivation of mindfulness, then, may reduce maladaptive efforts to control or remove anxiety (Hofmann et al., 2012; Hofmann, Sawyer et al., 2010). Through a mindfulness perspective, physiological arousal and negative thoughts are viewed as transient events and allowed to rise and fall naturally without eliciting secondary reactions that serve to increase anxiety (Roemer et al., 2008). Treatments incorporating mindfulness for the treatment of anxiety disorders have demonstrated significant improvements in anxiety symptoms and pathological worry, as well as overall stress and quality of life, although it is unclear whether such treatments outperform traditional treatments (e.g., Craigie et al., 2008; Kim et al., 2009; Koszycki et al., 2007). Mindfulness-based interventions for SAD have also proven effective (e.g., Bögels et al., 2006; Piet et al., 2010). Such interventions could be tailored for fear of blushing by emphasizing the importance of awareness and acceptance of physiological symptoms.

Finally, for patients who desire more information about the nature of fear of blushing and its treatment, just one empirically based book on psychological approaches for fear of blushing has been published. *Coping with Blushing* (Edelmann, 2004) describes physiological components of blushing, contains a number of personal accounts from patients with a fear of blushing and describes how fear of blushing may be overcome through the use of relaxation techniques and cognitive restructuring. Though the book does not cover some of the therapeutic techniques described in this chapter (e.g., TCT, SST), it is a good starting point for those who wish to do additional reading on the topic.

REFERENCES

Alden, L. E., & Bieling, P. (1998). Interpersonal consequences of the pursuit of safety. *Behaviour Research and Therapy*, 36, 53–64.
American Psychiatric Association. (2000). *Diagnostic and statistical manual of mental disorders*, 4th edn, text rev. Washington, DC: Author.
Amies, P. L., Gelder, M. G., & Shaw, P. M. (1983). Social phobia: a comparative clinical study. *British Journal of Psychiatry*, 142, 174–9.
Amir, N., Beard, C., Taylor, C., Klumpp, H., Elias, J., Burns, M., & Chen, X. (2009). Attention training in individuals with generalized social phobia: a randomized controlled trial. *Journal of Consulting and Clinical Psychology*, 77, 961–73.
Baker, S. R., & Edelmann, R. J. (2002). Is social phobia related to lack of social skills? Duration of skill-related behaviours and ratings of behavioural adequacy. *British Journal of Clinical Psychology*, 41, 243–57.
Beidel, D. C., Rao, P. A., Scharfstein, L., Wong, N., & Alfano, C. A. (2010). Social skills and social phobia: an investigation of DSM-IV subtypes. *Behaviour Research and Therapy*, 48, 992–1001.

Beidel, D. C., Turner, S. M., & Morris, T. L. (1998). *Social effectiveness therapy for children: A treatment manual.* Unpublished manuscript, Medical University of South Carolina.
  (1999). Psychopathology of childhood social phobia. *Journal of the American Academy of Child and Adolescent Psychiatry*, 38, 643–50.
  (2000). Behavioral treatment of childhood social phobia. *Journal of Consulting and Clinical Psychology*, 68, 1072–80.
Beidel, D. C., Turner, S. M., & Young, B. J. (2006). Social effectiveness therapy for children: five years later. *Behavior Therapy*, 37, 416–25.
Beidel, D. C., Turner, S. M., Young, B. J., & Paulson, A. (2005). Social effectiveness therapy for children: three-year follow-up. *Journal of Consulting and Clinical Psychology*, 73, 721–5.
Bellack, A. S. (1983). Recurrent problems in the behavioral assessment of social skill. *Behaviour Research and Therapy*, 21, 29–41.
Bögels, S. M. (1994). Cognitive therapy versus applied social skills training for fear of blushing, trembling and sweating. Paper presented at the 24th Congress of the European Association of Behavioural and Cognitive Therapies, Corfu, Greece, September.
  (2006). Task concentration versus applied relaxation, in combination with cognitive therapy, for social phobia patients with fear of blushing, trembling and sweating. *Behaviour Research and Therapy*, 44, 1199–210.
Bögels, S. M., Alberts, M., & de Jong, P. J. (1996). Self-consciousness, self-focused attention, blushing propensity and fear of blushing. *Personality and Individual Differences*, 21, 573–81.
Bögels, S. M., Alden, L. E., Beidel, D. C., Clark, L. A., Pine, D. S., Stein, M. B., & Voncken, M. (2010). Social anxiety disorder: questions and answers for the DSM-V. *Depression and Anxiety*, 27, 168–89.
Bögels, S. M., & Mansell, W. (2004). Attention processes in the maintenance and treatment of social phobia: hypervigilance, avoidance and self–focused attention. *Clinical Psychology Review*, 24, 827–56.
Bögels, S. M., Mulkens, S., & de Jong, P. J. (1997). Task concentration training and fear of blushing: practitioner report. *Clinical Psychology and Psychotherapy*, 4, 251–8.
Bögels, S. M., & Reith, W. (1999). Validity of two questionnaires to assess social fears: the Dutch Social Phobia and Anxiety Inventory and the Blushing, Trembling and Sweating Questionnaire. *Journal of Psychopathology and Behavioral Assessment*, 21, 51–66.
Bögels, S. M., Sijbers, G. F. V. M., & Voncken, M. (2006). Mindfulness and task concentration training for social phobia: a pilot study. *Journal of Cognitive Psychotherapy*, 20, 33–44.
Bögels, S. M., & Voncken, M. (2008). Social skills training versus cognitive therapy for social anxiety disorder characterized by fear of blushing, trembling, or sweating. *International Journal of Cognitive Therapy*, 1, 138–50.
Chaker, S., Hofmann, S. G., & Hoyer, J. (2010). Can a one-weekend group therapy reduce fear of blushing? Results of an open trial. *Anxiety, Stress and Coping*, 23, 303–18.

Clark, D. M., Ehlers, A., Hackmann, A., McManus, F., Fennell, M., Grey, N., Waddington, L., & Wild, J. (2006). Cognitive therapy versus exposure and applied relaxation in social phobia: a randomized controlled trial. *Journal of Consulting and Clinical Psychology*, **74**, 568–78.

Clark, D. M., Salkovskis, P. M., Hackmann, A., Middleton, H., Anastasiades, P., & Gelder, M. (1994). A comparison of cognitive therapy, applied relaxation and imipramine in the treatment of panic disorder. *British Journal of Psychiatry*, **164**, 759–69.

Clark, D. M., & Wells, A. (1995). A cognitive model of social phobia. In R. G. Heimberg, M. R. Liebowitz, D. A. Hope & F. R. Schneier (Eds.), *Social phobia: diagnosis, assessment and treatment*. New York: Guilford Press, 69–93.

Clark, J. V., & Arkowitz, H. (1975). Social anxiety and self-evaluation of interpersonal performance. *Psychological Reports*, **36**, 211–21.

Colonnesi, C., Engelhard, I. M., & Bögels, S. M. (2010). Development in children's attribution of embarrassment and the relationship with theory of mind and shyness. *Cognition and Emotion*, **24**, 514–51.

Craigie, M. A., Rees, C. S., Marsh, A., & Nathan, P. (2008). Mindfulness-based cognitive therapy for generalized anxiety disorder: a preliminary evaluation. *Behavioural and Cognitive Psychotherapy*, **36**, 553–68.

Daly, J. A., Vangelisti, A. L., & Lawrence, S. G. (1989). Self-focused attention and public speaking anxiety. *Personality and Individual Differences*, **10**, 903–13.

Dijk, C., Buwalda, F. M., & de Jong, P. J. (2011). Dealing with fear of blushing: a psychoeducational group intervention for fear of blushing. *Clinical Psychology and Psychotherapy*. Advance online publication. doi: 10.1002/cpp.764.

Edelmann, R. J. (1990). Chronic blushing, self-consciousness and social anxiety. *Journal of Psychopathology and Behavioral Assessment*, **12**, 119–27. (2004). *Coping with blushing*. London: Sheldon Press.

Feske, U., & Chambless, D. L. (1995). Cognitive behavioral versus exposure only treatment for social phobia: a meta-analysis. *Behavior Therapy*, **26**, 695–720.

Garssen, B., & Hornsveld, H. (1992). Power analysis or the determination of the size of the sample. *Gedragstherapie*, **25**, 107–21.

Gerlach, A. L., Wilhelm, F. H., Gruber, K., & Roth, W. T. (2001). Blushing and physiological arousability in social phobia. *Journal of Abnormal Psychology*, **110**, 247–58.

Ginsburg, G. S., Riddle, M. A., & Davies, M. (2006). Somatic symptoms in children and adolescents with anxiety disorders. *Journal of the American Academy of Child and Adolescent Psychiatry*, **45**, 1179–87.

Gould, R. A., Buckminster, S., Pollack, M. H., Otto, M. W., & Yap, L. (1997). Cognitive-behavioral and pharmacological treatment for social phobia: a meta-analysis. *Clinical Psychology: Science and Practice*, **4**, 291–306.

Hakamata, Y., Lissek, S., Bar-Haim, Y., Britton, J. C., Fox, N. A., Leibenluft, E., Ernst, M., & Pine, D. S. (2010). Attention bias modification treatment: a meta-analysis toward the establishment of novel treatment for anxiety. *Biological Psychiatry*, **68**, 982–90.

Hayward, C., Varady, S., Albano, A. M., Thienemann, M., Henderson, L., & Schatzberg, A. F. (2000). Cognitive-behavioral group therapy for social phobia in female adolescents: results of a pilot study. *Journal of the American Academy of Child and Adolescent Psychiatry*, **39**, 721–6.

Heimberg, R. G., Horner, K. J., Juster, H. R., Safren, S. A., Brown, E. J., Schneier, F. R., & Liebowitz, M. R. (1999). Psychometric properties of the Liebowitz Social Anxiety Scale. *Psychological Medicine*, **29**, 199–212.

Herbert, J. D., Gaudiano, B. A., Rheingold, A. A., Moitra, E., Myers, V. H., Dalrymple, K. L., & Brandsma, L. L. (2009). Cognitive behavior therapy for generalized social anxiety disorder in adolescents: a randomized controlled trial. *Journal of Anxiety Disorders*, **23**, 167–77.

Hodson, K. J., McManus, F. V., Clark, D. M., & Doll, H. (2008). Can Clark and Wells' (1995) cognitive model of social phobia be applied to young people? *Behavioural and Cognitive Psychotherapy*, **36**, 449–61.

Hofmann, S. G. (2004). Cognitive mediation of treatment change in social phobia. *Journal of Consulting and Clinical Psychology*, **72**, 392–9.

(2007). Cognitive factors that maintain social anxiety disorder: a comprehensive model and its treatment implications. *Cognitive Behaviour Therapy*, **36**, 195–209.

Hofmann, S. G., Asnaani, A., & Hinton, D. E. (2010). Cultural aspects in social anxiety and social anxiety disorder. *Depression and Anxiety*, **27**, 1117–27.

Hofmann, S. G., Moscovitch, D. A., & Kim, H. J. (2006). Autonomic correlates of social anxiety and embarrassment in shy and non-shy individuals. *International Journal of Psychophysiology*, **61**, 134–42.

Hofmann, S. G., & Otto, M. W. (2008). *Cognitive-behavior therapy of social anxiety disorder: evidence-based and disorder specific treatment techniques.* New York: Routledge.

Hofmann, S. G., Sawyer, A. T., Fang, A., & Asnaani, A. (2012). Emotion dysregulation model of mood and anxiety disorders. *Depression and Anxiety*, **29**, 409–16.

Hofmann, S. G., Sawyer, A. T., Witt, A., & Oh, D. (2010). The effect of mindfulness-based therapy on anxiety and depression: a meta-analytic review. *Journal of Consulting and Clinical Psychology*, **78**, 169–83.

Hope, D. A., Gansler, D. A., & Heimberg, R. G. (1989). Attentional focus and causal attributions in social phobia: implications from social psychology. *Clinical Psychology Review*, **9**, 49–60.

Hope, D. A., Heimberg, R. G., & Bruch, M. A. (1995). Dismantling cognitive-behavioral group therapy for social phobia. *Behaviour Research and Therapy*, **33**, 637–50.

Jerremalm, A., Jansson, L., & Öst, L. (1986). Cognitive and physiological reactivity and the effects of different behavioral methods in the treatment of social phobia. *Behaviour Research and Therapy*, **24**, 171–80.

Kabat-Zinn, J. (2003). Mindfulness-based interventions in context: past, present, and future. *Clinical Psychology: Science and Practice*, **10**, 144–56.

Kelly, M. M., Walters, C., & Philips, K. (2010). Social anxiety and its relationship to functional impairment in body dysmorphic disorder. *Behavior Therapy*, **41**, 143–53.

Kim, Y. W., Lee, S. H., Choi, T. K., Suh, S. Y., Kim, B., Kim, C. M., Cho, S. J., Kim, M. J., Yook, K., Ryu, M., Song, S. K., & Yook, K. H. (2009).

Effectiveness of mindfulness-based cognitive therapy as an adjuvant to pharmacotherapy in patients with panic disorder or generalized anxiety disorder. *Depression and Anxiety*, **26**, 601–6.

Koszycki, D., Benger, M., Shlik, J., & Bradwejn, J. (2007). Randomized trial of a meditation-based stress reduction program and cognitive behavior therapy in generalized social anxiety disorder. *Behaviour Research and Therapy*, **45**, 2518–26.

Leary, M. R., & Meadows, S. (1991). Predictors, elicitors, and concomitants of social blushing. *Journal of Personality and Social Psychology*, **60**, 254–62.

McEwan, K. L., & Devins, G. M. (1983). Is increased arousal in social anxiety noticed by others? *Journal of Abnormal Psychology*, **92**, 417–21.

Mandler, G., Mandler, J. M., & Uviller, E. T. (1958). Autonomic feedback: the perception of autonomic activity. *Journal of Abnormal and Social Psychology*, **56**, 367–73.

Marks, I., & Mathews, A. (1982). Brief standard self-rating scale for phobic patients. *Behaviour Research and Therapy*, **17**, 263–7.

Mattick, R. P., & Peters, L. (1988). Treatment of severe social phobia: effects of guided exposure with and without cognitive restructuring. *Journal of Consulting and Clinical Psychology*, **56**, 251–60.

Meleshko, K. G., & Alden, L. E. (1993). Anxiety and self-disclosure: toward a motivational model. *Journal of Personality and Social Psychology*, **64**, 1000–9.

Melfsen, S., Kühnemund, M., Schwieger, J., Warnke, A., Stadler, C., Poustka, F., & Stangier, U. (2011). Cognitive behavioral therapy of socially phobic children focusing on cognition: a randomised wait-list control study. *Child and Adolescent Psychiatry and Mental Health*, **5**(1), 5.

Mersch, P. P., Emmelkamp, P. M., Bögels, S. M., & Van der Sleen, J. (1989). Social phobia: individual response patterns and the effects of behavioral and cognitive interventions. *Behaviour Research and Therapy*, **27**, 421–34.

Mohlman, J. (2004). Attention training as an intervention for anxiety: review and rationale. *Behavior Therapist*, **27**, 37–41.

Mulkens, S., Bögels, S. M., de Jong, P. J., & Louwers, J. (2001). Fear of blushing: effects of task concentration training versus exposure in vivo on fear and physiology. *Journal of Anxiety Disorders*, **15**, 413–32.

Mulkens, S., de Jong, P. J., Dobbelaar, A., & Bögels, S. M. (1999). Fear of blushing: fearful preoccupation irrespective of facial coloration. *Behaviour Research and Therapy*, **37**, 1119–28.

Newman, M. G., Hofmann, S. G., Trabert, W., Roth, W. T., & Taylor, C. B. (1994). Does behavioral treatment of social phobia lead to cognitive changes? *Behavior Therapy*, **25**, 503–17.

Öst, L. (1987). Applied relaxation: description of a coping technique and review of controlled studies. *Behaviour Research and Therapy*, **25**, 397–409.

Öst, L., Jerremalm, A., & Johansson, J. (1981). Individual response patterns and the effects of different behavioral methods in the treatment of social phobia. *Behaviour Research and Therapy*, **19**, 1–16.

Pelissolo, A., Moukheiber, A., Lobjoie, C., Valla, J., & Lambrey, S. (2012). Is there a place for fear of blushing in social anxiety spectrum? *Depression and Anxiety*, **29**, 62–70.

Piet, J., Hougaard, E., Hecksher, M. S., & Rosenberg, N. K. (2010). A randomized pilot study of mindfulness-based cognitive therapy and group cognitive-behavioral therapy for young adults with social phobia. *Scandinavian Journal of Psychology*, 51, 403–10.

Rodebaugh, T. L., Holaway, R. M., & Heimberg, R. G. (2004). The treatment of social anxiety disorder. *Clinical Psychology Review*, 24, 883–908.

Roemer, L., Orsillo, S. M., Salters-Pedneault, K. (2008). Efficacy of an acceptance-based behavior therapy for generalized anxiety disorder: evaluation in a randomized controlled trial. *Journal of Consulting and Clinical Psychology*, 76, 1083–9.

Scheier, M. F., & Carver, C. S. (1983). Self-directed attention and the comparison of self with standards. *Journal of Experimental Social Psychology*, 19, 205–22.

Schmidt, N. B., Richey, J. A., Buckner, J. D., & Timpano, K. R. (2009). Attention training for generalized social anxiety disorder. *Journal of Abnormal Psychology*, 118, 5–14.

Scholing, A., & Emmelkamp, P. M. G. (1993). Cognitive and behavioural treatments of fear of blushing, sweating or trembling. *Behaviour Research and Therapy*, 31, 155–70.

(1996). Treatment of fear of blushing, sweating, or trembling: results at long-term follow-up. *Behavior Modification*, 20, 338–56.

Segal, Z. V., Williams, J. M. G., & Teasdale, J. D. (2002). *Mindfulness-based cognitive therapy for depression: a new approach to preventing relapse*. New York: Guilford Press.

Spence, S. H., Donovan, C., & Brechman-Toussaint, M. (2000). The treatment of childhood social phobia: the effectiveness of a social skills training-based, cognitive-behavioural intervention, with and without parental involvement. *Journal of Child Psychology and Psychiatry*, 41, 713–26.

Stopa, L., & Clark, D. M. (1993). Cognitive processes in social phobia. *Behaviour Research and Therapy*, 31, 255–67.

Takahaski, T. (1989). Social phobia syndrome in Japan. *Comprehensive Psychiatry*, 30, 45–52.

Taylor, S. (1996). Meta-analysis of cognitive-behavioral treatment for social phobia. *Journal of Behavior Therapy and Experimental Psychiatry*, 27, 1–9.

Van Dam-Baggen, R., & Kraaimaat, F. (2000). Group social skills training or cognitive group therapy as the clinical treatment of choice for generalized social phobia? *Journal of Anxiety Disorders*, 14, 437–51.

Veale, D. (2004). Body dysmorphic disorder. *Postgraduate Medical Journal*, 80, 67–71.

Voncken, M. J., & Bögels, S. M. (2008). Social performance deficits in social anxiety disorder: reality during conversation and biased perception during speech. *Journal of Anxiety Disorders*, 22, 1384–92.

(2009). Physiological blushing in social anxiety disorder patients with and without blushing complaints: two subtypes? *Biological Psychology*, 81, 86–94.

# 15 Psychophysiological aspects of rosacea

*Peter D. Drummond and Daphne Su*

### Introduction

Rosacea is a chronic and progressive disorder characterized by extremely sensitive skin, burning and stinging sensations, and persistent flushing of the cheeks, nose, chin or forehead accompanied by acne-like facial papules or pustules (Elewski et al., 2010; Wilkin, 1994). Primary diagnostic features include one or more of the following signs: frequent transient flushing; persistent redness; papules and pustules; and prominent facial capillaries. Secondary features may include: burning or stinging sensations; elevated red plaques; rough and scaly 'dry' skin; facial swelling; ocular discomfort; lid inflammation and red eyes; and skin thickening (Wilkin et al., 2002). A standard classification system for rosacea, developed by the National Rosacea Society Expert Committee on the Classification and Staging of Rosacea, lists four subtypes: *erythematotelangiectatic rosacea*, characterized by persistent flushing, central facial redness and small blood vessels near the surface of the skin; *papulopustular rosacea*, characterized by persistent facial redness and red bumps (papules), some filled with pus (pustules); *phymatous rosacea*, associated with thickened skin, particularly around the nose (rhinophyma); and *ocular rosacea*, where the main features are red, dry irritated eyes and eyelids (Wilkin et al., 2002). Patients may have more than one subtype, or may progress from one subtype to another.

As flushing often aggravates other symptoms of rosacea, many people with rosacea avoid vasodilator agents such as alcohol and foods high in histamine or nitrate content or that are highly spiced. They also avoid soaps, lotions and creams that irritate the skin or that dilate blood vessels directly, exercise, exposure to environmental stimuli that increase skin blood flow (e.g., extremes of heat or cold, strong winds and sunlight), and psychological factors that may aggravate symptoms (e.g., stress, anxiety and emotions such as anger and embarrassment) (Culp & Scheinfield, 2009; Scharschmidt et al., 2011). They may also avoid interacting with other people due to concerns about their appearance.

Not surprisingly, then, the symptoms of rosacea can impact severely on self-esteem and quality of life.

This chapter begins with an overview of the epidemiology and etiology of rosacea. We then examine the link between psychological stress and rosacea, with a particular focus on the role of blushing.

## Epidemiology of rosacea

Estimates of the prevalence of rosacea vary considerably across epidemiological studies, possibly due to the different population samples, different criteria used for diagnosis, or difficulties with differential diagnosis. Indeed, questions have been raised about whether rosacea is one disease entity or encompasses several diseases with different etiologies (Elewski et al., 2010). For example, dermatological conditions such as seborrheic dermatitis, keratosis pilaris, lupus erythematosus, perioral dermatitis, acne vulgaris and steroid side-effects may mimic features of rosacea (Culp & Scheinfield, 2009), and some may even be variants of rosacea (Kligman, 2004; Webster, 2009).

The first comprehensive epidemiological study of rosacea came from a Swedish study of the cutaneous effects of visual display units in 809 office employees (Berg & Liden, 1989). Of these, eighty-one (10 per cent) had rosacea – 13.7 per cent of women and 5.4 per cent of men. Facial flushing was the most common symptom but 1.8 per cent of the study population also had papules and pustules. A large-scale study of common skin diseases in German workers who participated in skin cancer screening trials provided another insight into the prevalence of rosacea in the workplace (Schaefer et al., 2008). In contrast to the Swedish study, rosacea was detected in 2.3 per cent of men and 2.0 per cent of women. Whether the disparity between these studies was due to different diagnostic criteria or to sampling differences is uncertain. However, a recent cross-sectional study of 348 people aged over 30 years selected randomly from the Estonian working population suggests that symptoms of rosacea are relatively common, as 22 per cent had one or more of the primary features of rosacea included in the classification criteria of the American National Rosacea Society Expert Committee (Abram, Silm & Oona, 2010). Symptoms were most frequent in people with photosensitive skin types and increased after the age of 40 years, but were similar in women and men. Surprisingly, one third of the study participants who met diagnostic criteria for rosacea had not noticed their skin changes.

The prevalence of papulopustular rosacea was investigated recently in an Irish study (McAleer et al., 2010). To explore effects of chronic ultraviolet radiation exposure, 500 hospital workers were compared with 500 island inhabitants with outdoor occupations and lifestyles. Skin damage due to sun exposure was also rated clinically. Skin sensitivity to sun exposure was similar in the two populations, but skin damage was greater in islanders than in hospital workers. Papulopustular rosacea was detected in 2.6 per cent of hospital workers and 2.8 per cent of islanders, and was unrelated to skin damage from sun exposure.

Analysis of patients who attend dermatological outpatient clinics suggests that the gender distribution of patients with rosacea varies at different stages of life. In a cross-sectional study of 50,237 patients who attended a general state hospital dermatological outpatient clinic in Athens, Greece, between 1995 and 2002, 615 (1.2 per cent) were diagnosed with rosacea (Kyriakis et al., 2005). Stratification by age and gender indicated that attendance for treatment of rosacea was unusual in either sex below 35 years of age. Between 36 and 50 years of age, rosacea affected a greater proportion of women than men (2.4 per cent and 0.7 per cent respectively). However, rosacea increased abruptly in men after 50 years of age and reached a peak of 3.9 per cent in the 76–80 age group. Rosacea detection rates were greater in winter (1.4 per cent) and spring (1.5 per cent) than in summer (0.7 per cent) or autumn (1.0 per cent).

Rosacea is more visible in fair- than in dark-skinned people, but people of any ethnic group may be afflicted (Webster, 2009). For example, in a retrospective study of patients who attended an outpatient dermatology clinic between 1990 and 2003 in Tunis, North Africa, rosacea affected 0.2 per cent of cases (Khaled et al., 2010) compared with 1.2 per cent in the Greek study (Kyriakis et al., 2005). The sex ratio of rosacea in this study was 71 per cent female to 29 per cent male. Highly pigmented skin may be protective against rosacea, as a sun-reactive skin type that usually or always burns after first exposure to midday sunshine for 30 minutes was identified as an independent risk factor for rosacea in a community sample of Estonians (Abram, Silm, Maaroos et al., 2010).

Together, these epidemiological studies indicate that rosacea is a reasonably common dermatological disease that typically affects women aged between 30 and 50 years. It is most often observed in people of north and west European descent but occasionally develops in people with dark skin. In northern European countries, prevalence estimates of rosacea range between 1 and 10 per cent. Skin sensitivity to sun exposure appears to be a risk factor for rosacea, but may not contribute directly to the papulopustular stage of rosacea.

## Etiology and pathogenesis of rosacea

Some theorists have focused on explaining the prominent vascular disturbances that typically develop early in the course of rosacea (Kligman, 2004; Wilkin, 1994). For example, Wilkin (1981) demonstrated that hot liquids provoked flushing in patients with rosacea, and proposed that the exchange of heat from blood in the internal jugular vein or cavernous sinus to the arterial supply of the hypothalamus triggered thermoregulatory flushing. Brinnel and colleagues (1989) suggested that a fault in this countercurrent heat exchange system prevented diversion of cool venous blood from the facial circulation to intracranial structures in patients with rosacea, thereby provoking persistent facial flushing. In support of this hypothesis, facial flushing developed in four rosacea patients but not in two controls during body heating. Moreover, flushing was associated with signs of impaired blood flow through the emissary veins that channel cool blood from the face to intracranial sites, thus preventing selective brain cooling.

Increased blood flow through vessels in the superficial dermis of rosacea sufferers may lead to an accumulation of extracellular fluid in the tissues of the face (Søybe, 1950). In particular, Wilkin (1994) proposed that chronic progressive damage to lymphatic drainage vessels in rosacea (e.g., from sun exposure) may result in swelling and persistent inflammation which, in turn, could result in papule formation and provoke the growth of new blood vessels in the skin (angiogenesis). This explanation fits with histological signs of disorganization of the upper dermal connective tissue, elastosis, dilated vascular channels in the subpapillary venous plexus, accumulation of inflammatory infiltrate and oedema in the skin of rosacea patients (Marks & Harcourt-Webster, 1969).

To investigate mechanisms of facial flushing in rosacea, we recently assessed endothelial and axon-reflex vasodilatation in response to the transcutaneous iontophoresis of acetylcholine in patients and age- and sex-matched controls (Drummond & Su, 2012a). Acetylcholine induces the release of the vasodilator nitric oxide by binding to $M_2$ muscarinic receptors on the endothelial surface of blood vessels (Berghoff et al., 2002). Acetylcholine also binds to nicotinic receptors on cutaneous C fibres (Izumi & Karita, 1992), thereby initiating an axon reflex that culminates in the release of the potent vasodilators calcitonin gene-related peptide and substance P. In general, vasodilator responses to acetylcholine were similar in both groups. However, axon-reflex vasodilatation was greater in patients with severe than with mild rosacea, and stinging sensations (most likely relayed by nociceptive nerve fibres containing substance P) were greater in patients than in controls. These findings suggest that the nociceptive fibres that signal stinging sensations and that mediate axon-reflex vasodilatation in the facial skin may play a role in rosacea.

It now seems clear that dysregulation of the innate immune system lies at the heart of rosacea (Yamasaki & Gallo, 2009). This system responds to harmful environmental stimuli by releasing inflammatory mediators and anti-microbial peptides (cathelicidins) into the skin. In particular, cathelicidins provide a first line of defence against skin infection, modify local inflammatory responses, act directly on endothelial cells to trigger blood vessel growth, and activate adaptive immunity. Yamasaki and colleagues (2007) reported that people with rosacea expressed abnormally elevated levels of cutaneous cathelicidin, possibly due to a change in toll-like receptor 2, part of the pattern recognition system of the innate immune system (Yamasaki et al., 2011). In addition, the cathelicidin in rosacea patients took on an abnormal form that rapidly resulted in inflammation when injected into the skin of mice. The innate immune system is programmed to detect microbe infestation, tissue damage due to ultraviolet radiation, and physical and chemical trauma. Thus, stimuli that typically trigger weak inflammatory reactions may evoke the much larger changes associated with rosacea in susceptible people.

More controversial is the role of demodex folliculorum, a mite that lives within the sebaceous gland of hair follicles. Powell (2004) suggested that the mite may play a role in rosacea by triggering inflammatory or allergic reactions, or by acting as a vector for bacteria that attack the skin. Although the population of these mites is increased in the affected skin of rosacea patients, this may be a consequence rather than a cause of rosacea as the mites thrive in the conditions associated with papulopustular rosacea. Moreover, treatments that reduce symptoms do not necessarily eliminate the mites (Bonnar et al., 1993).

## Effects of rosacea on quality of life

Two recent Polish reports indicate that rosacea can have an array of adverse effects on quality of life. In the first paper, Salamon and colleagues (2008) evaluated quality of life in forty rosacea sufferers and forty healthy controls using the Short Form 36 Health Survey. Rosacea sufferers reported difficulties in terms of general health, vitality, emotional state, physical functioning, mental health and bodily pain. In a companion paper, Chodkiewicz and colleagues (2007) reported that patients with rosacea were less satisfied with their lives, felt that they received poor social support and had higher levels of anxiety and depression than healthy controls.

The impact of treating symptoms of rosacea on quality of life was investigated in a recent Turkish study of 308 patients referred to a hospital dermatology clinic for treatment of rosacea (Aksoy et al., 2010). Health-related quality of life was measured with the Dermatology Life Quality Index Questionnaire, a validated instrument that assesses the impact of dermatological disorders on quality of life in terms of symptoms and feelings, daily activities, leisure time, work and school, personal relationships and response to treatment (Ozturkcan et al., 2006). Rosacea had a greater impact on the quality of life of women than men, and was greater for younger than older people. The impact depended on the severity of symptoms; these negative impacts decreased after successful treatment of symptoms.

## Relationships between rosacea and emotional distress – cause or effect?

As Western cultures place a heavy emphasis on appearance, especially of the face, many dermatological patients encounter stigmatization such as verbal rejection or stares (Thompson & Kent, 2001). Thus, it is not surprising that disfiguring skin conditions impact heavily on psychological well-being (Bickers et al., 2006), potentially leading to psychiatric comorbidity (Gupta & Gupta, 2003; Millard, 2000). Skin disorders such as psoriasis, atopic dermatitis and acne may evoke a sense of hopelessness which is aggravated by a poor response to treatment (Carroll et al., 2005; Cohen et al., 1991; Hashiro & Okumura, 1997; Gupta et al., 1994; Kimball et al., 2005; Papadopoulos et al., 2000). Indeed, psychiatric disorders, particularly mood and anxiety disorders, may be present in 25–30 per cent of dermatological patients (Millard, 2000; Picardi & Abeni, 2001; Picardi et al., 2000, Picardi et al., 2004).

Although rosacea is one of the most visible skin disorders, the impact of rosacea on psychological well-being has received relatively little attention (Garnis-Jones, 1998). Nevertheless, emerging research suggests that many rosacea sufferers are distressed about their symptoms. For example, in a small-scale questionnaire study conducted by nurses, dissatisfaction with self-image increased in line with the severity of rosacea symptoms (Lindow et al., 2005). Similarly, in a study by Balkrishnan and colleagues (2006), an elevated fear of negative evaluation was detected in seventy-three women with severe skin conditions, including four with rosacea. Whether this applies more broadly to people with rosacea, or is most apparent in those who attend dermatology clinics, has yet to be explored.

More is known about the role of personality traits in rosacea. On the basis of Rorschach tests, White, Jones and Ingham (1956) concluded that rosacea patients referred for psychiatric assessment were characterized by emotional inhibition, and had 'an immature reaction to life with a rather infantile but strongly inhibited affective response. All adjustments seemed poor, and neurotic trends marked' (p. 88). In an independent clinical assessment, these patients appeared to lack self-confidence, relied heavily on their relatives or a few close friends for emotional support, blushed readily and felt ill at ease in social settings. Plesch (1951) also employed Rorschach tests in his psychiatric assessment of patients with rosacea or a fear of blushing. He identified neurotic tendencies in the majority of cases, along with nonspecific paranoid signs and castration and homosexual fantasies.

Whitlock (1961) doubted whether these psychiatric observations applied to the majority of patients seen in general dermatological practice. To confirm this clinical impression, the Maudsley Medical Questionnaire (a precursor of the Eysenck Personality Inventory) was administered to fifty rosacea patients and to a control group of another fifty patients who attended a dermatological outpatient clinic. No consistent differences were detected between rosacea patients and controls on questions concerned with social anxiety or neuroticism. However, in eight cases emotional disturbances (particularly a sense of shame coupled with feelings of resentment and injustice) appeared to be important in the evolution of rosacea.

Marks (1968) reported that rosacea patients did not differ from normal in their prior history of psychiatric disorders or emotional trauma. However, depression scores on a self-report inventory were elevated in the rosacea group. Gupta and colleagues (2005) audited data deposited in the National Ambulatory Medical Care Survey and the National Hospital Ambulatory Care Survey databases, based on visits to physicians' private rooms and hospital outpatient clinics across America between 1995 and 2002. A diagnosis of rosacea was associated with 2.3 per cent of all dermatology visits, predominantly Caucasian women aged between 40 and 70 years. Among the patients with rosacea, 1.04 per cent had a comorbid psychiatric diagnosis, primarily major depressive disorder. The prevalence of depressive illness in patients with rosacea was higher than expected (the odds ratio for depressive disease in rosacea patients was 4.81). This finding is important, because physicians are unlikely to make a psychiatric diagnosis during a visit for a dermatological complaint unless the psychiatric comorbidity requires urgent attention (Gupta et al., 2005).

Over the years, the National Rosacea Society of America has conducted informal online surveys (http://www.rosacea.org/rr/2007/spring/

article_3.php). In 2007, the survey was answered by 603 respondents. Of these, 76 per cent reported having low self-esteem, 69 per cent said they felt embarrassed by their facial redness and disfigurement and 65 per cent said they felt frustrated. These findings have been corroborated in small-scale surveys, in which rosacea sufferers reported that they avoided social interaction due to feelings of embarrassment and self-consciousness (Harlow et al., 2000; Nicholson et al., 2007).

Whether these views are shared by people who do not participate in internet surveys remains uncertain. Nevertheless, it appears that many patients seen in dermatology practices are distressed by their condition. In addition, social anxiety is associated with rosacea in some cases. Whether this might reflect referral bias was explored recently by Abram and colleagues (2009) in a study of seventy consecutive patients who attended a dermatologist. These patients were compared with fifty-six people with symptoms of rosacea selected from among the working population who had never sought medical care for their symptoms. Consistent with referral bias, dermatology patients more frequently had moderate or severe forms of rosacea and were more disturbed by their symptoms, even when mild, than the community sample. Depressive symptoms did not differ between the two groups, but were greatest in those most disturbed by rosacea.

We recently assessed social anxiety (fear of negative evaluation, social interaction anxiety and social phobia) and distress (self-reported depression, anxiety and stress) in nineteen participants with mild rosacea (defined as mild facial flushing and sporadic papules and pustules), another twelve with more severe flushing and/or a dense concentration of papules and pustules in the facial region, and eighty-six normal controls without rosacea (Su & Drummond, 2011). Five of the rosacea sufferers were recruited from dermatology practices and the remainder by advertisement in community newspapers, radio interview, an internet forum for rosacea sufferers, and undergraduate psychology classes. Participants with extensive facial papules and pustules had higher stress and social phobia scores than controls or others without papules or pustules. However, mild rosacea appeared to have little impact on social anxiety or distress. Stress scores reflected issues such as difficulty relaxing, nervous tension, or feeling irritable, agitated or impatient. The Social Phobia Scale employed in this study (Mattick & Clarke, 1998) included items such as 'I get nervous that people are staring at me as I walk down the street', 'I feel awkward and tense if I know people are watching me' and 'I would get tense if I had to sit facing people on a bus or a train'. Thus, some participants with severe rosacea apparently were self-conscious about their appearance. In the extreme, such concerns could result in avoidance of situations that might involve scrutiny by others.

## Role of blushing in rosacea

It has long been suspected that frequent blushing is an early sign of rosacea. According to Miller (1921, pp. 123–4), 'blushing which is produced by the slightest provocation forms one of the early symptoms of the disease, frequent repetition producing enlarged blood vessels and finally tissue hypertrophy'. This theme was explored further by Klaber and Wittkower (1939), who noted that redness or flushing in rosacea generally preceded the papulopustular stage by months or years. Most patients in this series said that rosacea was worse if they became hot, hurried or worried, and they regarded worry as the most important aggravating factor. In a psychological investigation of fifty patients and fifty controls, thirty-five patients (compared with eleven controls) described features of social anxiety as children, and this anxiety usually persisted into adulthood. Most patients reported that excitement or worry brought on hot flushes and that emotional stress intensified the severity of rosacea. Moreover, in thirty-three cases, the onset of rosacea was preceded by acute emotional trauma or prolonged emotional stress. Klaber and Wittkower postulated that feelings of guilt, inferiority or shame that provoked repetitive bursts of blushing increased vulnerability to rosacea, and eventually produced a 'permanent blush'.

Despite these intriguing observations, whether blushing plays a causative role in rosacea remains unresolved. We recently administered the Blushing Propensity Scale (Leary & Meadows, 1991) to our series of nineteen mild rosacea sufferers and twelve with more severe rosacea (Su & Drummond, 2011). Blushing propensity scores were greater in severe than in mild rosacea sufferers or controls, indicating that participants with severe symptoms thought that they blushed readily in a range of social situations. However, as scores on the Blushing Propensity Scale are associated with self-focused attention and heightened social anxiety (Bögels et al., 1996; Edelmann & Skov, 1993; Leary & Meadows, 1991; Neto, 1996), elevated scores could represent anxiety about blushing rather than blushing per se. Alternatively, interoceptive cues of blushing might be stronger than usual in people with severe rosacea, particularly if blushing aggravates symptoms and evokes uncomfortable stinging or burning sensations in the face.

The participants were also asked whether they recalled blushing strongly as a child. Irrespective of the severity of rosacea, recollections of childhood blushing were greater in rosacea sufferers (61 per cent) than in controls (27 per cent). Although these observations suggest that frequent childhood blushing is a correlate of rosacea, whether this is relevant to the etiology of rosacea is uncertain. On the one hand, blushing in childhood might reflect a predisposition for facial blood vessels to dilate readily. If this promotes inflammatory responses (e.g., in skin made susceptible to inflammation by sun damage), recurrent blushing might establish a cycle of vasodilatation and inflammation that evokes symptoms of rosacea. On the other hand, recollections of childhood blushing might be coloured by associated emotions. For example, blushing might have been remembered because of a predisposition to experience or recall strong emotional responses or to interpret those responses as threatening. This explanation is consistent with the observation that social anxiety frequently precedes rosacea (Klaber & Wittkower, 1939), and is present in adulthood in more severely affected rosacea sufferers (Su & Drummond, 2011). Alternatively, rosacea might retrospectively increase the salience of blushing, thereby assisting the recall of relevant childhood memories.

Ultimately, prospective studies will be required to tease out which, if any, of these explanations is correct. In the meantime, it would be interesting to investigate interactions between vasodilatation and inflammation in normal and damaged skin, to clarify the role of blushing and other forms of vasodilatation in the development and/or maintenance of rosacea symptoms. It may also be informative to explore the role of the neuroendocrine system in the production of rosacea symptoms, as stress hormones such as corticotropin-releasing factor activate cutaneous mast cells which, in turn, release vasoactive, nociceptive and pro-inflammatory mediators into the skin (Singh et al., 1999). These mediators could amplify the initial response to stress by acting on blood vessels, sensory nerves and resident immune cells to produce symptoms of rosacea.

In our biopsychosocial model of rosacea, we postulate that symptoms of rosacea might escalate during psychological stress due to a reciprocal relationship between facial flushing and stress (Figure 15.1). To investigate this component of the model, we recently compared blushing in rosacea sufferers and controls while they completed a series of embarrassing laboratory tasks (singing, giving an impromptu speech, and listening to recordings of these activities) (Drummond & Su, 2012b). Changes in forehead blood flow were similar in rosacea sufferers and controls. Even so, rosacea sufferers, particularly those with the most severe symptoms, thought that they blushed more intensely and were more embarrassed than controls during most of the tasks. The laser Doppler perfusion signal was greater in patients with severe than with mild symptoms throughout the experiment; nevertheless, increases in

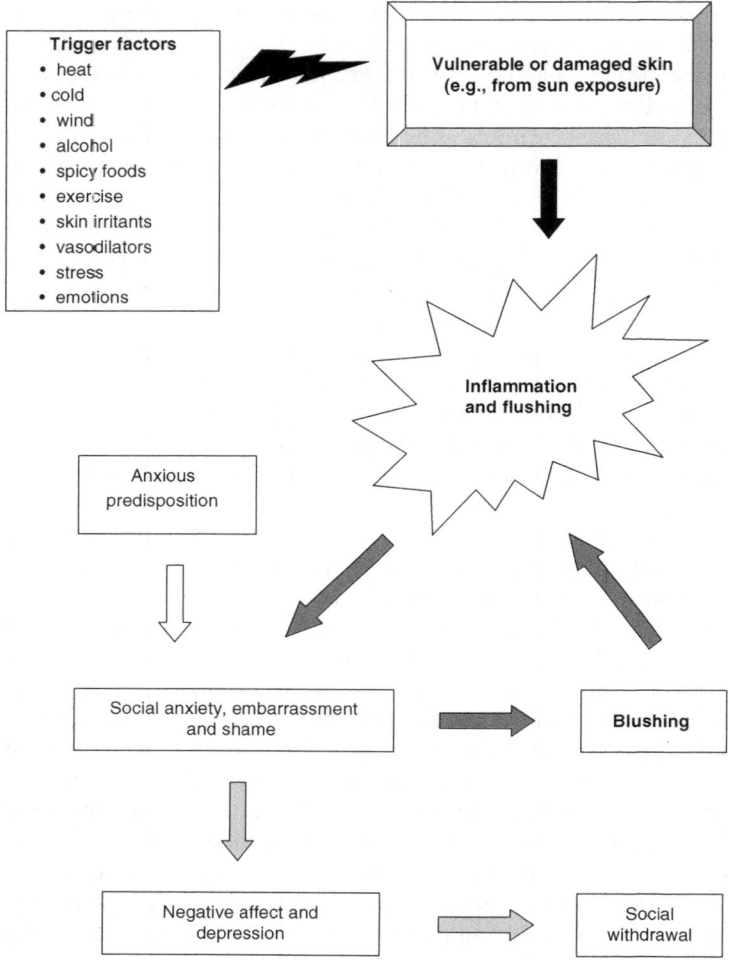

Figure 15.1 Hypothesized link between psychological factors and symptoms of rosacea. Trigger factors, including psychological stress and emotions such as embarrassment, guilt and shame, may act upon vulnerable or damaged skin to provoke inflammation and flushing in people with rosacea (shown by the lightning bolt and black arrow). Signs of rosacea, primarily inflamed and flushed skin, may promote social anxiety and associated emotions which, in turn, evokes blushing and aggravates facial flushing. This cycle may escalate (dark grey arrows), particularly in people with an anxious predisposition (clear arrow). In addition, the facial disfigurement associated with rosacea may result in negative affect and depression which, in turn, results in social withdrawal and decreased quality of life (light grey arrows).

blood flow (expressed as the percentage change from baseline) were similar in both groups during the embarrassing laboratory tasks. These findings suggest that rosacea sufferers are concerned about blushing; however, the findings do not support the notion that this heightened concern intensifies blushing, at least in the short term. Nevertheless, further investigation is warranted to establish whether a reciprocal loop between facial flushing and psychological stress contributes to symptoms of rosacea in the longer term. In addition, basal levels of flow could be important, as increases in flow might have different physiological and/or psychological implications when coming off a high rather than a low base. For example, high levels of flow could contribute to inflammation by initiating endothelial vasodilatation or axon reflexes. In addition, increases in flow coming off a high base might be more visible (and thus potentially more distressing) than increases coming off a low base.

### Role of psychological treatment in rosacea

Psychological interventions can help to alleviate the distress associated with dermatological symptoms and other forms of disfigurement (Fried, 2002; Papadopoulos, 2005; Robinson et al., 1996). For example, a twelve-week individually administered psychotherapy programme consisting of relaxation training, imagery training and cognitive behavioural stress management techniques resulted in significant reductions in stress levels and symptoms of psoriasis (Zachariae et al., 1996). Similarly, application of mindfulness techniques during an extended course of phototherapy or photochemotherapy accelerated the rate of clearance of psoriatic lesions (Kabat-Zinn et al., 1998). Positive outcomes have also been reported for patients with atopic dermatitis after training in relaxation, self-control of scratching, and stress management (Ehlers et al., 1995).

Many investigators have highlighted the importance of managing rosacea using appropriate medication, with relaxation and other stress reduction methods as treatment adjuncts (e.g., Bikowski, 2000; Bikowski & Goldman, 2004; Elewski et al., 2010; Gupta & Chaudhry, 2005). However, to our knowledge, benefits of psychological treatment have not been investigated systematically for patients with rosacea. We recently explored this issue in three rosacea sufferers who were concerned about the social implications of episodic or persistent facial flushing (Su & Drummond, 2011). In each case, blushing triggered persistent facial flushing in association with additional symptoms of anxiety (e.g., a racing heart, sweating, trembling hands, confusion or intrusive thoughts). In addition, social anxiety and avoidance centred on concerns about being regarded negatively for blushing excessively. Encouragingly, all three patients appeared to benefit from cognitive behavioural techniques (relaxation training, challenging negative beliefs, task concentration training and graded exposure to feared activities) in terms of an increased repertoire of activities and reductions in social anxiety. In particular, relaxation training promoted an overall sense of control over physiological disturbances, and helped to shift the focus of attention from the face to other parts of the body. Controlled studies on larger cohorts of rosacea sufferers are now required to verify and extend these preliminary observations, and to identify the active components of treatment.

## Directions for future research

Although there is no consensus on whether psychological factors increase vulnerability to rosacea, an association between rosacea and social anxiety is widely recognized. It seems likely that this association stems largely from concern about facial disfigurement. In addition, however, social anxiety may be involved more directly in the pathogenesis of rosacea. One possible scenario is illustrated in Figure 15.1. According to this scheme, trigger factors such as psychological stress might act upon skin rendered vulnerable to persistent inflammation and flushing (e.g., by sun damage) in people with rosacea. Emotional responses that provoke blushing may then aggravate inflammation and flushing in vulnerable skin. If blushing and/or flushing due to inflammation also exacerbate social anxiety, this could establish a cycle of symptom escalation that is interrupted only by escape from and subsequent avoidance of provocative situations.

Hence, psychological treatments that help to break this vicious cycle could provide substantial benefits for people with rosacea. For example, procedures that help alleviate a fear of blushing, such as task concentration training and cognitive therapy (Bögels, 2006; Bögels & Voncken, 2008), might also be of benefit to patients with rosacea. Moreover, as rosacea is associated with disfigurement and physical discomfort, cognitive behavioural strategies and mindfulness training could provide additional benefits. It would be particularly interesting to determine whether these treatment approaches help to relieve the physiological signs of rosacea. Conversely, it would be interesting to evaluate the effects of rosacea treatments on chronic blushing. For example, a heightened inflammatory response may increase vulnerability not only to rosacea but also to blushing (Drummond & Lazaroo, 2012). If so, anti-inflammatory agents that reduce flushing in rosacea might also reduce the skin redness that sometimes is associated with frequent or severe episodes of blushing.

# REFERENCES

Abram, K., Silm, H., Maaroos, H. I., & Oona, M. (2009). Subjective disease perception and symptoms of depression in relation to healthcare-seeking behaviour in patients with rosacea. *Acta Dermato-Venereologica*, **89**(5), 488–91.

(2010). Risk factors associated with rosacea. *Journal of the European Academy of Dermatology and Venereology*, **24**(5), 565–71.

Abram, K., Silm, H., & Oona, M. (2010). Prevalence of rosacea in an Estonian working population using a standard classification. *Acta Dermato-Venereologica*, **90**(3), 269–73.

Aksoy, B., Altaykan-Hapa, A., Egemen, D., Karagoz, F., & Atakan, N. (2010). The impact of rosacea on quality of life: effects of demographic and clinical characteristics and various treatment modalities. *British Journal of Dermatology*, **163**(4), 719–25.

Balkrishnan, R., McMichael, A. J., Hu, J. Y., Camacho, F. T., Shew, K. R., Bouloc, A., Rapp, S. R., & Feldman, S. R. (2006). Correlates of health-related quality of life in women with severe facial blemishes. *International Journal of Dermatology*, **45**(2), 111–15.

Berg, M., & Liden, S. (1989). An epidemiological study of rosacea. *Acta Dermato-Venereologica*, **69**(5), 419–23.

Berghoff, M., Kathpal, M., Kilo, S., Hilz, M. J., & Freeman, R. (2002). Vascular and neural mechanisms of ACh-mediated vasodilation in the forearm cutaneous microcirculation. *Journal of Applied Physiology*, **92**(2), 780–8.

Bickers, D. R., Lim, H. W., Margolis, D., Weinstock, M. A., Goodman, C., Faulkner, E., Gould, C., Gemmen, E., & Dall, T. (2006). The burden of skin diseases, 2004: a joint project of the American Academy of Dermatology Association and the Society for Investigative Dermatology. *Journal of the American Academy of Dermatology*, **55**(3), 490–500.

Bikowski, J. B. (2000). Rosacea: a tiered approach to therapy. *Cutis*, **66**(4 Suppl.), 3–6.

Bikowski, J. B., & Goldman, M. P. (2004). Rosacea: where are we now? *Journal of Drugs in Dermatology*, **3**(3), 251–61.

Bögels, S. M. (2006). Task concentration training versus applied relaxation, in combination with cognitive therapy, for social phobia patients with fear of blushing, trembling, and sweating. *Behaviour Research and Therapy*, **44**(8), 1199–210.

Bögels, S. M., Alberts, M., & de Jong, P. J. (1996). Self-consciousness, self-focused attention, blushing propensity and fear of blushing. *Personality and Individual Differences*, **21**(4), 573–81.

Bögels, S. M., & Voncken, M. J. (2008). Social skills training versus cognitive therapy for social anxiety disorder characterized by fear of blushing, trembling, or sweating. *International Journal of Cognitive Therapy*, **1**(2), 138–50.

Bonnar, E., Eustace, P., & Powell, F. C. (1993). The Demodex mite population in rosacea. *Journal of the American Academy of Dermatology*, **28**(3), 443–8.

Brinnel, H., Friedel, J., Caputa, M., Cabanac, M., & Grosshans, E. (1989). Rosacea: disturbed defense against brain overheating. *Archives of Dermatological Research*, **281**(1), 66–72.

Carroll, C. L., Balkrishnan, R., Feldman, S. R., Fleischer, A. B. Jr, & Manuel, J. C. (2005). The burden of atopic dermatitis: impact on the patient, family, and society. *Pediatric Dermatology*, **22**(3), 192–9.

Chodkiewicz, J., Salamon, M., Miniszewska, J., & Wozniacka, A. (2007). [Psychosocial impact of rosacea]. *Przeglad Lekarski*, **64**(12), 997–1001.

Cohen, C. G., Krahn, L., Wise, T. N., Epstein, S., & Ross, R. (1991). Delusions of disfigurement in a woman with acne rosacea. *General Hospital Psychiatry*, **13**(4), 273–7.

Culp, B., & Scheinfeld, N. (2009). Rosacea: a review. *P&T: A Peer-Reviewed Journal for Formulary Management*, **34**(1), 38–45.

Drummond, P. D., & Lazaroo, D. (2012). The effect of niacin on facial blood flow in people with an elevated fear of negative evaluation. *European Neuropsychopharmacology*, **22**(3), 200–4.

Drummond, P. D., & Su, D. (2012a). Endothelial and axon reflex vasodilatation to acetylcholine in rosacea-affected skin. *Archives of Dermatological Research*, **304**(2), 133–7.

(2012b). Blushing in rosacea sufferers. *Journal of Psychosomatic Research*, **72**(2), 153–8.

Edelmann, R. J., & Skov, V. (1993). Blushing propensity, social anxiety, anxiety sensitivity and awareness of bodily sensations. *Personality and Individual Differences*, **14**(3), 495–8.

Ehlers, A., Stangier, U., & Gieler, U. (1995). Treatment of atopic dermatitis: a comparison of psychological and dermatological approaches to relapse prevention. *Journal of Consulting and Clinical Psychology*, **63**(4), 624–35.

Elewski, B. E., Draelos, Z., Dreno, B., Jansen, T., Layton, A., & Picardo, M. (2010). Rosacea – global diversity and optimized outcome: proposed international consensus from the Rosacea International Expert Group. *Journal of the European Academy of Dermatology and Venereology*, **25**(2), 188–200.

Fried, R. G. (2002). Nonpharmacologic treatments in psychodermatology. *Dermatologic Clinics*, **20**(1), 177–85.

Garnis-Jones, S. (1998). Psychological aspects of rosacea. *Journal of Cutaneous Medicine and Surgery*, **2**(Suppl. 4), S4–16–19.

Gupta, A. K., & Chaudhry, M. M. (2005). Rosacea and its management: an overview. *Journal of the European Academy of Dermatology and Venereology*, **19**(3), 273–85.

Gupta, M. A., & Gupta, A. K. (2003). Psychiatric and psychological co-morbidity in patients with dermatologic disorders: epidemiology and management. *American Journal of Clinical Dermatology*, **4**(12), 833–42.

Gupta, M. A., Gupta, A. K., Chen, S. J., & Johnson, A. M. (2005). Comorbidity of rosacea and depression: an analysis of the National Ambulatory Medical Care Survey and National Hospital Ambulatory Care Survey – Outpatient Department data collected by the U.S. National Center for Health Statistics from 1995 to 2002. *British Journal of Dermatology*, **153**(6), 1176–81.

Gupta, M. A., Gupta, A. K., Schork, N. J., & Ellis, C. N. (1994). Depression modulates pruritus perception: a study of pruritus in psoriasis, atopic dermatitis, and chronic idiopathic urticaria. *Psychosomatic Medicine*, **56**(1), 36–40.

Harlow, D., Poyner, T., Finlay, A. Y., & Dykes, P. J. (2000). Impaired quality of life of adults with skin disease in primary care. *British Journal of Dermatology*, **143**(5), 979–82.

Hashiro, M., & Okumura, M. (1997). Anxiety, depression and psychosomatic symptoms in patients with atopic dermatitis: comparison with normal controls and among groups of different degrees of severity. *Journal of Dermatological Science*, **14**(1), 63–7.

Izumi, H., & Karita, K. (1992). Axon reflex flare evoked by nicotine in human skin. *Japanese Journal of Physiology*, **42**(5), 721–30.

Kabat-Zinn, J., Wheeler, E., Light, T., Skillings, A., Scharf, M. J., Cropley, T. G., Hosmer, D., & Bernhard, J. D. (1998). Influence of a mindfulness meditation-based stress reduction intervention on rates of skin clearing in patients with moderate to severe psoriasis undergoing phototherapy (UVB) and photochemotherapy (PUVA). *Psychosomatic Medicine*, **60**(5), 625–32.

Khaled, A., Hammami, H., Zeglaoui, F., Tounsi, J., Zermani, R., Kamoun, M. R., & Fazaa, B. (2010). Rosacea: 244 Tunisian cases. *La Tunisie Médicale*, **88**(8), 597–601.

Kimball, A. B., Jacobson, C., Weiss, S., Vreeland, M. G., & Wu, Y. (2005). The psychosocial burden of psoriasis. *American Journal of Clinical Dermatology*, **6**(6), 383–92.

Klaber, R., & Wittkower, E. (1939). The pathogenesis of rosacea: a review with special reference to emotional factors. *British Journal of Dermatology and Syphilis*, **51**(12), 501–24.

Kligman, A. M. (2004). A personal critique on the state of knowledge of rosacea. *Dermatology*, **208**(3), 191–7.

Kyriakis, K. P., Palamaras, I., Terzoudi, S., Emmanuelides, S., Michailides, C., & Pagana, G. (2005). Epidemiologic aspects of rosacea. *Journal of the American Academy of Dermatology*, **53**(5), 918–19.

Leary, M. R., & Meadows, S. (1991). Predictors, elicitors, and concomitants of social blushing. *Journal of Personality and Social Psychology*, **60**(2), 254–62.

Lindow, K. B., Shelestak, D., & Lappin, J. (2005). Perceptions of self in persons with rosacea. *Dermatology Nursing: Dermatology Nurse's Association*, **17**(4), 249–54, 314; quiz 263.

McAleer, M. A., Fitzpatrick, P., & Powell, F. C. (2010). Papulopustular rosacea: prevalence and relationship to photodamage. *Journal of the American Academy of Dermatology*, **63**(1), 33–9.

Marks, R. (1968). Concepts in the pathogenesis of rosacea. *British Journal of Dermatology*, **80**(3), 170–7.

Marks, R., & Harcourt-Webster, J. N. (1969). Histopathology of rosacea. *Archives of Dermatology*, **100**(6), 683–91.

Mattick, R. P., & Clarke, J. C. (1998). Development and validation of measures of social phobia scrutiny fear and social interaction anxiety. *Behaviour Research and Therapy*, **36**(4), 455–70.

Millard, L. (2000). Dermatological practice and psychiatry. *British Journal of Dermatology*, **143**(5), 920–1.

Miller, F. P. (1921). Etiology of acne rosacea through a viscero-neurologic mechanism. *American Journal of the Medical Sciences*, **161**(1), 120–4.

Neto, F. (1996). Correlates of social blushing. *Personality and Individual Differences*, 20(3), 365–73.

Nicholson, K., Abramova, L., Chren, M. M., Yeung, J., Chon, S. Y., & Chen, S. C. (2007). A pilot quality-of-life instrument for acne rosacea. *Journal of the American Academy of Dermatology*, 57(2), 213–21.

Ozturkcan, S., Ermertcan, A. T., Eser, E., & Sahin, M. T. (2006). Cross validation of the Turkish version of dermatology life quality index. *International Journal of Dermatology*, 45(11), 1300–7.

Papadopoulos, L. (2005). Psychological therapies for dermatological problems. In C. Walker & L. Papadopoulos (Eds.), *Psychodermatology: the psychological impact of skin disorders*. Cambridge University Press, 101–15.

Papadopoulos, L., Walker, C., Aitken, D., & Bor, R. (2000). The relationship between body location and psychological morbidity in individuals with acne vulgaris. *Psychology, Health and Medicine*, 5(4), 431–8.

Picardi, A., & Abeni, D. (2001). Stressful life events and skin diseases: disentangling evidence from myth. *Psychotherapy and Psychosomatics*, 70(3), 118–36.

Picardi, A., Abeni, D., Mazzotti, E., Fassone, G., Lega, I., Ramieri, L., Sagoni, E., Tiago, A., & Pasquini, P. (2004). Screening for psychiatric disorders in patients with skin diseases: a performance study of the 12-item General Health Questionnaire. *Journal of Psychosomatic Research*, 57(3), 219–23.

Picardi, A., Abeni, D., Melchi, C. F., Puddu, P., & Pasquini, P. (2000). Psychiatric morbidity in dermatological outpatients: an issue to be recognized. *British Journal of Dermatology*, 143(5), 983–91.

Plesch, E. (1951). A Rorschach study of rosacea and morbid blushing. *British Journal of Medical Psychology*, 24(3), 202–5.

Powell, F. C. (2004). Rosacea and the pilosebaceous follicle. *Cutis*, 74(3 Suppl.), 9–12, 32–4.

Robinson, E., Rumsey, N., & Partridge, J. (1996). An evaluation of the impact of social interaction skills training for facially disfigured people. *British Journal of Plastic Surgery*, 49(5), 281–9.

Salamon, M., Chodkiewicz, J., Sysa-Jedrzejowska, A., & Wozniacka, A. (2008). [Quality of life in patients with rosacea]. *Przeglad Lekarski*, 65(9), 385–9.

Schaefer, I., Rustenbach, S. J., Zimmer, L., & Augustin, M. (2008). Prevalence of skin diseases in a cohort of 48,665 employees in Germany. *Dermatology*, 217(2), 169–72.

Scharschmidt, T. C., Yost, J. M., Truong, S. V., Steinhoff, M., Wang, K. C., & Berger, T. G. (2011). Neurogenic rosacea: a distinct clinical subtype requiring a modified approach to treatment. *Archives of Dermatology*, 147(1), 123–6.

Singh, L. K., Pang, X., Alexacos, N., Letourneau, R., & Theoharides, T. C. (1999). Acute immobilization stress triggers skin mast cell degranulation via corticotropin releasing hormone, neurotensin, and substance P: a link to neurogenic skin disorders. *Brain, Behavior, and Immunity*, 13(3), 225–39.

Søybe, P. (1950). Aetiology and pathogenesis of rosacea. *Acta Dermato-Venereologica*, 30, 137–58.

Su, D., & Drummond, P. D. (2011). Blushing propensity and psychological distress in rosacea sufferers. *Clinical Psychology and Psychotherapy*. Advance online publication. doi: 10.1002/cpp.763.

Thompson, A., & Kent, G. (2001). Adjusting to disfigurement: processes involved in dealing with being visibly different. *Clinical Psychology Review*, 21 (5), 663–82.
Webster, G. F. (2009). Rosacea. *Medical Clinics of North America*, 93(6), 1183–94.
White, J. M., Jones, A. M., & Ingham, J. G. (1956). A Rorschach study of the neurodermatoses. *Journal of Psychosomatic Research*, 1(1), 84–93.
Whitlock, F. A. (1961). Psychosomatic aspects of rosacea. *British Journal of Dermatology*, 73(4), 137–48.
Wilkin, J., Dahl, M., Detmar, M., Drake, L., Feinstein, A., Odom, R., & Powell, F. (2002). Standard classification of rosacea: report of the National Rosacea Society Expert Committee on the Classification and Staging of Rosacea. *Journal of the American Academy of Dermatology*, 46(4), 584–7.
Wilkin, J. K. (1981). Oral thermal-induced flushing in erythematotelangiectatic rosacea. *Journal of Investigative Dermatology*, 76(1), 15–18.
  (1994). Rosacea: pathophysiology and treatment. *Archives of Dermatology*, 130 (3), 359–62.
Yamasaki, K., Di Nardo, A., Bardan, A., Murakami, M., Ohtake, T., Coda, A., Dorschner, C., Bennart, P., Descargues, A., Hovnanian, A., Morhenn, V. B., & Gallo, R. L. (2007). Increased serine protease activity and cathelicidin promotes skin inflammation in rosacea. *Nature Medicine*, 13(8), 975–80.
Yamasaki, K., & Gallo, R. L. (2009). The molecular pathology of rosacea. *Journal of Dermatological Science*, 55(2), 77–81.
Yamasaki, K., Kanada, K., Macleod, D. T., Borkowski, A. W., Morizane, S., Nakatsuji, T., Cogen, A. L., & Gallo, R. L. (2011). TLR2 expression is increased in rosacea and stimulates enhanced serine protease production by keratinocytes. *Journal of Investigative Dermatology*, 131(3), 688–97.
Zachariae, R., Oster, H., Bjerring, P., & Kragballe, K. (1996). Effects of psychologic intervention on psoriasis: a preliminary report. *Journal of the American Academy of Dermatology*, 34(6), 1008–15.

# 16  Conclusions, what we don't know and future directions for research

## W. Ray Crozier and Peter J. de Jong

Scientists are addressing the blush in a systematic and sustained way for the first time since Darwin's pioneering chapter on the blush in *The Expression of the Emotions in Man and Animals* (1872); we hope that this volume has demonstrated that considerable progress has been made in addressing the issues he raised. Yet in many respects the blush remains a puzzle and we consider these issues in this final chapter on the basis of empirical research that directly bears on the blush and evidence from related fields that is covered in a number of chapters in this volume.

### The nature of the blush

For a long time, the scientific literature about the nature of the blush was heavily dominated by theoretical speculations and anecdotal observations, whereas solid empirical evidence was virtually absent. Clear progress has been made in this respect during the last two decades as is evidenced by the studies reported throughout this volume. Perhaps most importantly, an increasing number of studies has started to measure participants' actual blushing in 'live' social situations, thereby drawing on multiple methods such as collecting self-reports and observer-reports of blushing, and making physiological recordings of vasodilatation, blood flow and temperature changes of the skin.

Another important step forward is that several of these studies have experimentally manipulated key features of the situations and/or critical components of participants' physiological systems, thus allowing the testing of critical assumptions about the characteristics and function of the blush response as well as its neurophysiological underpinnings. Accordingly, some studies have used experimental manipulations to induce embarrassment or other sources of arousal, and/or employed a pharmacological manipulation via administering drugs that have predictable effects upon sympathetic nervous system activation. Other studies have subjected participants to experimentally controlled moral transgressions or social predicaments, or provided participants with false feedback about their blushing. Studies have used these methods to investigate the psychophysiology of the blush (Chapter 2), its communicative function (Chapter 12), and the characteristics of individuals with heightened fear of blushing (Chapter 13).

Drummond (Chapter 2) confirms the critical involvement of the sympathetic nervous system in social blushing. On the basis of the experimental work and clinical observations discussed in this and other chapters in this volume it seems safe to conclude that the acute accumulation of red blood cells in the superficial venous plexus of the facial skin is regulated primarily by sympathetic vasodilator nerves that give rise to an increase in arterial supply. Together with a β-adrenergic vasodilator mechanism that increases the capacity of facial veins to hold blood, this may eventually result in the typical blush response. The acute neural vasodilator responses that mediate flushing seem part of the classic 'fight or flight' response. Yet, it remains a puzzle what (defensive) function is actually served by the social blush and how this particular response has evolved in our phylogenetic history.

Research in vertebrates such as dogs has shown that blood is typically directed towards the face during confrontational defence, and is coupled with facial muscles involved in snarling and biting. It seems unconvincing to argue that in the typical blush-eliciting context the blusher is predisposed to behave in a dominant manner and needs to be prepared for aggressive (anger) responses. Throughout all the chapters of this volume blushing is typically associated with submission and appeasement instead of dominance and aggression. However, in the typical blush-eliciting situations, flight responses do not seem to be helpful and would probably (also) contribute further to loss of face. Perhaps, then, the activation of the sympathetic nervous system is due to the paradoxical situation that on the one hand the actor experiences a strong urge to flee, whereas on the other hand the actor needs to inhibit this initial tendency as such a response would make things even worse. As discussed by van Hooff (Chapter 5), in primates such situations tend to elicit a crouched body posture away from the adversary that is often accompanied by a silent, bared-teeth display; a ritualized expression of fear in which screaming is suppressed. The opposite of a threat display logically serves an appeasing function and may require an acute increase in facial blood flow for metabolic requirements or for thermoregulatory purposes. Perhaps, then, such a type of suppressed fear signal forms the evolutionary basis for social blushing. Clearly, this speculation is only a first step towards arriving at a satisfactory answer on the still open question of how exactly the blush response has evolved and what

## Social blushing: unique physiological response or unique elicitors?

Colour and temperature metaphors, notably references to redness and heat of the face, are common when describing emotion. We talk of blushing with embarrassment, shame and guilt; flushing with pride or pleasure; reddening with anger and indignation. We are hot with embarrassment, burn with indignation. Such expressions have a long history and there is evidence that they are widely shared across cultures (Casimir & Schnegg, 2002). Research needs to go beyond these ordinary language expressions to determine whether there are different forms of facial reddening involving different mechanisms, with different relations to emotions. Germane to this, Drummond points to the apparent similarities between changes in facial blood flow elicited by embarrassing situations and those that elicit joy or anger. This suggests that similar physiological mechanisms may be involved in very different emotions. Perhaps, then, the interpretation and functional meaning of the same visible clues (i.e., reddening of the face) critically depend on contextual factors. It is possible that reddening with anger reflects similar physiological mechanisms to the flush with pleasure or the blush with guilt. Differential interpretation and attributional processes in the actor as well as in the observers may therefore be due to the type of elicitor.

In addition, there is reason to speculate that apparently different types of blush responses may essentially reflect similar underlying psychological processes. For example, Leary, Britt, Cutlip and Templeton (1992) distinguished the classic blush from the 'creeping' form and Drummond (Chapter 2) reports evidence of a prolonged, slowly spreading blush in a sample of participants answering an advertisement offering treatment for fear of blushing. Clearly, this creeping blush is not under direct nervous control and seems therefore dissimilar to the typical blush that is characterized by an acute reddening of the cheeks. Yet, it may well be that at least on some occasions this slow reddening is a by-product of an acute blush, elicited by hormonal effects of released neurotransmitters that end up in the bloodstream. Moreover, it might reflect a heightened sensitivity to catecholamines in people with social anxiety, perhaps as a psychophysiological consequence of recurrent blushing. Further research is also warranted that carefully investigates the specificity of the blush response as a function of individual differences. Clearly, such research promises to make a significant contribution to our understanding of social blushing.

Research into the nature of the blush has been greatly facilitated by the development of measurement techniques such as photoplethysmography and laser Doppler flowmetry as described by Cooper and Gerlach (Chapter 3). All psychophysiological measures have their limitations, if only for the reason that the apparatus inevitably changes the social situation that the research participants encounter. This raises questions about the reliability and validity of these measures. Inter-correlations of measures of blushing taken on the same occasion are typically modest at best. Cooper and Gerlach discuss the care that has to be taken using psychophysiological measures of blushing: for example, the sensitivity of photoelectric sensors to movement and extraneous sources of light. Also, caution needs to be taken in interpreting results since these might be influenced by characteristics of measurement instruments rather than substantive issues. For example, the conclusion that people can be seen to blush before they are aware that they are doing so might be a function of properties of the measures of blood flow and temperature: participants might be aware straight away that their temperature is increasing but there is a delay in the thermistor's capacity to record any change in temperature at the surface of the skin.

The analysis by Cooper and Gerlach clearly indicates that it is important to use multiple measures, not only to improve reliability but also because the various response parameters may reflect differential aspects, each of which may inform us about other aspects of the blush (e.g., perceived intensity vs actual increase in blood flow vs observed intensity of the blush). Unfortunately, thus far none of the available techniques provides a straightforward measure of the objective visibility of the blush. Such an index seems especially relevant in the face of testing further the alleged communicative functions of the blush. Although Chapter 3 does highlight some promising approaches to capturing the skin's colour that are being developed in the area of computer graphics, the currently available techniques are insufficiently flexible and too slow to reliably measure *changes* in facial colourization, which is a crucial feature when dealing with the facial blush. Moreover, simpler approaches such as off-line analysis of video recordings of people's faces do not provide a straightforward alternative. For example, most modern video cameras automatically adjust lens and white balance, which may affect the recording of the blush. Clearly, then, for research into the social implications of the blush, further development of objective measurements of its visibility would be extremely welcome.

Conclusions

## The blush as signal

The blush does seem to be uniquely human but, as van Hooff (Chapter 5) concludes from studies investigating behavioural displays related to changes in motivational variations of primate species, the functions it serves may not be. He modifies Darwin's assertion that the blush is a uniquely human expression to suggest that its functions of 'safeguarding social bonds and acceptance' are not uniquely human at all. Moreover, Chapter 5 discusses the possibility that in primates as well momentary skin colour variations may signal short-term variations in motivational state. Some authors even argue that the ability to distinguish emotional states on the basis of subtle fluctuations in the redness of the face may explain the emergence of red perception in the primate branch of mammals.

Unfortunately, thus far research on (blood) colour signalling in primates has predominantly focused on longer-term changes; it might therefore be fruitful to investigate more systematically transient changes in colouring in primates and to see how these responses might relate to variations in motivational processes and affect behaviours among conspecifics. Detailed observation would be one way to improve insight into the influence of state-dependent colour changes on conspecific behaviours in primates. Yet this may be complicated by the fact that what our human colour sense can distinguish might well differ from what various primate species can distinguish. One way to circumvent this problem would be to manipulate the ability to detect the relevant reddish colours (e.g., by manipulating the frequencies of ambient light) and to see how that affects intergroup behaviours. Such primate studies might also inform us about the function of the blush in humans.

In the meantime, we have already obtained a clearer picture of the signalling functions of the human blush, via a series of recent experimental studies that have tested people's reactions to the visible blush and the interpretations they make of the blusher's character and conduct (see Chapter 12). Like the experience and expression of embarrassment, a blush has been shown to be socially useful even though, or perhaps precisely because, it can be an unpleasant experience for the blusher.

Leary and Toner (Chapter 4) and de Jong and Dijk (Chapter 12) review research into the social remediation function of blushing in deflecting potentially negative evaluations of the blusher's behaviour by conveying the blusher's awareness of his or her inappropriate or silly behaviour. In other words, the blush would signal the blusher's acknowledgment of wrongdoing and would serve as an apology aimed at inhibiting others' aggression or avoiding social ostracism. Leary and Toner not only present empirical evidence supporting these properties of the blush but also findings indicating that people behave as if they are aware of these effects of their blushing. Blushers' beliefs about whether or not an observer is aware that they are embarrassed or that they are blushing influences their subsequent expression of embarrassment and their self-presentation to the observer.

An important question that is addressed in these chapters is how the blush achieves its face-saving and/or remedial effects. Does it achieve this by displaying embarrassment, shame or guilt so that others present can draw inferences about the blusher's motives – that is to say, would any display of embarrassment or shame produce the same outcome? A salient feature of the blush that is mentioned in several chapters is that it is involuntary, uncontrollable and cannot be feigned. This seems to make the blush a particularly convincing medium of communication, more convincing than, say, a verbal confession of embarrassment or a facial expression that might not be sincere. In line with this, Chapter 12 presents findings indicating that indeed blushing might be experienced as more sincere than other signs of embarrassment or shame. Moreover, Chapter 12 provides evidence that blushing also leads to more positive observers' judgments when the blush is displayed on top of other relevant facial expressions, indicating that the blush has complementary signal value. Perhaps because the available range of means of expressing shame/embarrassment via contraction of the relevant facial musculature is restricted, the blush might have useful complementary remedial value, especially when people have already reached a full-blown (muscular) expression of shame/embarrassment. Moreover, blushing might have complementary value by attesting to the apparent sincerity that one is ashamed and/or embarrassed, because it is impossible to control the blush intentionally. Clearly, future research is necessary to test the robustness of these findings and to test the validity of the proposed mechanisms that underlie this (surplus) effect of the blush on the observer's judgment.

How a blush is perceived and interpreted depends on its context, and research is attempting to understand this better. The available evidence led de Jong and Dijk (Chapter 12) to reach the preliminary conclusion that in situations that clearly imply some kind of misbehaviour such as a faux pas or transgression, the blush has face-saving properties and serves as a nonverbal submissive excuse. Yet, in many other situations that are more ambiguous with regard to the blushing actor's antecedent behaviours and/or their underlying intentions, the blush may have undesirable revealing effects. Germane to this, Crozier (Chapter 11) makes a convincing case that people's sudden awareness that something may be revealed that they prefer to keep hidden, might also be a powerful trigger for a blush to occur. Accordingly, people's concern that something may come into the open, may elicit the ironic effect of unveiling the hidden information via the display of a blush.

It should be acknowledged that most studies of the alleged signal value of the blush have relied on self-report data and imagined situations. Several theorists have argued that these approaches are problematic for emotion research and cast serious doubts on the validity of such scenario studies (e.g., Parkinson & Manstead, 1993). However, testing the influence of actual blushing on actual interpersonal behaviours is notoriously difficult as it requires that the experimental manipulation reliably elicits a (visible) blush in the actors, that at least one other individual is present who may observe the blush and whose judgments and/or behaviour may be influenced by the blush, and, finally, it requires a (controllable) social interaction during which the potential influence of the actor's blush response on the observer's behaviour can be reliably assessed. Based on these prerequisites a series of recent studies used a morally framed prisoner's dilemma game (PDG; de Jong et al., 2002; Dijk et al., 2011; see also Chapter 12). Although these studies provided behavioural evidence supporting the view that blushing following a transgression has remedial effects, PDGs represent a highly specific interpersonal context and it remains important, therefore, to test the influence of the blush in other social situations as well. One fruitful way to pursue this research would be to use virtual reality techniques since such an approach allows us to test participants' behaviour in response to blushing others in more common (naturalistic) social situations.

In spite of its apparent signal value, people may be unaware of the fact that other people have displayed a blush and/or that this blush may have affected their judgment. It seems reasonable to assume that in actual social situations the signal value of the blush may operate quickly and at an implicit level (Glashouwer et al., 2011). Knowing the neural basis of perceiving a blush might therefore help us to understand the mechanisms involved in this complex interpersonal response. It has been shown that specific brain networks are involved in the implicit judgment of faces in terms of trustworthiness. It would be interesting to see whether similar brain patterns are evident when participants observe blushing actors. Furthermore, by comparing the neural response to shame (without a blush) with the response to a blushing person we might be able to test if blushing, in particular, elicits neural responses that are associated with trustworthiness. This would also be relevant for the question whether or not blushing signals something that otherwise could not be signalled in these contexts.

A functional view of the blush as advocated in this volume also raises critical questions. If it serves as an admission of guilt, indicates appeasement or conveys a nonverbal apology for violation of a social norm, why should it also be triggered when we are praised or thanked in the absence of obvious norm violations? This raises a more general question about the evaluative nature of shame, embarrassment and blushing. Shame involves a breach of fundamental standards of conduct, a serious dereliction, a violation of moral rules. The social evaluation model of embarrassment (see Chapter 9) proposes that it is caused by the threat of negative evaluation by others. The notion that a blush is targeted at inhibiting others' aggression or social rejection implies a sense of wrongdoing on the blusher's part, as Leary and Toner (Chapter 4) point out in their review of psychological theories. Why, then, do embarrassment and blushing occur when we are praised, congratulated, thanked or rewarded, or when we are wished 'Happy Birthday'? One explanation could be derived from the dramaturgical account of the blush discussed in the chapters of Scott and Miller. That is, perhaps in these relatively infrequent situations a blush is elicited because people experience a *loss of script*: people may find themselves flustered and unsure of what to do or say as a result of an unanticipated event or revelation.

A further apparently problematic feature for a functional approach is the observation that blushing can also be elicited when we are simply the object of scrutiny or at least believe we are so. In response, Leary and colleagues (1992) suggest that blushing occurs when the attention we receive is undesired, and not necessarily negative. Other interpretations have been proposed, in terms of exposure of private aspects of the self (Crozier, Chapter 11). On the basis of the developmental perspective outlined by Stegge in Chapter 6, it seems relevant to differentiate between exposure embarrassment and evaluative embarrassment. Stegge argues that exposure embarrassment may occur as soon as the self becomes an object to the self (e.g., at 2 years of age). The presence of an audience is critical for the occurrence of this shame-related affect, but at this early age this seems to involve concern about being observed rather than about being evaluated. As soon as children become able to judge the self against behavioural standards of conduct, evaluative embarrassment may start to occur. Perhaps, then, the ontogenetic older form of embarrassment (i.e., exposure embarrassment) remains relevant and may help explain why merely being the centre of unwanted attention often gives rise to a blush. Such an explanation also seems pertinent to Darwin's claim that the blush results from scrutiny by others, and the finding discussed by Drummond (Chapter 2) that embarrassed participants showed a relatively large increase in blood flow on the observed side of their face.

# Conclusions

How might the blush have evolved to fulfil a communicative function? Van Hooff (Chapter 5) discusses the evolution of trichromatic colour vision that enables the discrimination of reddish hues and which is found in marsupials, monkeys and apes. He considers the hypothesis that it evolved to permit discrimination of changes in skin colour that are associated with sexual states and dominance, and can serve as socio-sexual signals. In particular, primates show colour variation in the facial and anal-genital area that contributes to adaptive displays. The evolved sensitivity to reddish hues may also have set the stage for submission-associated facial flushing to become an appeasement display in humans when they encounter a social threat and are unable to leave the situation and/or are unwilling to forgo their relationship with the others involved. The benefits provided by its involuntary nature (i.e., sincerity) may have resulted in its continuing adaptive value even after the evolution of language has offered other means of expressing submission.

From this perspective it might also be relevant to extend the research on the social implications of the blush to the more general impact of phasic changes of people's skin colour on interpersonal behaviours. Since the human visual system seems equipped with an exceptional sensitivity to two dimensions of skin reflectance modulation – one associated with haemoglobin oxygen saturation and one associated with haemoglobin skin concentration (Changizi *et al.*, 2006) – this seems to provide the opportunity to detect both the level of blood accumulation in the skin (e.g., because of blood pooling or increased circulation) and the type of blood (venous or arterial). So it would be interesting to see whether perhaps more subtle changes in skin colour may affect interpersonal behaviours more generally. It might be especially relevant to differentiate between the impact of the more reddish colour of arterial blood – which may be associated with a more dominant, aggressive mental state – versus the impact of the more greenish colour of venous blood, that seems most relevant for social blushing. Moreover, it might be that the impact of the blush also depends on the level of blood accumulation. In some contexts, a subtle, mild reddening might have a positive influence, whereas under the same conditions a strong coloration might have detrimental social consequences (cf. Miller's argument in Chapter 9 that when the expressed intensity of embarrassment is not attuned to the type of elicitor, the expression of embarrassment becomes counterproductive). The same might be true for the social implications of other types of blood-related reddening of visible body parts, such as the blush that sometimes occurs in more prolonged social evaluative contexts and that seems to creep across one's skin, especially around the neck. The (implicit) impact of the various types of state-dependent facial coloration might even open a completely new avenue of research into the social implications of signalling more subtle emotional and/or motivational states in interpersonal contexts.

Yet there remains the issue of human variation in the visibility of the blush, since the reddening is less visible in people of dark skin tone whereas lighter skin is thought to be an adaptation after the emergence of *homo sapiens* in Africa (Jablonski, 2006). Had the blush evolved prior to this adaptation and, if so, how could it have served a communicative function when all members of the species were dark skinned and the blush would have been less visible? We don't know enough about human evolution to answer these questions. However, they definitely suggest the need to undertake cross-cultural research into the communicative functions and psychological meanings of the blush. It would therefore be important to test the influence of skin complexion on the communicative properties of the blush. In this regard we should also not neglect to study those individuals whose complexion makes a blush more visible. It would also be important to explore whether people whose blushing cannot be accurately detected may have acquired other displays and/or signalling strategies. Germane to this, previous experimental research showed that after a clear-cut predicament, participants typically engaged in (alternative) self-presentational tactics to improve their damaged social image when they were led to believe that the experimenter *did not* notice their blushing (Leary et al., 1996). It would be interesting to see whether the strength of such motivated expression of embarrassment and/or shame may also vary as a function of relatively stable (e.g., skin complexion) or temporary (e.g., ambient light) differences in the visibility of one's blushing.

## Blushing with embarrassment

Embarrassment and the blush are closely connected in ordinary language and in psychological theory. The claim that the blush is the 'hallmark of embarrassment' (Buss, 1980, p. 129), in the sense of being specific to it, seems to be over-stated, although little research has addressed this directly. Historical and cross-cultural analyses of emotion vocabulary suggest that people also blush with shame (as Darwin proposed). There is little consensus in psychological theories about the relations between shame and embarrassment, as Darby and Harris show in Chapter 7.

Embarrassment has been studied for many years yet there still exist competing theories of its nature, notably evaluation theory and dramaturgical theory (Darby & Harris, Chapter 7; Miller, Chapter 9), each of which captures some aspects of embarrassment. As each chapter shows, attempts have been made to test predictions from the two theories. Less attention has been paid to the part played by blushing in embarrassment; while we do blush when embarrassed we do not know whether this is always the case or whether some kinds of circumstances trigger one but not the other. They can both be unpleasant experiences even though they can both produce useful outcomes, as the signal account of blushing suggests. Miller (Chapter 9) outlines some of the biases that lead us to exaggerate the consequences of our embarrassment, and how this may motivate all kinds of dysfunctional behaviours such as avoidance of seeking medical help. It would be useful to investigate the contribution of blushing to these biases: for example, a blush makes it harder to cover up embarrassment and leaves us vulnerable to closer scrutiny and to teasing, but may also be helpful in the sense that it may elicit behaviours in others that may resolve the embarrassing component of a particular situation. More generally, it would be important to acquire insight into the ways in which the experience of embarrassment with blushing differs from embarrassment without it.

The interviews reported by Scott (Chapter 10) offer a closer look at people's experience of blushing and the strategies they use to conceal it. She argues that the blush is not only a reaction to stress but is a 'performance' in its own right, which has consequences for the blusher and his or her social encounters. Her research focuses on shy participants: Darwin had suggested that shyness is one of the major causes of blushing, but this has seldom been investigated. In her chapter Scott argues that those who self-identify as shy experience the blush as doubly stigmatizing: it involves both the fear of a discreditable stigma being revealed (i.e., one's perceived social incompetence), and the display of a signal that is in itself discrediting because it exposes uncertainty and lack of poise. Accordingly, shy people anticipate negative social consequences because of their blushing. Yet, what seemed to evoke actual social disapproval was not their blushing per se, but rather the strategies they used to manage it, and the further actions this led on to. In Chapter 10 Scott found that many actors felt so self-conscious about blushing, and fearful of the consequences of this discrediting attribute being visible, that they made further deviant moves. As a result, these people may enter a vicious cycle confirming their perceived social incompetence and promoting the chance of actual disapproval by others. This analysis seems highly consistent with the experimental work of Dijk, Voncken and de Jong (2009), showing that false blush feedback during a social interaction task resulted in less favourable social judgments of the 'blusher' by their interaction partners (see also Chapter 13). Scott argues that shy actors and their audiences ultimately share the same goal of interactional harmony. In her view, the designation of some shy blushers as outsiders is therefore just a socially constructed definition of the situation. Although the blush may be especially cumbersome for shy people, the positive implication of this constructional view is that socially constructed definitions are always open to reinterpretation and revision. Clearly, this also points to important clues that may help to improve further the currently available therapeutic interventions as described in chapters 14 and 15.

## Blushing, embarrassment and anxiety

If the blush is a response to cues for threat of social exclusion how does it relate to other responses to social threats? Darby and Harris (Chapter 7) and Miskovic and Schmidt (Chapter 8) provide contrasting accounts of the psychobiology of embarrassment and social anxiety, respectively. The psychophysiology of fear and anxiety has attracted much more research than equivalent studies into embarrassment and blushing. It has drawn upon animal research (less relevant, surely, to the study of the blush) and upon developments in functional neuroimaging methods, which have yet to be applied to blushing. For example, neuroimaging studies have examined responses to threatening stimuli, including facial expressions. As Miskovic and Schmidt indicate, quite precise links have been made between the prefrontal cortex and specific divisions of the amygdala, on the one hand, and emotional experience and behaviours, on the other. Equivalent research into the blush is still missing. In order to improve our understanding of the blush it would be valuable to fill this gap. Research should investigate the neurophysiological signature of the blush response and explore whether the brain networks sustaining the blush differ from the brain responses that have been identified in the context of (social) anxiety, and whether different systems of arousal are involved. Is a blush a sign of social anxiety, as Buss (1980) and others have claimed, or is it a sign of a different emotion, perhaps shame or embarrassment, with its own psychophysiology?

For most of us, blushing is usually a transient response and any unpleasantness that is associated with it is mild, but for many others it creates considerable anxiety and reduces the quality of their life. Fear of blushing is often a component of social anxiety disorder, although there is also evidence for the existence of a category of people for whom fear of blushing is the single symptom (Pelissolo *et al.*, 2012). In particular, individuals in the latter category regard their blushing as the main source of their anxieties, and not just as a symptom. People with fear of blushing

# Conclusions

commonly attribute their fear to a heightened tendency to blush. This raises the question whether indeed they do blush more frequently or intensely than others do.

Most studies (reviewed by Drummond in Chapter 2 and Dijk and de Jong, Chapter 13) seem to show that fearful individuals differ from their peers only in a biased perception of their blushing. These findings clearly converge on the conclusion that a bias towards overestimating the intensity of their reddening is involved in blushing phobia. Yet it seems premature to conclude on the basis of these findings that blushing-fearful individuals do not (also) blush more intensely or more often than people without fear of blushing. Most of these studies used very embarrassing blush-eliciting tasks which might have undermined the sensitivity for distinguishing reactions of those high and low in anxiety. In accordance with this, Chapter 13 reports growing evidence suggesting that, especially in more common social situations at least, a subgroup of fearful individuals tend to blush relatively easily and/or relatively intensely. This accords well with the clinical impression that some blushing-phobic individuals tend to blush very easily in common social situations that usually do not elicit a blush in other people.

Even if future research were to support the conclusion that blushing-phobic individuals are characterized by a heightened tendency to blush, this does not imply that blushing-fearful individuals are the victim of a hyper-responsive physiological 'blush' system. Although such a somatic explanation is quite common among people with fear of blushing, it seems inconsistent with findings indicating that following successful treatment people not only report lower levels of fear but also a lower frequency of displaying a blush (see Chapter 13). Accordingly, Dijk and de Jong argue in Chapter 13 that more malleable psychological mechanisms rather than hard-wired physiological features may best explain blushing-fearfuls' liability to blush. In line with the evaluation theory discussed by Miller in Chapter 9, these authors argue that a relatively high sensitivity to other people's judgment, together with a tendency to attribute relatively restrictive social standards to other people (e.g., about what is appropriate and what is not), may explain their liability to blush. Thus, perhaps, people who fear blushing just blush more easily because they have (think they have) more reasons to blush than low blushing-fearful controls. A critical next step would be to test whether modifying blushing-fearfuls' conception of the prevailing social standards would indeed attenuate their tendency to blush.

The research reviewed in Chapter 13 provides ample evidence to suggest that all kinds of negative cognitions and biased judgments are at the heart of blushing phobia. As a relatively new development, several authors have designed computer tasks to directly target these types of cognitive biases (for a clinical comment see March, 2010). A rapidly growing number of studies has shown that such cognitive bias modification (CBM) procedures focusing on judgmental biases have the potential to yield clinically significant and prolonged reductions in anxiety symptoms (e.g., Amir *et al.*, 2008). If indeed cognitive biases play a critical role in the maintenance of blushing phobia, similar CBM procedures may be tailored to reduce symptoms of blushing phobia as well.

Current research explores further the role of information-processing biases and dysfunctional beliefs in the origin and maintenance of blushing fears. In the meantime, more clinically oriented research has aimed to identify the most effective interventions to help sufferers overcome their fear. In Chapter 14, Capozzoli, Vonk, Bögels and Hofmann review the small number of studies that have researched psychological methods using randomized controlled trials with samples of participants who are high in fear of blushing. The methods they have applied have not been specifically developed for blushing but represent modified protocols that have been successfully used in the treatment of social anxiety disorder: social skills training, relaxation techniques, task concentration training, exposure therapy and cognitive therapy. In a similar vein, psychological methods including relaxation training, imagery training and cognitive behavioural stress management techniques have been used successfully in the treatment of rosacea, to help patients cope with the distress that the condition brings (Drummond & Su, Chapter 15). Although the currently available psychological treatment options have been shown to be moderately successful, there is ample room for further improvement. Perhaps interventions could become even more successful if they were tailored to target more directly the mechanisms that are specifically involved in blushing phobia. The various contributions of this volume provide several starting points for such tailored interventions.

Some people prefer a medical approach such as endoscopic thoracic sympathectomy to remedy their symptoms. The effects of such surgical intervention have also been investigated in clinical trials as a treatment for fear of blushing. This procedure has proved successful in eradicating blushing but there are frequently unwanted side-effects, including compensatory sweating, which are reported by a substantial proportion of patients (Drummond, Chapter 2). Given that anxiety seems to be the primary concern of patients it might be thought that interventions to reduce anxiety would be more appropriate than surgery to prevent blushing, particularly given that the procedure has an unwanted impact on thermoregulation and destroys a functional emotional display that may help out in socially awkward situations. A, perhaps extreme, comparison might be with the condition of body dysmorphic disorder where some patients seek amputation of a healthy limb, feeling 'alienated' from it or believing that it is diseased (e.g., Bayne & Levy, 2005). The duty to take patients' wishes into account and the possibility that they might take drastic action themselves pose ethical problems for doctors, yet its causes surely lie in the patient's beliefs or body schema and these should be the target of intervention, and typically are in psychological treatments.

## Sex and the blush

The sexual element in blushing is under-researched. Darwin speculated on the similarity between the blush and sexual arousal, and concluded that this is because of each sex's interest in what the other sex thinks of their appearance. The sexual nature of the blush is emphasized in psychoanalytical theory (see Leary & Toner, Chapter 4). As in typical psychoanalytic interpretation of psychological phenomena the underlying meaning of the phenomenon is disguised and displaced, as a mechanism for protecting the ego. For example, displacement of the sexual excitement from the genitals to the face is said to occur because of fear of castration.

A blush and sexual arousal are both instances of increased blood flow to a part of the body that can be produced simply by mental activity and can be uncontrollable. But is there a more fundamental association between sex and the blush? For example, the blush might have evolved in sexual selection as a signal to communicate sexual availability and readiness to mate. In chimpanzees the rumps of females become swollen and bright red when they are sexually receptive. In other species, males provide colourful displays to signal their positive qualities to prospective mates, the peacock's vivid display of tail plumes being a prime illustration of this. It is often speculated that a blush functions in a similar way in humans, where the blush has long been regarded as a sexually attractive feature, particularly in women. However, it seems important to note that these colour displays in animals typically reflect tonic effects (see also van Hooff, Chapter 5), very different from the phasic blush response in humans. Also the application of rouge that is often interpreted as pointing to the link between social blushing and sexual attractiveness seems not to be directly related to social blushing. Clearly, the acute blush is only one way in which our blood circulation may act as a signalling device. One could speculate that a particular, more enduring reddish complexion may be associated with a healthy physical condition related to reproductive success. Since this would then be specifically relevant for women of child-bearing age, such a type of skin colour might have become an important proximal factor to attract men. The application of rouge would then just reflect an attempt to profit from this evolved preference for particular skin colours. To complicate matters, it could of course also be that typically in women with a 'healthy' skin complexion, a phasic blush would be highly visible.

The sexual connotation of the blush may be fuelled further by the finding that sexual encounters and conversations with sexual connotations are common circumstances in which a blush is triggered (see Crozier, Chapter 11). Rather than postulate an inherent link between sex and the blush it could be argued that the connection is due to the shame and embarrassment about sexual matters that characterizes Western societies at least. Sexual matters might trigger a blush because of cultural and religious attitudes to sexuality and sexual morality in the context of the association between guilt and shame and sexual activity and exposure of the naked body and the genitals that is common to many religious doctrines. Exposure of the body and discussion of sexual matters are 'taboo' in many societies, which may be why they give occasion to blush. The shame and embarrassment that these matters cause is evident in contemporary Western society and they act as a constraint upon behaviour, often to the individual's cost. Thus, Darby and Harris (Chapter 7) and Miller (Chapter 9) review the problems caused by embarrassment about health matters concerning medical examinations and sexual practices. From this perspective, there is nothing intrinsic in the relation between sex and the blush and it can be explained by the mediating factors of embarrassment and shame. Nevertheless, shame, the blush, nakedness and sex are associated in many societies remote from the major world religions: for example, instances of shame and blushing brought about by being seen engaged in sexual intercourse or toileting identified by Strathern (1977) in a study undertaken in Papua New Guinea.

Finally, it is often assumed that women blush more readily than men do, but the evidence is neither compelling nor consistent (see Drummond, Chapter 2). Comparison of studies reveals variation in tasks and measures that may be relevant to discrepancies in findings. More research into this variation in experimental designs would be productive. There are methodological issues with self-report studies (what benchmark are respondents comparing themselves against when they report on how frequently they blush?) and further research is needed to clarify these. Nor should the question of the relation between blushing and gender be restricted to the identification of gender differences in the frequency or intensity of blushing in a single type of blush-eliciting context. Where and when men and women blush, and the meanings that these blushes have for the blusher and others present, are worthy of research. Clearly, then, potential gender differences in people's tendency to blush warrants further examination.

## Conclusion

The blush presents many challenges to researchers. Yet it is a significant element of social life and greater understanding will contribute to many areas of the human sciences. This is the first volume to bring together leading international researchers to focus on the blush and related topics of social anxiety, embarrassment and rosacea. We hope the volume has fulfilled its aims to review the current state of knowledge and to stimulate further enquiries.

REFERENCES

Amir, N., Weber, G., Beard, C., Bomyea, J., & Taylor, C. T. (2008). The effect of a single-session attention modification program on response to a public-speaking challenge in socially anxious individuals. *Journal of Abnormal Psychology*, **117**, 860–8.

Bayne, T., & Levy, N. (2005). Amputees by choice: body integrity identity disorder and the ethics of amputation. *Journal of Applied Philosophy*, **22**(1), 75–86.

Buss, A. H. (1980). *Self-consciousness and social anxiety*. San Francisco: Freeman.

Casimir, M. J., & Schnegg, M. (2002). Shame across cultures: the evolution, ontogeny and function of a 'moral emotion'. In H. Keller, Y. H. Poortinga & A. Schölmerich (Eds.), *Between culture and biology: perspectives on ontogenetic development*. Cambridge University Press, 270–300.

Changizi, M. A., Zhang, Q., & Shimojo, S. (2006). Bare skin, blood and the evolution of primate colour vision. *Biology Letters*, **2**, 217–21.

de Jong, P. J., Peters, M., De Cremer, D., & Vranken, C. (2002). Blushing after a moral transgression in a prisoner's dilemma game: appeasing or revealing? *European Journal of Social Psychology*, **32**(5), 627–44.

Dijk, C., Koenig, B., Ketelaar, T., & de Jong, P. J. (2011). Saved by the blush: being trusted despite defecting. *Emotion*, **11**, 313–19.

Dijk, C., Voncken, M., & de Jong, P. J. (2009). I blush, therefore I will be judged negatively: influence of false blush feedback on anticipated others' judgments and facial coloration in high and low blushing-fearfuls. *Behaviour Research and Therapy*, **47**, 541–7.

Glashouwer, K. A., de Jong, P. J., Dijk, C., & Buwalda, F. M. (2011). Individuals with fear of blushing explicitly and automatically associate blushing with social costs. *Journal of Psychopathology and Behavioral Assessment*, **33**, 540–6.

Jablonski, N. G. (2006). *Skin: a natural history*. Berkeley: University of California Press.

Leary, M. R., Britt, T. W., Cutlip, W. D., & Templeton, J. L. (1992). Social blushing. *Psychological Bulletin*, **112**, 446–60.

Leary, M. R., Landel, J. L., & Patton, K. M. (1996). The motivated expression of embarrassment following a self-presentational predicament. *Journal of Personality*, **64**, 619–36.

March, J. S. (2010). Attention bias modification training and the new interventions research. *Biological Psychiatry*, **68**, 978–9.

Parkinson, B., & Manstead, A. S. R. (1993). Making sense of emotions in stories and social life. *Cognition and Emotion*, **7**, 295–323.

Pelissolo, A., Moukheiber, A., Lobjoie, C., Valla, J., & Lambrey, S. (2012). Is there a place for fear of blushing in social anxiety spectrum? *Depression and Anxiety*, **29**, 62–70.

Strathern, A. (1977). Why is shame on the skin? In J. Blacking (Ed.), *The anthropology of the body*. London: Academic Press, 99–110.

# Index

accusation of blushing
 triggers blush, 67, 204, 215
acute negative public self-attention, 64, 233
age changes in blushing, 113–15
Alden, L. E., 67, 274, 291
amygdala, 149–52, 165, 166, 167, 169
anger, 23–4, 32
animal displays
 appeasement, 87
 courtship, 79
 guilt, 89–90
 ritualization, 79, 82, 86, 93
 sources, 79
 submission, 87, 89–91, 94
apology
 blush as, 65, 78, 91, 94, 123, 196, 203, 236, 250, 258, 260, 271, 331, 334
 in embarrassment, 196
appeasement, xii, 122, 131, 171, 203, 236, 271, 328
appeasement display, 91, 124, 170, 214, 236, 252, 328, 334, 335
Asendorpf, J. B., 103, 124, 125
audience
 effect of size on blushing, 23, 127
 necessary for embarrassment, 103, 121, 190–1, 334
 role in embarrassment, 112
audience provocation, 188–9, 197
autism, 129, 130
avoidance of embarrassment, 132–8, 194–5

beta-adrenoceptors, 5, 15, 25–6, 32, 50, 127, 243
blood pressure
 in embarrassment, 125–6
blush
 as a mask, 235–6
 as embodied performance, 209
 believed to reveal incompetence, 208, 209, 215, 280

'hallmark' of embarrassment, 8, 185, 193, 199, 222, 231, 233, 237, 336
 implications for self-identity, 218
blushing propensity
 and effects of betablocker on blushing, 25–6
 and fear of blushing, 269–71
 and feedback about blushing, 33
 and measures of blushing, 25–7
 and remedial function of blush, 51
 and social anxiety, 30, 51
Blushing Propensity Scale (BPS), 25, 31, 32, 50–1, 52, 269, 270, 300, 316
Blushing, Trembling and Sweating Questionnaire (BTS-Q), 50, 51–2, 268, 300
bodily embarrassment, 137
Bögels, S. M., 10, 19, 20, 25, 27, 28, 43, 44, 50, 51, 52, 53, 166, 212, 267, 268, 269, 270, 272, 273, 274, 276, 280, 286, 287, 291, 293, 294, 295, 296, 297, 298, 300, 301, 302, 316, 320, 340
brain cooling, 21–2
Burgess, T. H., 3, 4, 64, 242, 244, 245
Buss, A. H., 7, 8, 51, 70, 107, 108, 126, 153, 185, 193, 222, 336

Casimir, M. J., 101, 231, 329
Castelfranchi, C., 51, 65, 101, 203, 231, 236, 243, 245–6, 247, 271
Changizi, M. J., 19, 85, 86, 243, 335
childhood blushing, 7, 100, 111, 299, 316–17
children's understanding of blush, 111–13
Clark, D. M., 170, 171, 274, 291, 293, 294, 295, 297, 299
classification of circumstances
 of blushing, 222–3, 226, 229, 230
 of embarrassment, 186–9, 195, 222
cognitive bias modification, 280

345

colour patterns in organisms
   and reproductive status, 82–3, 341
   and social rank/status, 81–2, 83
   as social signals, 82–3
   automimicry, 81, 83
   in primates, 80–3
colour perception
   and social signals, 85, 243
   identification of emotional states, 19, 86
   species differences, 83–5
   trichromatic vision, 84–5, 335
communicative function of blush, 64–8, 86, 101, 203, 250, 251
comparison of psychological theories, 73–4
compensatory sweating, 21
complexion differences, 23, 63, 236, 259, 310, 336
compliments, 69, 230, 234
conspicuousness, 63, 187, 189, 191, 204, 206, 210, 229, 236
coyness blushing, 92
creeping blush, 29, 223, 329, 330, 335
Crozier, W. R., 9, 71, 72, 73, 77, 91, 108, 110, 113, 122, 198, 203, 204, 206, 210, 213, 215, 226, 249, 250, 269, 273, 332, 334, 342
cultural differences
   in blushing, 3, 237, 329, 336, 342
   in bodily embarrassment, 137
   in fear of blushing, 67
   in shame-related lexicon, 231

Darby, R. S., 7, 123, 137, 138, 336, 338, 342
Darwin, C., xi, 2–4, 5, 6, 8, 15, 24, 64, 77, 94, 100, 101, 138, 222, 231, 233, 235, 237, 238, 243, 245, 331, 341
de Jong, P. J., 9–10, 23, 51, 52, 53, 66, 67, 91, 101, 123, 194, 198, 203, 214, 246, 251, 254, 256, 260, 267, 269, 270, 271, 272, 274, 276, 277, 278, 279, 286, 287, 294, 296, 297, 298, 300, 316, 331, 332, 333, 337, 339
de Waal, F. B. M., 2, 88, 90, 242, 248
Dijk, C., 9–10, 23, 29, 43, 52, 66, 67, 91, 94, 101, 194, 198, 203, 209, 212, 254, 256, 259, 260, 267, 268, 270, 272, 275, 276, 277, 278, 280, 298, 331, 332, 333, 337, 339
dramaturgic model
   compared to social evaluation model of embarrassment, 121–2, 190–2
   of embarrassment, 121, 189–90, 336
dramaturgical theory
   and self-presentation, 203
   of blushing, 203, 204, 209–10, 334
Drott, C., 21
Drummond, P. D., 5, 10, 16, 18, 19, 20, 21, 22, 23–4, 25, 26, 27, 28, 30, 31, 32, 33, 41, 42, 43, 44, 45, 46, 47, 50, 52, 63, 67, 69, 127, 193, 248, 259, 269, 270, 311, 315, 316, 317, 319, 320, 328, 329, 334, 339, 340, 342

Edelmann, R. J., 25, 28, 31, 46, 63, 93, 124, 126, 140, 196, 204, 215, 222, 234, 242, 269, 273, 286, 291, 297, 302, 316
Ekman, P., 124
embarrassability, 31, 192–3
embarrassment
   and impression formation, 66–7
   and measurement of blushing, 22–3
   consequences, 193–4
   historical changes in meaning, 232
   in childhood, 103
   motivates dysfunctional behaviours, 337
   motivates prosocial behaviour, 122–3
   nonverbal displays, 124–5
Emmelkamp, P. M., 267, 280, 286, 291, 296
empathic blushing, 23, 70
empathic embarrassment, 189
endoscopic thoracic sympathectomy, 20–1, 340–1
evaluative embarrassment, 103, 109, 110, 334
exposure, 109, 110–11, 224, 229, 234, 236, 260, 276
exposure embarrassment, 103, 104, 109, 334
exposure theory, 9, 71–4, 110, 204, 223–6, 234–5

Facial Action Coding System (FACS), 124
facial colour analysis, 48–9
facial skin temperature
   measurement, 22–3, 46–8
   relation to visible blush, 46–7, 65, 127–8
   thermistor measure, 5, 46, 47, 330
fear of blushing
   and rosacea, 314
   and social phobia, 267–8
   automatic associations, 277–8, 279
   biased judgments, 67, 194, 272–3, 297, 339
   consequences, 268
   core concerns, 267, 275–6
   empirical studies of blushing, 28–30

# Index

feedback about blushing, 29
information-processing biases, 279–80, 340
judgments of standards, 271–2
measurement, 46, 52
prevalence, 268
propensity to blush, 269–71, 339
self-focused attention, 272–5, 293, 294
sensitivity to others' judgments, 271–2
fear of embarrassment, 132, 193–4, 197
biased judgments in, 276–7
fear of negative evaluation, 31, 192, 272, 315
feedback effects on blushing, 26–7, 29, 33
Ferguson, T. J., 101, 102, 105, 111, 114
Fessler, D. M. T., 89, 90, 231, 236
flushing
and anger, 32
and blushing, 29, 32, 33, 45
and sexual excitation, 83
in rosacea, 10, 308–9, 311, 315, 316, 317, 319, 320
in social anxiety disorder, 31
in thermoregulation, 21
post-surgical, 21
with rage, 19, 20
Fox, N. A., 148, 152, 153, 154, 158
Frank, R. H., 243, 244, 260
Frijda, N., 236, 249
frontal and temporal lobes
in embarrassment, 130
frontotemporal lobe degeneration (FTLD), 128–9

Gawronski, B., 278
gaze aversion, 31, 70, 87, 103, 114, 124, 125, 139, 140, 167, 236
gender differences
in blushing, 22, 92, 342–3
in bodily embarrassment, 137
in responses to blushing, 214
in rosacea, 309–10, 313
in seeking medical attention, 134–5
Gerlach, A. L., 5, 19, 20, 27, 39, 42, 50, 51, 53, 125, 127, 267, 270, 287, 301, 330
Gilovich, T., 69, 71, 193, 194
Goffman, E., 70, 121, 203, 205, 208, 209, 210, 211, 212, 213, 214, 217, 218, 243, 257
guilt
and blushing, 2, 66, 91, 222, 245, 250, 254, 329, 332
and rosacea, 316
and shame, 231, 342

Harris, C. R., 7, 122, 123, 124, 125, 126, 131, 133, 134, 137, 138, 195, 336, 338, 342
Harris, P. R., 64, 233
heart rate
and fear of blushing, 20
in embarrassment, 7, 125–7
in temperamental shyness, 154
Hofmann, S. G., 10, 31, 42, 67, 125, 127, 148, 170, 171, 270, 286, 295, 297, 299, 302, 340
humour, 139, 185, 196, 197, 235

illusion of transparency, 194
infrared thermography, 48
involuntary nature of blush, xi, 2, 5, 51, 65, 91, 101, 113, 207, 210, 211, 252, 332, 335
Izard, C. E., 102, 106, 113, 140, 223

Kagan, J., 104, 148, 149, 152, 153, 154
Keltner, D., 101, 109, 111, 122, 123, 124, 125, 129, 131, 138, 139, 140, 222, 232, 246, 250, 252, 271

laser Doppler flowmetry, 5, 22, 24, 25, 42, 43, 48, 317, 330
Leary, M. R., 6, 7, 19, 25, 29, 32, 50, 66, 68, 70, 92, 94, 101, 106, 109, 110, 132, 193, 195, 204, 206, 215, 223, 224, 230, 234, 243, 247, 248, 259, 267, 269, 271, 273, 316, 329, 331–2, 334, 336, 341
Lewis, H. B., 224, 226, 237
Lewis, M., 70, 103, 104, 105, 109, 110, 113, 115, 139, 140, 191, 231

Manstead, A. S. R., 123, 196, 197, 249, 251, 254, 333
measurement. See facial skin temperature; infrared thermography; laser Doppler flowmetry; photoplethysmography; physiological measures of blush
medical embarrassment, 132–8, 194–5
Mellander, S., 5, 15, 32, 50, 243
Miller, R. S., 8, 70, 108, 120, 121, 125, 138, 139, 185, 186, 188, 189, 190, 191, 192–3, 195, 196, 197, 198, 215, 222, 230, 246, 335, 336, 337, 339, 342
Miskovic, V., 7, 154, 157, 158, 166, 168, 170, 249, 338
Mulkens, S., 25, 42, 46, 52, 53, 267, 268, 269, 270, 271, 272, 274, 286, 287, 294, 296, 297, 300

## Index

Neto, F., 25, 269, 272, 316
neuroanatomy
  of embarrassment, 128–31
  of social anxiety, 149–53
neuroticism, 24, 314
niacin, 31–2, 45
nitric oxide, 33, 311
nonverbal display
  of embarrassment, 139–40
  of shame, 139–40

observational measures of blushing, 52–4
Öhman, A., 147, 148, 166, 171
optimistic bias in embarrassment, 131
orbitofrontal brain damage, 129–31
others' negative response
  to blushing, 215–18, 254, 256
  to performance of shy role, 216–17
others' positive response
  to blushing, 198, 213–15, 252–3, 254, 256–7, 332
  to embarrassment display, 123–4, 197–8
overpraise, 69, 189

parasympathetic nervous system, 18–19, 20, 126–7
Parrott, W. G., 121, 138, 190, 222
Peters, M. L., 23, 52, 53, 66, 67, 198, 246, 254, 256, 271, 272, 276
photoplethysmography, 22–4, 40–6, 127, 330
physiological measures of blush
  caveats, 43–6, 46–7
  effects of facial movement, 44
  parameterization, 42–6
Poggi, I., 51, 65, 101, 203, 231, 236, 243, 245–6, 247, 271
psychoanalytic explanations, 64, 238
psychological interventions for fear of blushing
  applied relaxation, 292–3
  cognitive behavioural therapy, 280, 296, 298
    for children, 299
  cognitive therapy, 291, 293, 296, 297–8
  exposure therapy, 293, 295–7
    for children, 298–9
  mindfulness-based cognitive therapy, 295
  social skills training, 291–2, 298
    for children, 299
  task concentration training, 287, 293, 294–5
  treatment effectiveness, 292, 300–1, 340

Rapee, R. M., 27, 52, 53, 67
remedial function of blush, 65–8, 196, 250, 251, 252, 253, 254, 257, 331
remedial theory of blushing, 67–8, 73–4
responses to embarrassment, 195–8
Rochat, P., 108, 233, 236
rosacea
  etiology, 311–12
  nature of, 308
  prevalence, 10, 309–10
  psychiatric comorbidity, 313–14
  psychological interventions, 319–20
  role of blushing, 316–19
Rubin, K. H., 154
rule violation
  and blushing, 64, 65, 245, 246–7, 254, 271
  and fear of blushing, 296
  and shame, 232, 245, 334

Sabini, J., 121, 122, 132, 138, 190, 232, 233
safety behaviours, 274, 295, 296, 299
Salzen, E., 93, 236
Scheff, T. J., 113, 211, 213, 226, 233, 236, 237
Schmidt, L. A., 7, 148, 152, 153, 154, 156, 158, 163, 165, 166, 167, 168, 170, 249, 338
Schnegg, M., 101, 231, 329
Scholing, A., 267, 280, 286, 296
Scott, S., 8–9, 204, 205, 206, 207, 210, 214, 217, 337–8
self-conscious affect, 102–5
  development, 110
self-conscious emotions, 89, 94, 100, 128, 129, 130, 204, 210, 219, 245
self-consciousness, 25, 63, 89, 90, 209, 211, 212, 215, 233, 273, 315
  and blush, 209
  and shyness, 206–8, 209
  in adolescence, 102, 105–6
  in childhood, 102
  produced by blush, 209
Self-Consciousness Scale, 51
self-focused attention, 25, 272–5, 293, 299, 316
self-presentation strategies, 211–12, 216–17, 337
Semin, G. R., 123, 196, 197, 251
Setchell, J. M., 81, 82
sexual elements of blush, 341–2
shame
  about blushing, 211
  and exposure, 224–5
  and positive attention, 234–5

## Index

and rosacea, 314, 316
blush as sign of, 91
blush with, 3, 230, 231, 232, 237, 244–6, 336
display, 251, 253
distinct from embarrassment, 138–40, 230, 231–3, 246, 252
identification of, 129
in computer avatars, 66
motivates behaviour, 101
shame-related affect, 101–2, 105, 115, 334
Shearn, D., 5, 19, 23, 40, 42, 44, 47, 54, 70, 124, 125, 127, 246
Shields, S. A., 63, 108, 243, 248, 259, 267
shy blush
and self-consciousness, 209
as stigmatizing, 205, 208–12
shy self, the, 207
shyness
and blushing, 3, 208, 222
and social anxiety disorder, 31, 148, 153
as self-conscious emotion, 101
perception of facial expressions, 167
temperamental, 153–4, 165
signal
blush as, 92, 93–4, 242–4, 249–53, 257, 259, 331–3
Silver, M., 121, 190, 232
Simon, A., 63, 108, 243, 248, 259, 267
sincerity of blush, 249, 253, 257, 259, 260, 332, 335
smile control, 124, 139, 140
smiling, 65, 102, 103, 104, 124–5, 139, 140
social anxiety
and blushing, 170–1
and blushing propensity, 30
and rosacea, 315–16, 317, 319, 320
EEG studies, 165, 167–8
nature of, 147–8
neuroimaging studies, 152, 165–9
perception of facial expressions, 165–7
psychophysiological studies, 170
social anxiety disorder (SAD)
and blushing, 27–8, 31–2, 286
and blushing phobia, 212
measurement of blush, 46
pattern of brain activity, 165
scores on Blushing, Trembling and Sweating Questionnaire, 51
self-focused attention, 293, 299
social anxiety spectrum, 148
treatments of, 287, 291–3, 295–9, 301–2
with and without fear of blushing, 28, 286–7

social evaluation model
compared to dramaturgic model of embarrassment, 121–2, 190–2
of embarrassment, 121, 138, 190–3, 334, 336
spotlight effect, 69, 106, 193–4
staring
as trigger of blush, 69–70
Stegge, H., 7, 101, 102, 105, 108, 110, 112, 114, 334
Strathern, A., 231
Su, D., 10, 22, 30, 311, 315, 316, 317, 319
submissiveness, 91, 165, 170, 171, 248, 259, 328, 335
sweating, 47
as measure of blush, 49–50
excessive, 21
gustatory, 21
symbolic interactionism, 204, 205, 213
sympathetic nervous system, 4, 16–17, 19–21, 27, 28, 125–6, 127, 248, 327, 328–9

Tangney, J. P., 120, 138, 139, 140, 190, 204, 246, 250
Taylor, G., 224, 225, 231, 233
theory of mind, 90, 94, 128, 129, 130
thermoregulation, 4, 21–2, 39–40, 50, 243, 311, 328, 340
Tinbergen, N., 78, 79, 243, 249
trustworthiness
blush indicates, xii, 66, 91, 101, 198, 203, 251, 254, 256, 257, 260, 333
in human evolution, xii
judged from face, 260, 333

undesired social attention
and blush, 109, 204, 224, 234, 248, 334
undesired social attention theory, 68–71, 73–4, 234, 247–8

van Hooff, J. A. R. A. M., 6, 87, 88, 90, 92, 94, 249, 328, 331, 335, 341
vasodilatation, 5, 17, 18–20, 24, 27, 31, 33, 50, 63, 83, 86, 127, 235, 236, 238, 243, 311, 317, 328
Voncken, M. J., 19, 20, 27, 28, 44, 46, 53, 67, 194, 212, 270, 274, 276, 286, 287, 291, 295, 297, 298, 300, 301, 302, 320, 337

Wilkin, J., 20, 243

*Francis de Sales and
Jane de Chantal*

Saints by Our Side

# *Francis de Sales and Jane de Chantal*

By Wendy M. Wright

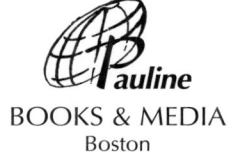

BOOKS & MEDIA
Boston

Library of Congress Cataloging-in-Publication Data

Names: Wright, Wendy M., author.
Title: Francis de Sales and Jane de Chantal / by Wendy M. Wright.
Description: Boston, MA : Pauline Books & Media, 2017. | Series: Saints by our side | Includes bibliographical references.
Identifiers: LCCN 2016028408| ISBN 9780819827388 (pbk.) | ISBN 081982738X (pbk.)
Subjects: LCSH: Francis, de Sales, Saint, 1567-1622. | Chantal, Jeanne-Françoise de, Saint, 1572-1641. | Christian saints--Biography. | Friendship--Religious aspects--Christianity.
Classification: LCC BX4655.3 W753 2017 | DDC 282.092/2 [B] --dc23

LC record available at https://lccn.loc.gov/2016028408

The Scripture quotations contained herein are from the *New Revised Standard Version Bible: Catholic Edition,* copyright © 1989, 1993, Division of Christian Education of the National Council of the Churches of Christ in the United States of America. Used by permission. All rights reserved.

Excerpt from John Paul II's *Letter on the Fourth Centenary of the Episcopal Ordination of St. Francis de Sales* copyright © Liberia Editrice Vaticana. All rights reserved. Used with permission.

Cover design by Rosana Usselmann

Cover art: Paintings executed in the 1950s by a Chicago artist, Ludwig Scheuerle. Used with permission of the Sisters of the Visitation, Toledo, Ohio.

All rights reserved. No part of this book may be reproduced or transmitted in any form or by any means, electronic or mechanical, including photocopying, recording, or by any information storage and retrieval system, without permission in writing from the publisher.

"P" and PAULINE are registered trademarks of the Daughters of St. Paul.

Copyright © 2017, Wendy M. Wright

Published by Pauline Books & Media, 50 Saint Pauls Avenue, Boston, MA 02130-3491

Printed in the U.S.A.

www.pauline.org

Pauline Books & Media is the publishing house of the Daughters of St. Paul, an international congregation of women religious serving the Church with the communications media.

1 2 3 4 5 6 7 8 9                                      21 20 19 18 17

# Contents

INTRODUCTION
Coming to Know Saints Francis de Sales
and Jane de Chantal . . . . . . . . . . . . . . . . . . . . . . . . . . . . . 1

CHAPTER ONE
The World of the Salesian Saints . . . . . . . . . . . . . . . . . . . . . . 5

CHAPTER TWO
Formative Years . . . . . . . . . . . . . . . . . . . . . . . . . . . . . . 11

CHAPTER THREE
Turbulent Times . . . . . . . . . . . . . . . . . . . . . . . . . . . . . . 17

CHAPTER FOUR
Forging New Paths . . . . . . . . . . . . . . . . . . . . . . . . . . . . . 23

CHAPTER FIVE
An Unforeseen Future . . . . . . . . . . . . . . . . . . . . . . . . . . . 31

CHAPTER SIX
Their Stories Converge .................................. 41

CHAPTER SEVEN
Spiritual Friendship ..................................... 55

CHAPTER EIGHT
Birth of a Community.................................... 67

CHAPTER NINE
Conflict and Growth .................................... 85

CHAPTER TEN
Trials .................................................. 95

CHAPTER ELEVEN
Ending and Beginning Anew ............................ 105

CHAPTER TWELVE
Final Years of Faithful Service........................... 109

Epilogue ............................................... 117

Prayer in Honor of
Saints Jane de Chantal and Francis de Sales ............... 119

Reflection Questions ................................... 121

Chronology............................................ 123

Notes ................................................. 131

Introduction
. . . . . . . . . . . .

# Coming to Know Saints Francis de Sales and Jane de Chantal

My decades-long familiarity with Saints Francis de Sales and Jane de Chantal began in the late 1970s when I was at the end of my graduate studies at the University of California at Santa Barbara and was searching for a dissertation topic. To write about a woman seemed natural as the retrieval of Christian women's texts and stories from the past had just begun in earnest in the English-speaking world. I was attracted to women with a contemplative bent, but sensed that I would need to feel a certain affinity with my subject. Six-year-old visionaries, women who eschewed marriage, and heroic martyrs were wonderfully fascinating, but my personal experience did not match that of these women. Plus I needed to find someone who was not overstudied so that I could break new ground, but whose writings were not so inaccessible that they would require decades of research in remote archives. As I surveyed the historic tradition, I kept coming across the name of Jane Frances Frémyot, baroness de Chantal, mostly as a footnote in accounts of Francis de Sales, the seventeenth-century, French-speaking bishop from the duchy of Savoy and author of the *Introduction to the Devout Life*. In fact, Francis himself tended to be something of a footnote in general histories of Christianity written in the 1970s, since figures from the era of the Catholic Reformation—with the exception perhaps of Carmelites Teresa of Àvila and John of the Cross—were not much studied at the time.

Jane drew me. She had been happily married, raised four children, and led a householder's life but also had a leaning toward a more contemplative existence. Due to the untimely death of her husband and her fated meeting with Bishop de Sales, she embraced religious life. Those events changed everything for her. I felt that I could identify both with her contemplative impulses and her identity as wife and mother, as well as with her experience as a working woman, since Jane was the busy foundress of a burgeoning community.

Thus I met Francis through Jane. My dissertation focused on their spiritual friendship as seen through the lens of Jane's growth and transformation. Because much of her correspondence with her mentor and friend has been lost, I had to reconstruct a good deal of their shared experience by reading his letters of spiritual guidance to her. This allowed me to, as it were, sit at his feet and learn in a special way. I also read a great deal of his voluminous correspondence to others and his writings for the public. All that reading was deeply formative for me. I quite simply came to love the spiritual perspective they shared. That perspective emerges from the rich soil of early-modern Catholic-Christian humanism. It is optimistic, balanced, heart-centered, and relational, applicable to many different persons in diverse circumstances, eras, and lifestyles. It has weathered the test of time well and continues to inspire us today.

Over the years I have had opportunities to continue to study Francis, Jane, and Salesian spirituality from a variety of perspectives. Although I have written extensively, I am delighted to be asked to pen a joint biography, quite a different task than considering simply the two saints' relationship. It has given me a perspective from which I have never viewed the two of them before. For while the spiritual bond of friendship is at the heart of both their lives, Francis de Sales and Jane de Chantal were also persons with very different life experiences and personalities. Their shared relationship did not fully define either of them. They were regarded by their contemporaries and by posterity in distinct ways. It is with delight that I turn again to the story of these two most attractive saints and see that story anew. It is a story that survives the centuries and speaks poignantly and powerfully in our present age.

## Chapter One

# The World of the Salesian Saints

Francis de Sales[1] arrived in the world on August 21, 1567, two months premature. His young mother, Françoise de Sionnaz; her older husband, François de Nouvelles; and the rest of the de Sales household feared for his life. According to one oral tradition, this tiny, frail infant—who was the heir to his family's feudal estates—was hastily named and baptized as an emergency measure. According to other sources, a few days or a day later baby Francis, swathed in protective cotton bunting, was baptized in the local parish of Saint Maurice and entrusted to an experienced wet-nurse. He was then brought to the countryside chateau of Monthoux where the air was thought to be more healthful and the vulnerable child's survival more assured.

Meanwhile, the patrimony to which Francis as the first-born male was destined—the seigneuries of both his father and his mother, Sales and Boissy, respectively—was also of concern to the young mother.[2] His birth had been preceded by her fervent prayers for a successful conception, since the issue of a male child was culturally expected of her. Soon after her marriage, she had placed her heartfelt petition into the divine heart as she knelt before the legendary Shroud of Turin, which was on temporary display in the Church of Notre Dame de Liesse in the nearby lakeside town of Annecy. She had even gone so far as to privately dedicate the hoped-for infant to the future service of God. After Francis was born, however, his mother's concerns became focused on the tiny child's well-being. He flourished in the country air and eventually rejoined his family.

That family quickly grew—Françoise would eventually give birth to thirteen more children. Throughout his life Francis gave much affection and loyalty to his beloved family. He is remembered as being an intelligent, obedient, and deeply affectionate child. His parents carefully nurtured him to grow into an exemplary gentleman who adhered faithfully to the Roman Catholic faith. They led by good example, attending the parish church and religious rites regularly and treating their servants and the poor with generosity and courtesy.

As he matured Francis showed a talent for study, but as heir he was also expected to excel at swordsmanship, hunting, fencing, and riding. His father, especially, insisted on his being raised on a bracing regime of wholesome food, outdoor play, and sleeping alone in the dark. This latter practice, designed to improve character and foster courage, was challenging for the sensitive boy. Years later, in a letter to a correspondent, the adult Francis would admit his terrible fear of the dark. It is characteristic of him that, even as a child, he met this challenge as a spiritual one.

> When I was young I was afflicted with this fantasy [that malign spirits lurked] and in order to rid myself of it, I forced myself little by little to go alone, my heart armed with confidence in God, into those places that frightened me. Finally I became so strong that the darkness and solitude of night became my delight.[3]

This remembered childhood fear of the dark and its resolution gives us a first intimation about the spiritual practices that would come to typify the adult man's spirituality. Characteristically, these disciplines would involve formation of the imagination. Fear, in this prepubescent case, was countered by directly confronting the terrorizing imaginative construct with another more confident one.[4]

The picturesque alpine town of Annecy to which his mother, the young Madame de Boissy, had traveled from her estates in the countryside, was geographically remote from the great cities of sixteenth-century Europe. But Annecy had long been at the crossroads of continental political affairs. The remains of ancient Roman settlements existed alongside the fortified chateau long used by the Dukes of Savoy. In the not distant past the troops of the Holy Roman Empire and the Kingdoms of France and Spain had crossed through the high mountain passes that led to Annecy and claimed outlying Savoyard territories as strategic outposts. Savoy was a proud independent duchy fifty miles south of Geneva, extending into the Piedmont region. Savoy was bordered on the west by the Kingdom of France and on the southeast by the Italian city states. Its capital, Turin, was home to one of the more sophisticated aristocratic courts of the era. Two Savoyard dukes,

Emmanuel Philibert (reigning from 1553–1580) and Charles Emmanuel I (reigning from 1580–1630) would rule and command the diplomatic loyalty of the house of Sales throughout Francis' lifetime.

Besides being an integral player on early modern Europe's dynastic and territorial chessboard, Savoy, and the town of Annecy especially, was significant from a religious point of view. When Francis entered the world in 1567, the great Christian reformations had been reshaping the ecclesial and spiritual map of Europe for three-quarters of a century. Europe was divided between countries and regions that embraced the changes initiated by those who came to be known as Protestants and those that still looked to Rome for religious guidance. Just three years before Francis' birth the Council of Trent, which had crafted the reforming agenda of the Roman Catholic Church, had closed its final session. Trent's decrees would gradually reshape the religious world in which the boy would mature. Among the reformers who had broken with Rome and initiated various new programs, theologian John Calvin had fled France and taken refuge in the city of Geneva. In 1541, he spearheaded a theocratic revolution of Church and civil society based on principles laid out in his *Institutes of the Christian Religion*. Opponents of Calvin's programs, including the Roman Catholic bishop whose see was historically centered in Geneva, were forced out. One year after the birth of Francis, Annecy became the official seat of the exiled prelate. The modest wooden church of Saint Pierre became the truncated diocese's cathedral, located in the center of the city beside one of the town's many picturesque canals.

The dukes of Savoy claimed fervent loyalty to the Church of Rome. Geneva had long been part of the diocese. Not only was it now Calvinist, but territories that had once belonged to the duchy had also been lost and evangelized for the Protestant faith. Further, the distinctive political-religious turmoil that had for decades torn at the fabric of the Kingdom of France was soon to escalate and create fissures in neighboring lands. Most European political territories, generally following the lead of their rulers, had aligned themselves with either the Church of Rome or with one of the branches of Protestantism. France found itself in an incendiary situation with a divided population. Powerful French noble families lined up to oppose each other and marshal support either for the Huguenots, as French Calvinists were called, or those who championed a thoroughly Catholic France.

In the midst of this civil unrest, the crown had been weakened in 1560 by the death of the young monarch Francis II and the ensuing regency of the Queen Mother, Catherine de Medici, who stood in for her underage son, Charles. Catherine and her advisors attempted to assuage religious tensions by recognizing Roman Catholicism as the state religion while forbidding any injury or injustice to French citizens who had differing religious loyalties. The compromise did not hold, and in 1562 the first battle of the French Wars of Religion broke out. These ferocious military conflicts were fueled by the rival noble factions. For decades the prolonged and vicious strife would continue to fuel violent confrontations and harden religious loyalties. Unaware of all this, the tiny, frail Savoyard infant entered this world, which would shape him in unexpected ways.

CHAPTER TWO

• • • • • • • • • • • •

# Formative Years

A decade after the onset of the Wars of Religion, French civil tensions had reached crisis level. King Charles IX had reached his majority. As his mother, Catherine, had done, he attempted to rein in religious sectarian violence. He arranged a marriage between his Catholic sister, Marguerite of Valois, and a Protestant cousin, Henry of Navarre, who was in a remote line to the French throne. The royal wedding, set for August 18, 1572, drew to Paris thousands of aristocrats of both religious persuasions and opposing political perspectives. Rivalries were revived, and on Saint Bartholomew's feast (August 24), just days after the wedding, a prominent Protestant nobleman was assassinated. His body was thrown into the street and mutilated, igniting a five-day killing spree that spread throughout the capital and into the French provinces, claiming the lives of up to ten thousand people.

On January 23 of that same year, a mere nine months before the Saint Bartholomew's Day massacre, a second child, a daughter, was born to the Catholic Burgundian lawyer, Benigne Frémyot, and his wife, Marguerite de Berbesey. They named the baby girl Jane in honor of Saint John the Almoner, whose feast was celebrated that day.[1] Later, at her confirmation, she added the name Frances, so that throughout her adulthood she went by Jane Frances.[2]

Jane; her elder sister, Marguerite; and her younger brother, André, grew up amid the urban bustle of prosperous mercantile Dijon. Their mother had died while giving birth to André, when Jane was just eighteen months old. The Parliament, where her father served as president, was situated directly across the street from their residence. The children were educated at home by tutors and cared for by an aunt and nurse, but they also received the fruits of their father's broad humanist views on history, morality, and the law. Father and daughter had close ties, and the character traits that Jane displayed later in life—her courage, clear-headedness, and resilience—may be said to have been passed down through the paternal line.

———•◆•———

Meanwhile, as Jane matured amid the urban bustle of Dijon, about three hundred kilometers away, high in the remote mountainous regions of Savoy, Francis was being groomed by his prominent family to enter the complex political world to which he was heir. With three cousins and a tutor, Monsieur Déage, Francis was sent at the age of six to be schooled in La Roche-sur-

Foron, about nine miles from home. Two years later he transferred to the Chappusien school in Annecy. (It is speculated that his father's support of the Duke of Savoy and opposition to the Duke of Nemour's plan to use the castle of Sales as a launching site for the invasion of Calvinist Geneva made the transfer prudent for his son.) In 1577, at the age of ten, he received his first Communion and was confirmed in the Church of Saint Dominic in Annecy.

Nestled on the southern shore of picturesque alpine Lake Annecy, the hilly town was laced through with canals. They flowed down toward the lakeshore from the prominent hill upon which the ancient ducal palace was perched, affording a panoramic view of the entire region. Narrow cobblestone streets wound through closely set shops, residences, and churches. The convent of the Poor Clares was just a brisk walk from the Cathedral of Saint Pierre. Another turn took one across a moat to the city prison marooned on a tiny, triangular island in the middle of the canals. Summer brought lakeside breezes and cascades of wildflowers dotting the surrounding hills, while winter spread a chalk-white blanket of deep alpine snow as far as the eye could see. Although in less than a year, Francis would leave the pastoral beauty of Savoy for the intense urban experience of France's glittering capital, Paris, "*chere* Nessy" ("dear little Annecy") would always be closest to the adult de Sales' heart.

When the appointed time came to leave "*chere* Nessy," the eleven-year-old, again accompanied by his tutor and his similarly-aged cousins, was sent to Paris to continue his education. His father and other Savoyard aristocrats had traditionally attended the college of Navarre (a college being roughly equivalent to a secondary school in the modern United States). But Francis had ideas of his own. He preferred the Jesuit college of Clermont. Its schoolmasters' reputation for educational excellence, holiness, and dedication to the Catholic reform appealed to the devout young student. So, Claremont it was. The Savoyards set up in the center of the turbulent, student-filled Latin Quarter. The Christian humanist curriculum at the Jesuit school was designed to include the best of the new learning: the Greek and Latin classics and their languages, rhetoric, geography, philosophy, mathematics, the study of Scripture, the Church fathers, and moral and dogmatic theology. Along with this intellectual formation, the skills a gentleman should acquire, such as fencing, were taught. In addition, boys who had a predisposition to piety beyond the ordinary were invited to join the Marian sodality where more intense engagement with Jesuit formation in the form of the daily *examen,* the Ignatian *Spiritual Exercises,* and fervent devotion to Our Lady was introduced. Francis became a student leader in Clermont's sodality.

Clearly, his seriousness had attracted the attention of his mentors. What perhaps could not have been anticipated was the spiritual crisis that would erupt somewhere between 1586 and 1587. Francis was an avid learner, devouring all the wisdom offered him. He drank deeply at the springs of humanist culture, setting his sights, as the *Spiritual Exercises* directed him, on the greater glory of God and becoming a disciple of Christ. His spiritual vision was further shaped by a course he took on the biblical *Song of Songs* with Benedictine Scripture scholar Gilbert Génébrard. The lesson became more than academic: Francis was swept off his feet by an encounter with the intimate love of God. This would become foundational to Francis' theological vision. Somewhere in his studies he also encountered the teaching of the medieval Franciscan Duns Scotus on the incarnation, which proposed that out of an excess of love God had intended to become human from the beginning of time and not merely, as was alternately taught, as a corrective in response to human sin.

These elements of thought, deeply internalized and experienced in prayer, emerged in the young de Sales as a vision of a world of interconnected hearts: the heart of God connected to human hearts through the gentle, humble heart of Jesus (see Mt 11:29) and human hearts joined together in loving relation as they become what they are intended to be—at one with and in the heart of God.

In the teeming, intellectually charged atmosphere of the capital, he also learned of the politically-freighted theological quarrels of the day that had generated so much violence. Although some French Catholic citizens took a pragmatic and reasoned approach to the Huguenot presence and the fraught royal succession, Catholic extremists (coming primarily from the Latin Quarter) could not abide what they viewed as faithlessness. They denounced the moderates as heretics damned to perdition. The threat of damnation coming from versions of Calvinist and other theologies that pointed in the direction of predestination were being avidly discussed. Francis seemed to have had access to his tutor's class notes where such ideas were presented. Add to this mix the heady brew of hundreds of adolescent boys exploring the limits of their potentials, and the conditions for a crisis were in place.

Francis would ultimately become known for his spiritual vision of divine-human love that would underpin his preaching and writing. But at this time, the swirling, turbulent brew of thoughts and emotions generated in the Latin Quarter threatened to overwhelm Francis, an acutely sensitive youth whose heart had been claimed by the God of Love. He was gripped by the chilling fear that he might not be destined to enjoy forever the presence of the God he had experienced as loving and beloved. For weeks he wrestled internally with this terror of alienation and ultimate separation. He fell ill, unable to sleep or eat. His tutor became alarmed. Francis saw no way out of this darkness.

Finally, entering the nearby Church of Saint Étienne de Grès he knelt before an ancient statue of the black Madonna, Our Lady of Good Deliverance, and prayed the hallowed Marian antiphon, the *Memorare:* "Remember most gracious Virgin Mary that never was it known that anyone who fled to your protection, implored your help, or sought your intercession was left unaided. . . ."

His emotional turmoil ceased. Casting himself upon the mercy of a God whose ultimate purposes he did not fully grasp, Francis resolved that even if he could not know the ultimate divine intent, he could and would choose in this life to love to the best of his ability. He resolved to follow the God who had revealed himself as Love incarnate. Such was the existential and affective resolution of Francis' mystical crisis. However, the intellectual dimension of the crisis was yet to be resolved. That resolution would take place several years later as he continued his educational journey in Italy.

Chapter Three
. . . . . . . . . . . .

# Turbulent Times

Francis' father, Monsieur de Boissy, had high hopes for his talented first-born, so after attending school at Clermont, in 1588 Francis was sent to the University of Padua, one of the elite academic institutions of the Catholic world. Like Paris, the Italian peninsula was teeming with intellectual energy. But with its strong Catholic identity, Italian spiritual energies were focused on reform from within the faith community. The towering presence of the reform-minded Bishop Charles Borromeo was felt everywhere. New experimental religious communities powered by a renewed spiritual vision sprang up: the charismatic Philip Neri's Congregation of the Oratory attracted secular priests to a renewed spirit of joyful service, the lay community founded by the Benedictine Oblate Frances of Rome lived in their homes, engaged in prayer and in serving the needs of society (a departure from the dominant enclosed monastic life available to women of the day). Francis took as his spiritual mentor the Jesuit Antonio Possevino. This erudite papal diplomat promoted the Catholic reform throughout Europe.

As the inheritor of the Sales-Boissy legacy, it was expected that Francis would study civil law, which he did. But again following his own deepest promptings, he also studied canon law and theology. In fact, the youth was beginning to discern a call to the priesthood. In Padua, he found an intellectual resolution of his crisis concerning salvation. The crux of the issue was the question of predestination. The teachings of such masters as Thomas Aquinas and Augustine of Hippo did not fully accord with what Francis felt he had gleaned from other sources. He especially drew from the theology of the Spanish Jesuit Luis de Molina, who taught that God intends salvation for all human beings, provides sufficient grace to all to that end, yet allows for human freedom that can turn from and reject that grace. Once again in ardent prayer de Sales begged pardon of the two august Church fathers, asked to be shown otherwise if he was mistaken, and adopted the optimistic views of Molina on the divine Lover's deepest plans for human salvation. It was during this time that Francis drew up for himself a rule of life that would serve to guide his daily activities and approach. This moderate but disciplined rule allowed him to integrate prayer into his routine and to direct his quotidian thoughts and actions toward the service of God.

———•◆•———

While de Sales was completing his studies at Padua, Italy, in France Jane Frémyot was continuing to mature. Her formal education was deemed complete when she was sixteen years old. She was then sent as a companion to her newly married sister Marguerite. She and her husband lived in their new home near Poitiers, an area less troubled than Dijon by the threat of civil war. Still, the scars inflicted by those religious wars left their mark all over the nearby landscape: desecrated churches, shrines, and monasteries. Jane accompanied her sister on the usual rounds of baronial life: entertainment, visits, and parties. Marguerite bore two children, and Jane then became absorbed in her duties as an aunt.

Soon, however, Jane's brother-in-law, the Baron des Francs, pressured her to marry. The Baron put forth a potential suitor whom Jane perceived, much to her brother-in-law's displeasure, as having concealed Protestant allegiances. She refused the suit, straining her relationship with the Baron and his family. It was soon revealed that her suspicions were accurate. Thankfully time would heal some of those familial wounds.

As Jane grew to adulthood, the divisions unfolding in the wake of current political events would reach even more deeply into her immediate family. These events had a complex background. Two decades earlier, Charles IX had reigned only a brief three years as King of France, and in 1574 he had been succeeded by his twenty-two-year-old brother Henry III. As the years passed Henry's failure to produce a male heir created space for powerful political factions funded by foreign powers to emerge: on one hand the fervent Catholic League supported by Spain, and on the other hand the Huguenot faction buttressed by England and by French aristocratic malcontents who opposed Henry's absolutist ambitions. A succession crisis erupted when

Henry's younger brother died. The only remaining heir to the French throne was now a Protestant cousin, Henry of Navarre. He claimed the throne as Henry IV in 1598 after Henry III was assassinated by Catholic fanatics who detested his decadent lifestyle and feared his pragmatic view of the succession. The new monarch eventually thought it prudent to abjure his Protestant faith ("Paris is worth a Mass" he is reputed to have quipped). But Catholic loyalists were appalled, leading to four years of bitter bloodshed between the forces of the Catholic League and those of Navarre, who eventually won a military victory.

Jane's immediate family was caught up in the escalating violence of that dangerous time. Many in the Dijon parliament had sided with the Catholic League and turned against the crown. Jane's father, Bénigne Frémyot, and a small group of followers refused to be disloyal to the king even at the risk of a Protestant becoming King of France. When Henry III was assassinated and Navarre put forth his claim to the throne, Frémyot was instrumental in pacifying resentful members of the Catholic League. He also brokered the new monarch's abjuration of his Protestant faith, for Frémyot too could not imagine France without a Catholic king.

In 1589, Frémyot went into exile with his supporters and formed a rival parliament at Semur, which gained the support of the Paris parliament. Frémyot's rivals were bent on intimidation. They kidnapped his son André, Jane's younger brother, and threatened to behead him if the older man refused to relinquish his position at Semur and return to Dijon. Eventually a truce was negotiated and the boy was released. As for Jane, for a time she joined her father in exile and became acquainted with many of the local landowners who supported him, including the older, widowed Baron Guy de Chantal. He would later play an important role in her story.

## Chapter Four

• • • • • • • • • • • • •

# Forging New Paths

For both Jane Frémyot and Francis de Sales, the year 1592 brought important changes. Jane had been living for a time within her sister's household when her father asked her to return to Dijon since the political tensions had calmed. Because of her own charms and her father's prestige, Jane became a highly eligible marriage prospect and was much courted. She settled on the choice her father offered, the handsome young Baron Christophe Rabutin de Chantal, the son of Guy de Chantal, one of Frémyot's supporters in the civil conflicts.

Jane's fiancé was an accomplished officer and swordsman, a sociable lover of the arts, an informed conversationalist, and, although not much drawn to pious devotion and often late for Mass, a confirmed and loyal Catholic. As was the legal custom, the two were married in a civil ceremony at Thostes and then in a religious celebration at the baron's fortified countryside castle at

Bourbilly. Jane's uncle, Baron Guy de Chantal, who was the prior of a Cistercian abbey not far from Dijon, presided at the marriage. The union was favorable from both families' perspectives. The Baron de Chantal as a "noble of the sword" had his lands and title, but the wars of religion had impoverished his estate, while Bénigne Frémyot, as a rising member of the professional class, had resources but lacked lands and title.[1] The alliance would secure the futures of both families.

As baroness, Jane threw herself into her new role. Christophe was a fine match and she was much in love with him. She greatly enjoyed his company and the rounds of social life, but was somewhat daunted when she realized that she would be responsible for the management of the estate, household, and lands. Christophe's mother had long attended to this task with devotion but, since her death a decade earlier, the estate's finances had been in disarray. Each morning the servants, laborers, and stewards reported to their mistress, and she gave them instructions for the day. She also oversaw the activities of the household herself. The baroness's concern extended beyond her own preserve and, as was the customary duty of the châtelaine (the female owner of an important household), Jane took it upon herself to assist the poor of the neighborhood. She gave alms and practiced nursing in the forms of herbal medicine and midwifery. She also kept a sort of soup kitchen open at the back of the castle during times of scarcity.

The young baroness was also concerned about the Catholic observance of her extended household. She employed a resident chaplain and reestablished the practice of daily Mass, which had lapsed in the late baroness's absence. Christophe was often away on various campaigns, and when he came home the household livened up and social gatherings sometimes overshadowed the religious events. When he left again, the routines of piety were renewed. Jane had a strong faith and allegiance to the Church, but she had never shown herself to be drawn to a vocation other than marriage. She was immensely happy with Christophe.

During the years the couple spent together Jane became pregnant six times. Four children survived infancy: a son, Celse-Bénigne (b. 1596); and three daughters, Marie Aimée (b. 1598), Françoise (b. 1599), and Charlotte (b. 1601). Thus in the last decade of the sixteenth century Jane Frances Frémyot, Baroness de Chantal, could reasonably be well assured that her future life was clearly and happily mapped out for her.

———•◆•———

At the same time Francis de Sales' fortunes were crystallizing. He graduated from the University at Padua, proficient in both civil and canon law. Then he traveled back to Savoy by way of the east coast of Italy in order to make a pilgrimage to the Holy House of Loreto, a shrine reputed to be the dwelling place of the Holy Family that had been miraculously brought there from the Holy Land. During his stay in Italy, Francis' sense of vocation had matured: he desired to enter the priesthood. This was not what his father had in mind, for Francis was expected to marry the daughter of the Duke's counsel. Despite his father's prior arrangements, Francis enlisted his mother to his cause. Together they persuaded Monsieur de Boisy that God had different plans for his talented son. In 1593 Francis renounced his hereditary title and declined the prestigious position of senator that the Duke had conferred on him. His two younger brothers, Louis (b. 1577) and Bernard (b. 1583), received respectively the titles Count of Sales, and Lord of Thuille and Baron of Thorens, which their elder brother had put aside.

As was typical for a well-placed and highly educated man of his day, the ecclesial authorities warmly welcomed Francis' declared vocation. By the end of December he had completed all the formal preparations for ordination to the priesthood. In that era formal seminary preparation was not yet required for ordination and a university degree, especially in canon law, was deemed sufficient. On December 18, 1593, he was ordained and celebrated his first Mass on December 21, which was then the feast of Saint Thomas the Apostle. Francis was then installed as Provost of the Cathedral and provost to the exiled Bishop of Geneva, Claude de Granier, who was in residence in Annecy. He thus became the chief dignitary of the Cathedral Chapter and assistant to the bishop.

De Sales plunged into his ministerial duties, of which preaching especially delighted him. He used all the rhetorical theory and skills he had learned as a student to draw his listeners closer into relationship with the God he knew intimately as Love Itself. Within a year those skills would be employed and tested in a new way. Through a series of wars and invasions in previous decades, the Swiss Calvinist Republic of Bern had taken political and religious control of the Chablais region, which had been part of Savoy. In 1593 diplomatic negotiations restored Chablais to Savoy. Charles Emmanuel, the impetuous duke, desired to consolidate his power and subdue a Protestant populace that was unhappy to be subsumed by the Catholic duchy. The young provost counseled instead a program of thoughtful evangelization rather than risk more bloodshed in another religiously fueled conflict.

In fact, Francis, along with his cousin, Canon Louis de Sales, with whom he had spent so many student years in Savoy and Paris, volunteered to undertake the dangerous mission. Although his father had been persuaded that God intended his son to take ecclesiastical office, Monsieur de Boissy was dead set against this new and perilous venture, as was Louis' family. Their fathers refused to provide funds or resources, including horses, for the journey in hopes that the two would be dissuaded. But Francis and Louis were undaunted. Following an all night prayer vigil on September 14, 1594 (the feast of the Exaltation of the Holy Cross), the companions set off on foot. They hiked thirty-one miles into Chablais, where they were welcomed by the supportive Baron d'Hermance at the fortress of Les Allinges at the edge of the mission territory.

The cousins lost no time launching their preaching mission. At first they attracted more hostility than listeners. Protestant pastors, who had great prestige, issued formal complaints and hurled accusations at the two. Ominous threats circulated throughout the population: at one site citizens threw stones as Francis and Louis preached, causing them to run for their lives. Still, they pressed on, hiking across the icy, snowbound territory even as winter approached. They ministered to the few enclaves of secret Catholics, preaching the compelling beauty of their faith, often encountering fierce opposition or risking bodily harm. Their approach starkly contrasted not only with the military coercion the duke promoted, but also with the fear-driven, zealous polemics adopted by most missionary preachers of the era. Francis' previous experiences with violent militant religiosity had convinced him that persuasion, not fear or force, had the best chance of succeeding with adversaries. It was also the way God desired, a God of infinite love who invites all to "learn from me; for I am gentle and humble in heart" (Mt 11:29). Francis used gentle pedagogy, graceful preaching, and carefully chosen, image-rich written words to cultivate respectful relationships. This approach, along with beautiful public liturgical celebrations, became his mode of pastoral practice, which he would continue to refine throughout his life.

The impressive Forty Hours devotion that he orchestrated at Annamasse in 1597 and in Thorens in 1598 illustrates his approach. This public celebration highlighted the Eucharist, the focal symbol of the Catholic renewal. Bishop de Granier joined his provost for the solemn Masses offered at the start and end of the extended celebration. Hundreds of heads of households processed through the villages and major cities of the region, stopping at churches where the Blessed Sacrament was adored.[2]

Over time the Chablais mission met with some success. Francis' first widely circulated written work emerged from it when he copied and secretly distributed his weekly sermons as brief tracts. These were compiled and later circulated as *The Controversies*. Three years later he drafted a "Brief Treatise on the Virtue of the Cross and the Way to Honor It," which was published in 1598 as *The Defense of the Standard of the Cross*. The provost's evangelizing efforts continued beyond Chablais when, commissioned by Pope Clement VIII, he met for cordial theological discussions with Theodore Beza (b. 1519), Calvin's successor in Geneva. Unsurprisingly, this did not result in the latter's conversion.

---

In 1598 de Sales was recalled from Chablais and the mission was given to the Capuchin Friars. Because Bishop de Granier's health was declining, he wished to nominate his younger charge for his episcopal seat. Francis protested, fearing that the successes in the mission field would be compromised if he left the new converts too soon. But he was eventually persuaded to accept the nomination. An *ad limina* visit to Rome was pending, when the bishop would give an account of life in his diocese to the Holy See. Francis was asked to lead the visit in place of his ailing superior.

They arrived in Rome during the festive Advent-Christmas season. Francis and his entourage, which included his dear friend from Annecy, the magistrate Antoine Favre, made pilgrimage visits to the Eternal City's holy sites. The first papal audience took place after Christmas and ended in a way Francis had not anticipated. He had a formal meeting with three distinguished examiners, including the Jesuit theologian Robert Bellarmine. They had been appointed by Clement VIII to determine if the young nominee would be a worthy co-adjutor (assistant) and successor to the bishop of Geneva. Clement and the panel are said to have been pleased with the surprised candidate's knowledge and modesty as he answered the questions posed to him.

Back in Savoy in his new position as co-adjutor, he found himself even busier than he had been in the mission field. Besides routine diocesan administration, preaching, and organizing the new parishes in the Chablais, Francis faced the vexing problem of the invasion of Savoy by the French King Henry IV. The conflict involved a treaty that had annexed a portion of Savoyard territory to France. Duke Charles Emmanuel had delayed executing the treaty, which gave the king no option but to insist on his rights militarily. The ensuing peace left Francis' episcopal see under the jurisdiction of two different monarchs, and added territories that were historically Calvinist. However, diplomatic responsibilities were part and parcel of ecclesial life in sixteenth- and seventeenth-century post-Reformation Europe. Much of Francis' energy would be spent throughout his life in negotiations that a later era would deem to be purely political.

## Chapter Five

# An Unforeseen Future

Francis' pastoral duties were closer to his heart than the necessary public, political role he had to play. For his model he chose the charismatic Cardinal and Archbishop of Milan, Charles Borromeo, who was widely admired as an exemplary reforming leader. Close to his people, Borromeo had spearheaded reforms of the Council of Trent in his diocese: he shored up ecclesial discipline, founded seminaries, began systematic catechetical instruction for children, preached tirelessly, and ministered to the poor, imprisoned, and sick.

The Milanese cardinal's younger admirer would likewise excel in these areas, especially preaching (although later he did not succeed in founding a seminary in his diocese). Francis, a gifted orator, was well schooled in the arts of rhetoric by his early Jesuit instructors. He became known as a preacher whose vivid images and metaphors captured the imagination of his listeners.

But his preaching style was not popular with other preachers of his day who led erudite sermons packed with clever theological references, designed to impress the elite. Instead, Francis became known as someone who preached heart to heart. He conveyed his own passionate love of God and his vision of a world of interconnected human-divine hearts to his eager audiences. Years later he would write a lengthy letter to Andre Frémyot, Archbishop of Bourges, tutoring his junior colleague in the art of preaching. Steeped in Scripture, leavened with love for both the Gospel and the least of the people to whom he spoke, Francis admonished Frémyot that:

> [A sermon] should be spontaneous, gracious, natural, deliberate, holy, thoughtful, and delivered slowly... in a word, we should speak affectionately and with devotion, simply and candidly and with confidence, convinced of and persuasive in the doctrine we teach. The best art is artless. Our words must catch fire, not because of our shouting or theatrical gestures but because of their inner authenticity. They must come from the heart more than the mouth. We may be good orators but the heart speaks to hearts and the tongue speaks only to the ears.[1]

As early as 1601 the co-adjutor was gaining a reputation as a sought after preacher. That year, the magistrates of the city of Annecy invited him to deliver the series of Lenten sermons that were popular social as well as spiritually edifying civic gatherings. Just before he stepped into the pulpit, he received a note that his father had died. Bravely, Francis delivered his prepared words and as he closed, asked his Savoyard congregation, who knew the deceased well, for their prayers.

Later that same year another sudden death would shatter the world of Madame de Chantal and her household. In October, Jane was spending the requisite weeks confined to bed after the birth of her fourth child and third daughter, Charlotte. Her much beloved thirty-five-year-old husband, Christophe, was also at home, having recently retired from active service at court. He was recovering from a serious case of dysentery. As Christophe gained his strength he grew restless with convalescence. He invited a neighbor who had stopped by to congratulate him on the newborn to join him on a deer-stalking walk in the woods. Crawling on their bellies through the underbrush, during the height of the chase, the strap of the neighbor's gun apparently caught on a branch, the gun accidentally discharged, and the scattered shot embedded itself in Christophe's torso and thigh. Sensing that his wounds were fatal, Christophe forgave his distraught friend. Then he sent the accompanying servants to fetch a priest and take a message to his wife. Although his message was not meant to alarm her, Jane rose from her confinement in distress and hurried to the nearby cottage where her husband had been carried on a stretcher.

They moved Christophe back to the castle, where he lay dying for over a week. Jane tearfully refused to believe in the end for which he was preparing: he put his affairs in order and made his will, which included a clause disinheriting any family member who might attempt to avenge his death. He counseled his wife to submit to the divine will. Even to the last, the twenty-eight-year-old baroness refused to accept the inevitable, her pleading prayers for his recovery rising in a torrent to God.

Months of intense mourning followed Christophe's death. In her grief and confusion Jane found herself longing for solitude. She was drawn to the idea that she should now give herself completely to God rather than follow the path of remarriage her relatives assumed she should. After all, her children were heirs to titles and an estate; their future and their fortunes should be suitably arranged. For some time Jane continued to faithfully fulfill her maternal and familial duties, while wrestling with her inner turmoil. Riding alone on horseback on the outskirts of her lands she replayed in her mind the stories of saintly widows that she had read. These holy women had vowed themselves to lives of chastity and devoted themselves to works of charity. Filled with a new ardor and a longing for God alone, she attempted to simplify her household and introduce more overtly pious daily practices. Even though she could not exactly name what she needed, she longed for someone to speak with, to help her discern God's will in the midst of conflicting expectations and emotions.

Spiritual direction was newly in vogue among pious laypersons in the great cities of France, which were caught up in the energies of the Catholic reform. But such direction was not widely available in the countryside. Still, Jane's longing for something like direction persisted. As she rode alone on her estates one afternoon, approaching the castle from the direction of a remote riverside sawmill, she saw an unusual sight. Someone seemed to be walking out of the wooded copse: a man of average height robed in a preacher's soutane, surplice, and biretta. A voice within her seemed to say, "This is the man beloved of God and among men into whose hands you are to commit your conscience."² The brief vision faded and, while she felt comforted, she did not know what to make of it.

Meanwhile, she threw herself and her household into a round of devotional and charitable activity, even as she pondered her future.

During a tour of nearby pilgrimage sites, she stopped at Notre Dame d'Etang. There she met a well-meaning Franciscan friar who had set himself up as a spiritual guide for religiously motivated noble women of the region, including several of Jane's acquaintances. At their urging, she asked him to be her spiritual director. Unfortunately, it was not a good match. The friar bound Jane by oath not to reveal her conscience to anyone else. He also saddled her with a strict regime of devotional exercises more suited to a solitary ascetic than a woman with a young family and extended household. Yet, Jane, straining Godward as she was, would embrace this regime wholeheartedly for two and a half years. Still, she recalled the lingering memory of the consoling vision near the sawmill at Bourbilly. The friar was not that man.

After Christophe's death, Jane and her children had found refuge with her own father in Dijon. But before long, in the autumn of 1602, a letter arrived from her elderly, widowed father-in-law, Baron Guy de Rabutin de Chantal. He ordered her and his grandchildren to come live with him at Montelon, the remote estate near Autun where he had retired after his late son's marriage. In this rural enclave he had become involved with a calculating housekeeper by whom he fathered several children out of wedlock. She had also been liberally spending his diminishing income on luxuries and extravagant entertainments. If

Jane did not come at once, the old baron declared he would disinherit her children. Despite her dismay, Jane dutifully obeyed, as was expected of a woman of her station.

For the next seven and a half years the widow de Chantal, once the lively, elegant, and undisputed mistress of her own baronial domain, lived in the physically cramped and morally compromised home at Montelon. The unscrupulous housekeeper continued to rule the household without any restraint from the baron. Basically confined to the upper story and back rooms of the dwelling, Jane's role became that of tutor to the extended family's children: her own (Celse-Bénigne, now seven; Marie Aimée, five; Françoise, four; and Charlotte, two); the housekeeper's brood; and a girl, Claudine, who somewhere along the way Christophe had fathered with another woman. (Jane would oversee Claudine's care for years and eventually arrange an advantageous marriage for her.) As she had previously done on her own baronial estates, the young widow also devoted herself to charitable work, providing the poor of the region with the medical care that was expected of a housewife and the legal advice that she had learned from her father. She set up a backdoor soup kitchen that operated in times of famine and want. So the difficult and confining perimeters of Jane Frances Frémyot, Baroness de Chantal's life were drawn for the foreseeable future.

---

In contrast, Francis' world was expanding. In early 1602 he went to Paris with a delegation from Savoy to the French court.

They had to negotiate the thorny issues around the reestablishment of Catholic parishes in the Calvinist valley of Gex. It had recently been ceded to France but remained under the ecclesial jurisdiction of the Diocese of Geneva. While his mission was diplomatic, Francis took time to seek out the luminaries of the Catholic renewal centered in the capital. An illustrious group met at the home of the spiritually gifted Madame Barbe Acarie (1566–1618). In her *salon* Francis came into contact with all the luminaries and leaders of the French spiritual reform.

During those months he was in much demand as a preacher. He preached during Lent at the Louvre and in several Parisian parishes. His meeting with Henry IV, which took place at Fontainebleau where the monarch chose to spend Easter, so charmed the French king that Henry offered to elevate Francis to a French bishopric. Francis declined the offer, desiring to remain in "his poor church of Geneva-Annecy."

September brought the news of Bishop de Granier's death. Grieved at the loss of this man whom he deemed a gentle shepherd, Francis spent the next several months preparing to take up his mentor's mantle. After making a retreat under the direction of the Jesuit Jean Fourier, who had been his spiritual guide at Clermont, Francis de Sales was ordained bishop on December 8, 1602, the feast of the Conception of the Virgin (now known as the Immaculate Conception). It took place at the Church of Saint Maurice at Thorens, the same church in which he had been baptized as an infant. Years later, he would recount to Jane his profound sense of the occasion.

> When I was anointed bishop, God took me to himself and away from my own self and then gave me back to my people,

that is to say, he changed me from being something in my own right to being something that existed only for their sake.³

After ordination as a bishop, Francis' pastoral activities intensified. The Council of Trent's reforming agenda and the continuing inspiration of Charles Borromeo guided his vision. First, he was to be for his priests and religious a model of simplicity and religious devotion. In this vein he had already renounced his own noble titles and inheritance. Now he took as his episcopal residence the ordinary apartments belonging to his friend Antoine Favre that were located directly across from Saint Pierre's, his cathedral in exile. His own rooms were modestly furnished.

Daily routine in the episcopal residence was devout but not rigidly so. Lifelong devotion to the Virgin Mary, solidified years before during his adolescent crisis in Paris, expressed itself in the daily household recitation of the Rosary. The bishop also instituted the diocesan celebration of several Marian feasts that were not obligatory at the time: the Purification, Annunciation, Assumption, and Nativity of Mary were designated as holy days of obligation. The Visitation and the feast of the Conception of Our Lady were considered feasts of devotion. He also instituted the thrice daily, public ringing of bells for the recitation of the Angelus.⁴

Concerned about religious ignorance among his flock, Francis introduced catechesis for children and laid down pedagogical guidelines for lay instructors to teach them. He launched what would become a several-year pilgrimage in order to personally visit each of the parishes of his far-flung diocese.

He traveled on horseback or on foot over the mountainous passes in all but the most impossible of seasons in the alpine environments of Savoy. At all opportunities he preached heart to heart, determined to draw every person he encountered into the beauty and mystery of the love of God.

The religious communities under his pastoral care were prompted to reform. Traditional practices such as simple meals, wearing the religious habit, and praying the divine office in common were reintroduced where they had fallen away. The Augustinian Canons Regular, Benedictines, Poor Clares, and Cistercians under his tutelage were called to more authentically live their particular charisms. During his first year in office, Francis' main emphasis was the administration and spiritual reform of his own diocese. Still, he also traveled to Turin, the capital of Savoy, to pay homage to the Duke. He also traveled to Gex and Belley, two French Calvinist regions assigned by treaty to his episcopal oversight.

CHAPTER SIX

· · · · · · · · · · · · ·

# Their Stories Converge

The year 1604 was to be a momentous one for both the widowed young Baroness de Chantal and the new Bishop of Geneva. For in that year their two divergent paths would cross, and they would begin to form one of the deepest and most creative spiritual friendships recorded in the Christian tradition.

During the previous years, Bénigne Frémyot, busy with his civil and legal work in Dijon, had been unaware of the full extent of his daughter's difficult situation at Montelon. She had chafed, but submitted to the restrictive demands her father-in-law placed on her and to the rigid religious regime her Franciscan guide had imposed. Although it was painful, she was determined to meet the imperious, insulting ways of her father-in-law's mistress with patience and exemplary goodness. In her typically dutiful way, Jane had not wanted to trouble her own father about her situation. She simply bravely soldiered on amid the reality in which she found herself. She would have liked to accept his invitation to return to Dijon for the Lenten sermons of 1603. But in deference to the elderly Guy de Chantal, she made instead the arduous daily early morning ride to the Cathedral of Autun to hear the sermons presented there. Then she urged her horse to get back in time for the baron's midday meal, fasting herself all the while.

When her father's invitation arrived from Dijon the following season, Jane accepted it. Almost everyone in town attended the popular Lenten sermons. In 1604, they were to be given by the much sought-after new Bishop of Geneva, whose reputation as an engaging preacher had attracted the Dijon magistrates. Madame de Chantal and her children arrived in her hometown just after the start of Lent. Friday, March 5, was the first day she attended the sermons. As her family was prominent, she was seated in the front row of the Church of Saint Chapelle, a short walk from her lodgings. When the Savoyard guest preacher stepped into the pulpit to begin his sermon, she recognized him as the figure she had seen years before in her vision near the sawmill at Bourbilly. For his part, Francis noticed the light-brown-haired woman in widow's garb who seemed to follow his words with acute attention. In fact, he too seems to have had a presentiment of her face many years previously. While kneeling in prayer in the chapel of his home at Sales, it had been revealed to him that someday he might found a religious congregation.

As the sermons continued, he inquired of his host, André Frémyot, about the woman who always sat immediately opposite the pulpit and listened so closely to his words. André was proud to reveal that she was his sister. For her part, Jane was pulled strongly by de Sales' presence as well as his mode of speaking heart to heart. Over the next weeks the two had opportunities to cross paths informally: Francis gave occasional talks on spiritual topics to a group of devout women that included Jane, and she saw him at her father's house when he visited. He gleaned from their passing conversations that she had a keen spiritual bent and that she did not desire to marry again, despite the fact that her extended family expected this of her. A charming anecdote from this period of their acquaintance has survived. Observing the fashionable ornaments attached to her widow's clothing, he quipped that if she did not intend to marry again perhaps she should take down the sign. Getting the drift of his humor, Jane promptly removed all the excess lace and tassels from her garments.

She longed to speak privately about her personal struggles to this person whom she sensed was a true man of God. Yet constrained by her vow to exclusive conversations with her guide from Notre Dame d'Etang, Jane hesitated. Finally she asked her brother to arrange a private interview. The two met on Wednesday of Holy Week and she spoke with Francis, admitting that she should not consult him, given her vow. For his part, the bishop was moved by the widow's simplicity, candor, and spiritual ardor. The exclusive vow, he felt, was highly irregular: a penitent should always feel free to speak with any priestly counselor. He even consulted another priest who concurred.

Presumably, at that first interview, she hinted about her insistent desire to give herself wholly to God. Perhaps she also spoke of the recurring and troubling doubts of faith that would plague her throughout her life. In any case, when Francis later overheard that she was planning a pilgrimage with her friends to the Shrine of Saint Claude in the Jura Mountains, he made it known that he had promised his mother that he would accompany her to the same shrine. Perhaps they could meet and continue their spiritual conversation at the sacred mountain site.

Jane later recounted that at the time she was reminded of a dream she had had before they met. She was seated in a carriage and glimpsed a church outside of which a joyous throng was gathered. She longed to join them but a voice cautioned, "You will never find the peace of a child of God unless you enter by the gate of Saint Claude."[1] This was the dream that had prompted her initial desire to visit the pilgrimage site.

Meanwhile, Francis volunteered to write and offer her whatever counsel he could. He left Dijon, accompanied by his brother Louis, on Monday, April 26. At the first stop he penned her a quick note that he sent back by messenger. "I think that God gave me to you; every hour makes me more sure of it, that is all I can say. Commend me to your guardian angel."[2]

Four months later the two did meet at Saint Claude. Jane arrived in the August heat with two childhood friends. Francis traveled with his mother, to whom he had always been devoted, and his youngest sibling, thirteen-year-old Jeanne. In the intervening months Jane, ever earnest, had consulted the rector of the Jesuit college near Dijon and satisfied herself that receiving advice from a new guide was fully within allowable practice.

The lengthy meeting of Francis and Jane at Saint Claude was to prove fortuitous. For her part, Jane seems to have poured out the longings of her heart: her widow's anguish and her confusion about her next step in life. Francis spent most of the following night in prayer. When they met the following day he, obviously fatigued from his night vigil, said he was now clear that the vows she had made were invalid and that he was prepared to formally take on the role of her spiritual guide.

Francis had long given general spiritual advice freely to all who requested it. But a formal relationship of spiritual direction was, in that era, quite serious. They both wrote and signed documents attesting to their respective commitments in the bond they were entering. Several years later, the bishop would describe this relationship in his book *Introduction to the Devout Life*, written for the many laypersons, especially women, who consulted him.

> Are you serious about following the path of devotion? Then look for a good man to guide and lead you: this is essential ... for such a director should be an angel. In other words, when you have found him do not simply place confidence in him or in human wisdom but in God who will bless you and speak to you through this man. God will put into his heart and mouth whatever is for your best. . . . Open your heart to him with fidelity and sincerity, revealing both what is good and bad in you without dissembling. By this means you will be consoled and strengthened in consolation and aided and healed in desolation.[3]

---

In the meantime, consoled by the affirmation and encouragement of her new guide, Madame de Chantal returned to Bourbilly to supervise the wine and corn harvest. Under her director's advice, she was for the foreseeable future to divide her time between Montelon and Dijon, with occasional forays to

Bourbilly. To paraphrase her director's words, she was to agreeably and humbly work toward the salvation of both her father and father-in-law. This meant she would be traveling frequently with her children—then ages eight, seven, six, and three—and constantly managing her estates and households.

During the next several years Jane would have only sporadic face-to-face contacts with Francis, but they would correspond regularly; this was the way he commonly gave direction to those who lived at a distance. Through his attentive direction she began to create for herself the foundation of a deep interiority that would sustain her for a lifetime. Her guide drew up for her a broad and supple rule of life that could facilitate growth into the interior freedom of a child of God. She was to envision her inner landscape in quasi-monastic terms: Monica, the patron saint of widows, was to be her novice-mistress and the Virgin Mary, her abbess. She was to begin the process of being remade in the image and likeness of the Savior whom she loved, to gain the interior freedom to respond to whatever God might have in store for her. And she must make peace with what had already occurred. That meant letting go of her anger at Christophe's hunting companion, an emotional task she had found difficult. Francis counseled her:

> You needn't try to find a particular time or opportunity to seek him out; but if he should come to you himself, I would like you to greet him with a gentle, gracious, and compassionate heart. Doubtless it will be uneasy and agitated and your blood will boil, but what of it?[4]

He was slowly urging her to learn to love beyond her present capacity. Similarly she was to make peace with this period of waiting, to surrender herself to the unfolding will of God, no matter what the future might hold. Her director loved her strong, ardent heart, but cautioned that the present, not merely the imagined future, was where God would most authentically meet her. She was, after all, a widow with family responsibilities.

> This straining eagerness then is a fault of yours; in this is the undefinable thing that is not satisfied in you, a certain lack of resignation. You do resign yourself, but it is with a *but*; for you want this and that, and you struggle to get it. A simple desire is not contrary of resignation, but a panting heart, fluttering wings, an agitated will, and many restless movements—all these undoubtedly add up to lack of resignation. Courage, my dear sister; if our will belongs to God, we ourselves are surely his. You have all that is necessary, but without feeling it; that is no great loss. Do you know what you ought to do? As your wings have not yet grown, try to find pleasure in not flying.[5]

Francis' letters to Jane reveal both the spiritual depth of his direction and his use of arresting images and scriptural allusions to convey what he intended to communicate, in this case the life-transformation in which she was engaged. Jane, who was accomplished in the sewing arts, would have understood his meaning.

> It seems that the Cross is a beautiful distaff of the holy bride of the Song of Songs—the devote Sulamite. The wool from the innocent Lamb that is carefully threaded there: that merit, example, and mystery.
>
> Now, reverently place this distaff at your left hand and spin continually with your spiritual considerations, aspirations, and exercises: in other words, by holy imitation. Spin, I say, and draw all this white and delicate wool into your

heart's spindle. The cloth that you make in this way will cover and save you from shame on the day of your death. It will keep you warm in the winter and, as the wise man says, you will fear neither cold nor snow. This is perhaps what that same wise man was thinking, when, praising this saintly housewife, he said that she sets her hands to the distaff and her fingers grasp the spindle. Because what is this audacious business which the spindle creates if not the mystery of the Passion spun by our imitation.[6]

The exchange of her present, troubled, and stony heart for a heart open to and responsive to God, a heart like that of Jesus, was the goal of her widow's novitiate. Francis was clear that this was the central task of the spiritual life. He was to write eloquently of this transformation in his manual for laypersons, the *Introduction to the Devout Life*.

I have wished above everything else to engrave upon your heart this holy, sacred motto, "Live Jesus!" I am sure that after that your life, which proceeds from the heart as an almond tree from its kernel, will produce all of its actions, which are its fruits, inscribed and engraved with the same word of salvation, and just as this sweet Jesus will live within your heart so he will also live in all your conduct. He will appear in your eyes, on your lips, your hands, and even the hair on your head. You will be able to say, in imitation of Saint Paul, "I live now, not I, but Christ lives in me."[7]

She was, to put it simply, being made anew. A simple regime of prayer was at the center of her daily practice: meditation on the events of Jesus' life as well as participation in the liturgies of the Church, all the while knowing that her main call at this point was to care for her children and her estates and to heed her father and father-in-law. During these years Jane remained firm in her aspirations even as her extended family presented eligible suitors and pressured her to accept their suits. Francis kept her focused on the slow and humble growth taking place within, even as she became infatuated with the sort of imageless and silent practices of prayer she encountered while visiting the Carmelite monastery in Dijon. It would become clear as time progressed that Jane was genuinely drawn to what she called a prayer of simple surrender that did not particularly involve the imagination or intellect. But the teaching coming from the Carmel was to actively suppress any mental images. Francis felt that was not ideal for his directee whose walk at that time was very much an earthy, human one.

―――•◆•―――

Jane's formation program reflected the wider wisdom of her director. Francis firmly believed that all persons, both women and men, no matter their background, occupation, or life situation, were called to a deep devotion and intimacy with God. In his view, the human heart was created precisely for this. Shaped in the image of God's own heart, the human heart was designed to beat in rhythm with the divine heartbeat. But wounded by sin, each heart needed, as it were, to be realigned, healed, and restored to its original state. This was accomplished through prayer and the practice of the virtues of the heart of Jesus who declares, "Come to me, all you that are weary and are carrying heavy burdens, and I will give you rest. Take my yoke upon you, and learn from me; for I am gentle and humble in heart, and you will find rest for your souls" (Mt 11:28–29).[8]

Thus the practice of what Francis called the "little virtues"—relational habits such as humility, gentleness, cordiality, simplicity, patience—constituted a program of formation that anyone, in any state in life could follow. Jane's "rule" was flexible and well suited to accommodate her duties. The formal devotional exercises Francis suggested were the background against which she cultivated a more habitual awareness of the divine presence and a readiness to respond to the needs of those around her.

> The essence of prayer is not to be found in always being on our knees but in keeping our wills closely united to God's in all events. The soul that holds itself ready and open to yield itself obediently on any occasion, and which receives these occasions lovingly as sent by God, can do this even while sweeping the floor.[9]

Amid the constraints and challenges of her present life, the young widow slowly learned to reconcile her persistent longing to "leave the world" and give herself entirely to God and the domestic life before her. Although his relationship with Jane was special in this regard, Francis commended to many of his correspondents this sort of devotion. It was adapted to the specifics of the laywoman's life—where the love of God was nurtured as much as attending to the needs of a sick child or the demands of an elderly in-law. At that time the bishop also corresponded with Madame Chamoisy, née Louise de Châtel, whom he knew from Annecy. She desired to know how she might cultivate a truly Christian life as she accompanied her husband to court, where he worked on behalf of the duke. It was notorious for luxury, loose morals, and fierce competition for power and position.

In his correspondence Francis often sent general spiritual counsel in the form of brief circulars. He gathered the fragments of advice he had offered to Madame Chamoisy and others and compiled them into what would later become his most popular work, the *Introduction to the Devout Life*. He maintained that everyone was called to devotion. To suggest otherwise was tantamount to heresy. The Gospel imperative was meant for all, not simply for priests and religious. But the form of that devotion would be shaped by the particulars of one's state in life. In Jane's case, Francis intuited that her chief challenge would be to patiently await whatever God had in store for her future while graciously resigning herself to her present circumstances.

---

The letters flowed frequently between Jane and her mentor in the year after her visit, but eventually the restless widow felt this was inadequate. With his approval she arranged to meet him in the spring of 1605 at his familial home at Sales where his mother and siblings lived. She traveled by way of Saint Claude and Gex, where one of the bishop's men met her with a short message: "Come joyfully, God is waiting for you. I pray that he may go close beside you forever."[10] From there Jane was escorted across the alpine valleys to Thorens via Geneva and to the castle Sales, where her director waited for her. Jane spent ten memorable days with him, his mother, and Francis' younger siblings in the bustling household. The two walked daily through Madame de Boissy's herb garden, down formal paths, and stopped to rest at the remains of a small pagan temple on a hillock within sight of the main house. Jane shared with Francis the rich jumble of feelings and thoughts that roiled within her. She left feeling more completely surrendered to her situation as a widow, in which she could give herself more completely to God.

Thus Jane continued her labors at Montelon. Especially vivid in later accounts are the reports of her care for her neighbors in need. The sick and lepers came for medical care to the small upstairs dispensary she set up. Those without proper clothing or food found her at the back door in a white apron ready to offer them clean patched garments or a bowl of soup. Her children in tow, she regularly made forays into nearby homes to visit the housebound or prepare the dead for burial.

Like his directee, the bishop's life was shaped by the duties of his present circumstances. This included pastoral visits, catechesis, the formation of his clergy, the reform of religious life, and preaching tours in the region. Amid all this, the bishop found time to collaborate with his dear friend, the jurist Antoine Favre, President of the Council of Geneva. They established a center for science and learning in Annecy, which they named the Florimontane Academy. As a man of prodigious intellectual gifts as well as pastoral acumen, Francis deemed it important to promote the cause of humanist culture. Meetings of scholars were held at Favre's home. The subjects ranged from theology, politics, philosophy, rhetoric, cosmology, and geometry, to languages, music theory, and the arts of navigation. Favre was eventually promoted to the presidency of the Savoy Senate and left Annecy for Chambery. Francis, overwhelmed with episcopal tasks, could not maintain the Academy by himself. In the following years, this Christian humanist vision was to take flesh not only in Francis' own pastoral ministry, but in the visionary venture that would emerge from his growing relationship with Madame de Chantal.

Chapter Seven
. . . . . . . . . . . .

# Spiritual Friendship

Two years after their previous encounter, Jane again met Francis face to face in Savoy, at the lakeside town of Annecy. She had increased in spiritual maturity, becoming accustomed to finding God in the circumstances of life. Still fervent by nature and continuing to sense that she was being called to some further self-donation, Jane had grown in interior freedom. She had a new capacity for flexibility and gentleness. Francis, for his part, was keenly aware of the depths of Jane's capacity for love and her willingness to generously respond to God's way of shaping her. Jane was learning to live with the gentle, humble heart of Jesus.

Part of that preparation had been to admit to an ongoing inner struggle that would last for most of her life. She experienced dryness, sadness, anxiety, and even unspecified doubts about the faith. Francis was not surprised. He knew that darkness and temptation are often part of the process of spiritual purification: God, as it were, creates space within the human heart into which divine love might dwell and replace secondary concerns. Francis taught her to simply direct her gaze to Christ instead of focusing on her difficulties or worrying about them. As he quaintly put it, instead of staying in the room where reason argued, she should leave by the side door of the will.

Their next meeting was planned for the end of May 1607. Francis' mother would again host Jane, but this time it would be in Annecy, his episcopal seat, rather than the family castle. Jane made the long, arduous journey on horseback propelled by anticipation. She was an accomplished rider, and at one point she rode all night through a thunderstorm so as to arrive on time. The mountainous terrain through which she passed was in the first flush of its wildflower blossoming. She saw for the first time the ancient hillside town of Annecy situated on the banks of a shimmering alpine lake. It was also the first time she encountered her mentor on his own ecclesial territory. She saw for herself how highly many others esteemed Francis. She also came to appreciate his affection for the town he referred to as "Cher Nessy" (dear little Annecy). Years later she would recall the impressions he made on those among whom he lived and worked.

> [He] was very approachable and of very easy access to anyone who wanted to talk to him. . . . He received all comers with the same expression of quiet friendliness, and never turned anyone away, whatever his station in life; he always listened with unhurried calmness and for as long as people felt they needed to talk. . . . His whole manner of speaking had great dignity and discretion but was at the same time humble, quiet, and candid; he never posed, was completely unaffected, and lacked any stiffness.[1]

Her observations indicate how others perceived that he lived the spiritual vision of the exchange of the human heart for the heart of Jesus.

> I don't think words can describe the sweetness and graciousness that God had put into his soul. He looked very gentle and meek; there was gentleness in his eyes and voice and movements, and he passed it onto the hearts of others. . . . When he was criticized for being too lenient with bad priests he said: "Isn't it better to convert them to penitence rather than punish them? After all, they haven't done anything to deserve the galleys or the scaffold." And he used to say that he would rather err on the side of leniency than of harshness. and that our Lord has told us to learn of him to be meek and humble of heart.[2]

Francis' pastoral sensitivity and inclusivity was especially noticeable. He was wont to pay particular attention to those whom others might deem insignificant or not sufficiently important to claim a bishop's time.

> . . . he welcomed every sort of person with a gracious and kind face and friendly words, so that even though he was the most serious and even majestic in his bearing, no one was afraid of going up to him and pouring out all their troubles with absolute confidence. And it was unheard of for anyone to come away disappointed and not love him with all honor and respect for his incomparable goodness and charity.
>
> His confessor told me that when he saw poor people in his fore court or gallery as he was leaving the house, he used to go up to them and take their papers so that they should not have to wait so long; and if he had happened to be with important visitors, he would send someone of his own household to see promptly to the business of the poor.[3]

Her observations suggest Francis was not only accessible, but prudent as well.

> He received women in every station of life at his house, he spoke to them, as everyone else, very cordially but without any word or demonstration of familiarity which was in the least unsuitable. Most of them came to discuss matters of conscience; while they were with him he always had the door of the room ajar. And as a rule one of his almoners or else a servant was within sight, and he said that the bishop should always have some cleric with him who could see what he was doing and bear witness if necessary. To sum up, he lived such a watchful, pure, and holy life that his reputation was always that of a most chaste, innocent, and untouched man.[4]

In their letters Francis and Jane had already discussed the question of her—embracing the religious life. In his gentle way Francis had enjoined her to exercise patience while also—honoring her heart's promptings. But now, on June 4, the topic emerged again. During his student years in Paris and Padua, Francis had become aware of a variety of new modes of Christian life emerging from the Catholic reform. Alongside such communities as the Society of Jesus and the Discalced Carmelites of Teresa of Ávila and John of the Cross, other innovative groups had sprung up. These included the Theatines, Barnabites, Ursulines, Piarists, and the Congregation of the Oratory. For some time Francis had seen a need for a community for faith-filled, Godward drawn women whose situations precluded them from entry into these other communities. They might be widows like

Jane, older women, or women of frail constitution or physical disability who would not be eligible for the new congregations with their austere rigors. As deep lovers of God, these women might not be drawn to the older unreformed orders, in which some members were placed there by family politics or societal conventions rather than a true vocation.

When they met, Francis told Jane that he had been considering her longstanding desire to give all to God. Attentive to her capacity to yield to the Spirit, he made several tentative suggestions: the Poor Clares, the Carmelites, or the sisters at the hospital in Beaune. She responded with gracious assent to each suggested possibility. Finally, he revealed the dream he had been nurturing of a modest congregation of women drawn together in the love of God and one another to "Live Jesus!" by having their own hearts exchanged for the heart of the gentle, humble, crucified One.

He envisioned a congregation that would require of its members only simple yearly vows, not binding solemn vows or the complete enclosure of a formal religious order. Physical austerities, much in vogue in reforming circles, would not be called for. Instead of severe fasting or bodily penances, the women of this new group would focus on interior mortification. Those little relational virtues such as humility, gentleness, cordiality, and simplicity, which Francis deemed the virtues of the divine heart, would be the hidden tools of the radical transformation asked of the true lover of God. Prayer would be at the heart of the community. But they would use the short, simplified Office of the Virgin rather than the formal monastic divine office. They would observe a general spirit of solitude and silence, but not have full enclosure and separation from the outside world. Women like Jane, after all, might be called away to attend to family business. And just as Jane had done at Montelon, these women could be expected, as circumstances required, to minister to the spiritual and temporal needs of their immediate neighbors. The community might also offer the option of retreat to married women who felt a need for periodic spiritual refreshment.

Jane was overjoyed to learn of her mentor's dream and affirmed his plan. But such a congregation could not be formed at once. An adequate preparation would take several years. Jane's children were still young. They would need to mature, and their futures had to be carefully arranged. Her father would have to agree to Jane's plan. And Francis would have to attend to the many financial, legal, and ecclesial logistics for such an undertaking.

So Jane returned to her former life buoyed by the prospect of an emerging new future. She traveled back home taking with her Francis' youngest sister, Jeanne, who was to attend school at a convent in Burgundy. Letters flew between the director and directee but as time passed and the distinct outline of the imagined congregation became clearer, their relationship deepened and leveled. Francis had from the outset been keenly aware of Jane's capacity for generous self-gift as well as her deep love of God. He had felt the Spirit moving between them as their respective dreams began to converge. Just seven months after their first meeting he had acknowledged their special bond.

> ... from the first time that you consulted me about your interior life, God granted me a great love for your spirit. When you confessed to me in greater detail, a remarkable bond was forged in my soul that caused me to cherish your soul more

> and more. This made me write to you that God has given me to you, not thinking that it would ever be possible for the affection that I felt in my spirit to be increased—especially by praying to God for you. But now, my dear daughter, a certain new quality has emerged which it seems I cannot describe, only its effect is a great interior sweetness that I have to wish for you a perfect love of God and other spiritual blessings. No, I am not exaggerating the truth in the least, I speak before "my heart's God" and yours. Each affection is different from others. The one I have for you has a certain quality which consoles me infinitely and, if all were known, is extremely profitable to me. Consider this an absolute truth and have no more doubts about it.[5]

That initial bond now deepened. Their two hearts were directed together toward the creation of a future institute, although they had to deal with several logistical issues and obstacles. Francis urged Jane to live graciously in the present; tomorrow was in God's hands. But unexpectedly the future pressed in of its own accord. When she had visited Annecy, Jane had been introduced to several members of Francis' large family. She found herself especially drawn to one of his younger brothers, Bernard. Francis' mother became aware of her fondness and used this as a pretext to put forward an idea she had been considering. Perhaps the two families might be joined through marriage. Bernard could wed Jane's eldest daughter, Marie-Aimée. The bishop was somewhat taken aback and Jane demurred, remaining graciously non-committal. She was aware of Marie-Aimée's youth (she was nine, and eleven was the earliest culturally acceptable age to wed), and the almost certain resistance of the grandfathers to the girl leaving France.

Nevertheless, events conspired to bring up the suggestion again. Back in Burgundy, Jane brought Francis' sister Jeanne to live with her as the school season closed. The child fell ill with an enteric fever and despite Jane's informed and determined ministrations, died in October 1607. Jane was devastated by the loss. Both Francis and his mother grieved deeply but accepted the news with resignation as God's will. Remembering Madame de Boissy's desire to join the two houses, Jane began to feel that a future union between Bernard and Marie-Aimée would be, as it were, an exchange for the sister and daughter the house of Sales had lost. In the context of the culture in which extended family identity was paramount, this was a natural thought. Gradually she also came to see that the marriage might serve as a bridge through which she too could begin her hoped-for new life. A newlywed Marie-Aimée would be too young to set up a household without a responsible older female relative nearby, so it would be appropriate for Jane to move to Savoy.

With Francis and Madame de Boissy's approval, she set about convincing her own father and her irascible father-in-law that it would be a fortunate union. Bénigne Frémyot agreed to the plan, though as yet he knew nothing of Jane's dreams of religious life. She faced opposition from the old Baron de Chantal whose domineering housekeeper had other ideas about whom Marie-Aimée should marry. In the ensuing awkward negotiations Frémyot became aware for the first time of his daughter's straitened circumstances at Montelon. He blamed himself for his blindness to Jane's predicament and overruled the objections raised by Guy de Chantal.

Once again, a journey to Annecy was planned. Francis was preaching the Lenten sermons at home and the bride-to-be needed to be introduced to the extended Sales family. Accompanied by Jane's two eldest daughters and by Charlotte de Brechard, a longtime friend who had recently put herself under Francis' direction, Jane's visit extended through Lent and culminated at Easter. For her the visit was about arranging both for her daughter's and (more privately) her own future. She and Charlotte de Brechard joined the Confraternity of the Holy Cross and, barefoot and draped in penitential garb, spent the entire night of Holy Thursday visiting all the churches of Annecy upon whose altars the Blessed Sacrament was reserved. On Good Friday she knelt privately before the bishop and renewed the vows of chastity and obedience that she had made after being widowed.

When she returned to France she revealed her plans to her father and sought his blessing. That was a great challenge because Bénigne Frémyot was deeply attached to his daughter and grandchildren. He was distressed to think that Jane would consider leaving him and her fatherless children. Jane also told her brother André, because women of this era were legally subject to all their adult male relatives. Her clear narrative of the way she, under Bishop de Sales' wise counsel, had discerned her new life impressed her brother. A decision was delayed until after her daughter's wedding, which took place in October 1609.

Bernard, his father's favorite, was twenty-five years of age, with fair hair and blue-eyes, and was esteemed for his valor and personal charm. He took as his wife the eleven-year-old

Marie-Aimée, a union of differing ages that would be unthinkable now, but that was not considered unusual in the era. (Francis' own mother, who had been promised in marriage at age seven, was her husband's junior by three decades.) Visitors to the elegant two-day celebration at Montelon recalled her as a happy, good looking girl who was tall for her age, even tempered, and intelligent. Like her new husband, she was inclined to piety. As a couple the two were well suited and agreeable to the match but, given the bride's age, it was decided that they would wait and not consummate their union until the following spring when they set up their home.

The extended familial gathering allowed for meetings between the bishop, Jane, and her father and brother. With Francis listening and lending the support of his presence, Jane gave an account of her years' long discernment that had now emerged as a call to enter a new sort of religious community. She had planned carefully for her children as well. Her finances were in perfect order and her late husband's estate was debt free. As to where this new group should be located, André suggested Autun, while Bénigne thought it should be Dijon. Then Francis spoke, outlining the dream he had been nurturing for an innovative community within his own diocese. As for Jane's children, Celse-Bénigne, her eldest, had reached the age when young men were typically sent away to school. His uncle André could watch over him. The young bride would need her mother nearby her new household in Savoy. The younger girls could be brought with their mother to the community. Child boarders were familiar figures in convents of the era.

*Spiritual Friendship*

Meanwhile, until the new community could be formed, Jane would be free to travel and attend to the needs of all her family members. As they had agreed, Bernard would come for his new bride, her mother, her sisters, and her companion Charlotte de Brechard the following spring of 1610 when they would relocate from Burgundy to Savoy. The eighty year old Baron de Chantal was not included in the deliberations, but when he learned of the impending move, burst out in an expression of belated affection for his daughter-in-law.

CHAPTER EIGHT

• • • • • • • • • • • •

# Birth of a Community

With their plans in place, Francis and Jane looked hopefully to the future. But besides organizing the new community, they also needed members. Charlotte de Brechard, Jane's longtime friend, emerged as a likely candidate. A single woman of mature age, Charlotte's childhood as the neglected daughter of a noble widower had led her as an adult to sympathize with the poor and outcast. That was how she had met Jane, who as a recent widow had thrown herself into charitable work. Before this, Charlotte had tried religious life with the Carmelites, but she couldn't endure the order's ascetic regime. Under Francis' direction her desire to enter religious life was channeled anew.

Francis had also met and recruited two other potential members. One was the youthful Jacqueline Favre, daughter of Antoine

Favre, with whom he enjoyed a rich friendship. Jacqueline had known and admired de Sales since childhood. A vivacious, pretty, and headstrong girl, she seemed destined to be a brilliant match for some eligible suitor. The popular teen enjoyed dancing at the elegant soirees held in her social circles, but at a party one evening, she suddenly had a vision of how futile life is when captured by worldly concerns. She vowed that she would dedicate herself to the service of God. Her intentions became clear when her father put forward a potential husband. Putting away her beautiful ball gowns with some regret, she told her father that she wished instead to join the bishop of Geneva in his new foundation.

Charlotte and Jacqueline would become with Jane the first choir sisters, that is, community members whose vows would specify a certain withdrawal from the world and recitation of the daily offices of common liturgical prayer. The Visitation congregation was never intended to be a community with an active apostolate, but it did have a flexible cloister and members could go out as familial circumstances required or need in the surrounding neighborhood might call them forth. Thus they would also need an "out-sister," someone whose primary duty would be to interface with the surrounding population and concern herself primarily with the logistics of the household. During his sojourn in the Chablais, Francis had met Anne Jacqueline Coste. She was a peasant woman who was helping to facilitate the underground movements of Catholics into and out of Geneva and the Protestant dominated region. Francis was struck with the courageous faith of this enterprising, unlettered woman. He invited her to Annecy and then invited her to become the community's out-sister.

The personnel were in place, but soon two untimely deaths spurred the planning forward. Charlotte, Jane's youngest daughter and close to her mother's heart because she was born just before Christophe's death in 1601, succumbed to a virulent fever despite Jane's careful ministrations. The sorrowful letter to Francis revealing this loss crossed in the mail with his own somber news: his beloved mother had suffered a stroke and died. This made it even more imperative that Jane leave France to accompany her newly married child to Savoy. Otherwise there would be no other knowledgeable maternal presence to oversee or aid the young bride.

In April Bernard de Sales traveled to Montelon to fetch his wife Marie-Aimée, as well as Jane and her daughter Françoise and their family friend Charlotte de Brechard. The poor from the region thronged the area outside the residence, lamenting Jane's departure. They would miss the kind baroness who had so graciously cared for their needs. The entourage journeyed to Dijon where Jane spent the Lenten season visiting all the people and places dear to her heart and making final arrangements with her father. On March 19 the entire Frémyot clan gathered in the hall of the home Jane was born in for the formal public leave-taking that was culturally expected of a prominent citizen. Jane said goodbye to each person awaiting her attention. Then she came to her son, Celse-Bénigne, for whom she had made careful arrangements to remain in the care of his uncle and grandfather. The adolescent boy launched a passionate appeal for her to stay. His dramatic words, which seemed to have been scripted in private, caught his mother by surprise. He had agreed to the arrangements which were typical for well-to-do young men of the era

(Francis and his cousins had been sent to Paris with a tutor at much younger ages). Tears welled up in Jane's eyes and when she stepped toward the open street-side door, Celse-Bénigne flung himself down across the threshold crying out, "I'm not strong enough to hold you back, but at least it shall be said that you trampled your own child underfoot."[1] The familial drama was in character, for the boy had always been temperamental and given to dramatic gestures. Jane had no choice but to choke back a sob and step over him. Loudly criticized by two rigidly pious onlookers for her lack of spiritual detachment (as might be expected if one read only the otherworldly lives of the saints popular at the time), she replied simply that after all, she *was* a mother.

The journey to Savoy took a week. The party was lodged with the Favre family since the de Sales household was in mourning for Madame de Boissy. Soon, Jane accompanied Marie-Aimée to Bernard's home in the countryside at Thorens and stayed a month to make sure the staff was appropriately trained. Several of the de Sales extended family lived nearby and they welcomed the youthful bride and her mother. Jane left Françoise in Annecy with Charlotte de Brechard in order to make plans for the fledgling congregation. Unfortunately, the donor who had expressed an interest in joining and had promised a property withdrew at the last minute. But a local Savoyard admirer of de Sales offered a lakeside house that could be easily modified to suit the needs of a religious community. The wine cellar downstairs was outfitted as a chapel and the small orchard behind the house became a cloister garden. The women would furnish their rooms from their own apartments.

Outside of Savoy significant political events were shaping history. France's Henry IV, who had so graciously welcomed Francis to Paris several years previously and had offered him a prelature in the capital, was assassinated in May 1610. Despite his conversion to Catholicism and his reputation as "good king Henry," he had many enemies. His 1589 Edict of Nantes was intended to foster religious tolerance by allowing the Huguenot minority designated civil and religious liberties. But radical Catholic loyalists could not accept his reign. Motivated by what he claimed were visions instructing him, Francois Ravillac, an occasional tutor and zealot, assaulted and stabbed the king as the royal carriage was detained on its way through the Paris streets. Louis XIII, who was just a child, assumed the throne under the regency of his mother Marie de Medici.

In provincial Savoy events were considerably less dramatic from an international perspective: the Savoyard ducal family had aligned itself diplomatically in opposition to the Spanish, a move that would have military repercussions in the near future. But more significant for the little group assembled around the exiled bishop of Geneva was the event that took place on June 10, the feast of the Holy Trinity. Joined by Charlotte de Brechard, Jacqueline Favre, and Anne-Jacqueline Coste, Jane knelt before Bishop de Sales, read aloud the rule of the new congregation that Francis had written, and exclaimed: "This is the place of our delight and rest."

A regular pattern of life was swiftly established at the little Gallery House, as it was called. The group was not meant to be a formal religious order exclusively dedicated to prayer, nor a congregation focused on an apostolic work such as teaching or nursing. Instead, the congregation was intended to be a place for women like Jane: widows, the frail or handicapped, whether youthful or older. It was not a call to intense asceticism but a deep drawing toward and love of God. They were to realize together the transformed vision of a world of intertwined human and divine hearts, the vision that undergirded all Francis de Sales' writings and pastoral ministry. At the center of this enterprise was the imperative to "Live Jesus!" to exchange one's heart for the heart of the crucified One who invited all: "Come to me, all you that are weary and are carrying heavy burdens, and I will give you rest. Take my yoke upon you, and learn from me; for I am gentle and humble in heart, and you will find rest for your souls" (Mt 11:28–29).

Daily life was simple. The shortened Little Hours of Our Lady punctuated the day as the women gathered at the prescribed times in the basement chapel. Other parts of the day were given to meals (two daily), the domestic work needed to run the house, spiritual reading and private prayer, assembly (time for community formation), and obedience (personal spiritual instruction). When two years of novitiate were completed, members might be assigned to go into the neighborhood and minister to the poor or ailing. This was very much an echo of the sort of charitable activity that the widow de Chantal had extended to her neighbors at Montelon. It was a localized active expression of the art of living Jesus, a loving attentiveness and heart-to-heart communication that God intended for human community. Accommodation was also made for outside women who might desire some prayerful respite from family responsibilities to share a short retreat on the premises.

Francis and Jane tended their fledgling congregation with care. Gathered beneath the pear trees behind the Gallery House —a space that became known as the "Conversations Garden"— the bishop often reflected with the sisters. They spoke about the "little virtues" that were the interior habits they were called to cultivate so that each one might realize the Pauline injunction: "It is no longer I who live, but it is Christ who lives in me" (Gal 2:20). Chief among de Sales' favored topics was the virtue of cordiality, which he explores as a form of spiritual friendship.

> . . . You will ask me now: what is meant by cordial friendship? It means that it is a friendship which has its foundation in the heart. As you have asked me, I will explain that cordial love with which the Sisters should love one another. This sort of love is nothing less than that of true and sincere friendship which can only occur between reasonable people. . . . This friendship must be grounded in the heart. . . . We are told by God to love our neighbor . . . but we must love our Sisters with all the expansiveness of our hearts, not simply as we love ourselves, as God commands us, but more than ourselves to observe the rules of Evangelical perfection which ask this of us. Our Lord has said: "Love one another as I have loved you" (see Jn 13:34; 15: 12).[2]

Francis guided the community with subtlety and balance, which gives insight into the phrase "inspired common sense," often used to describe Salesian spirituality.

> . . . This cordial love must be accompanied by two virtues: civility and gracious communication. Civility lends a certain agreeable tone to all the serious transactions and dealings we

have with one another. Gracious conversation allows us to enjoy less serious recreation and encounters with our neighbors. All virtues, as you know, have two contrary vices. Which are the extremes of the virtue. Civility is thus found between too much unrelenting seriousness and too much sentimentality and false flattery. . . . The virtue of gracious conversation requires that you share a holy and moderate joy . . . not boring your neighbor with your melancholy complaints or refusing to join in at the times set aside for recreation. . . . You must continue to hold on to the affection you have for your Sisters as equitably as possible. . . . All must know that they are loved with this cordial heart-felt love equally.[3]

Among the first decisions that the two founders had to make was what to call their community. For a time Francis favored bestowing the name and patronage of Saint Martha upon them: she was in his mind the image of the faithful housewife depicted in Luke, a traditional interpretation that contrasted Martha with her sister, Mary of Bethany, generally seen as the model of the contemplative life. But Jane herself preferred to place the congregation under the protection of the Virgin Mary who had long been her own intimate companion. Growing up motherless, Jane had turned to the Virgin as a maternal presence. Plus Francis had encouraged her in his early direction to make Mary the abbess of the interior monastery in which she was being formed for a life beyond widowhood. She felt her prayers to the Virgin in this regard were answered when Francis showed up one day suggesting that the congregation be named for the mystery of the Visitation. That scriptural story narrates the journey of the pregnant Mary to visit her cousin Elizabeth, who was herself surprised in her old age to be bearing a child. Their congregation would bear the title The Visitation of Holy Mary.

Over the years this Lucan moment unfolded its rich symbolic depth to the fertile imagination of Francis. He would come to see the Visitation as the archetype of the realization of the divinely intended world of intertwined hearts. Two ordinary people, to all observers engaged in the normal activity of caring for one another, in fact are caught up in the most mysterious and salvific of actions. The Savior is with them, carried in the womb. Francis saw this visitation as a recapitulation of the original visit that God made to humankind at the moment of the incarnation. This "kiss" of the incarnation, as he described it, was the divine lover's gesture that must take place over and over again in human interaction. When Mary embraced her older cousin, the child in Elizabeth's womb leapt: he recognized and was animated by the divine lover hidden within. For de Sales, the picture of the Visitation was completed by the presence of the two husbands, Joseph and Zachary, who were also touched and animated by the saving visit of the hidden Christ. Thus the spirit-filled visit gives life and grace wherever it is realized. In a 1611 letter to Jane, the bishop waxed eloquent about the mystery for which their community was named.

> I will leave you to imagine, my dear daughter, what a sweet odor this fleur-de-lis [Mary] spread about Zachary's house the three months she spent there. Imagine how they were busy about the place and how she, with few but fine words, poured out precious balm and honey on them with her sacred lips. What could she do but overflow with what she was filled with. She was full of Jesus.

> ... Oh, dear Jesus, be the child of our wombs, so that we
> will not breathe or feel anything but you.[4]

This hidden world of the Visitation, tucked away in the mountains of Savoy, was for the Genevan bishop and the widow de Chantal a microcosm of the transformed world God longed for, which had been revealed through the gentle, humble heart of the crucified One. On one level, they had established a unique religious institute. It was quite different from both the lax unreformed orders that admitted many who had no genuine vocation, and the formal rigorous Catholic orders founded or reformed in the past century. On another level, they had created a small, localized expression of the transformed Christian society that Francis envisioned, both through his own prayer and the crucible of his pastoral experience. The Visitation was his answer to the violence of the conflicts of his era among Christians and his response to zealous and divisive infighting of Catholic militancy.[5]

During those initial years of the Visitation of Holy Mary's existence, the friendship between Francis and Jane blossomed. From the outset each sensed that their relationship was providential. Their shared admiration grew as the years passed between Jane's early formation and the emergence of their shared dream. Now that they were working together for the new foundation, the deep and transformative affection of spiritual friendship came to maturity.

Francis and Jane knew that spiritual friendship was a pathway to intimacy with God. The ancient Greeks classified love into four types. Although they were intertwined, these types of love were seen as having different origins and ends. Medieval thinkers Christianized this view. All love, no matter if it was expressed as *agape* (universal), *eros* (between lover and beloved), *storge* (familial), or *philia* (friendship), had its beginning and proper end in God, who is Love Itself. *Philia* was the love characterized by mutuality and equality. Tradition spoke of a true friend as a second self. One could share confidences with such a friend, who could be trusted to call forth one's best self with honesty and discretion.

Francis had written in the *Introduction to the Devout Life* of the importance of discerning the quality of one's friendships, which could sometimes be based on self-serving or shallow motives. Yet he insisted that true spiritual friends—the intimate company and communication of those who shared a love of God and a love of one another in God—were utterly necessary for those who wished to live a devout life. Deeming the cultivation of such friendships a virtue, he practiced it himself. Antoine Favre, with whom he founded the Florimontane Academy, was a lifelong soul companion, as were others. But it was with Jane de Chantal that he shared one of the deepest and most fruitful friendships of his life. Early on he had written to her expressing the way in which this modality of love was drawing them together.

> I have never intended for there to be any connection between us that carries any obligation except that of love and true Christian friendship, whose binding force Saint Paul calls "the bond of perfection." And truly that is just, for it is indissoluble and will not slacken. All other bonds are temporary, even that of vows of obedience, which are broken by death and other occurrences. But the bond of love grows in time and takes on new power by enduring. It is exempt from the

severance of death whose scythe cuts down everything except love: "Love is a strong as death and more powerful than hell," Solomon says. . . . This is our bond, these are chains, which, the more they restrain and press upon us, the more they give us ease and liberty. Their power is only sweetness, their force only gentleness, nothing is so pliable, nothing so solid as they are. Therefore, consider me intimately linked with you and do not be anxious to understand more about it except that this bond is not contrary to any other bond, whether it be a vow or of marriage.[6]

The chains of this bond of perfection, which elsewhere he describes as chains of gold in contrast with chains of iron, bound the two friends more closely together as they labored to shape the vision of the congregation and ensure that it would be realized in practice.[7] The two met frequently in the Gallery House during these first years. But the bishop was also busy with his myriad diocesan obligations. He traveled frequently as well. Twice in 1611 he visited the region of Gex in an attempt to restore Catholic worship in that former Protestant region. The Gex affair earned him the disapproval of the courts of both France and Savoy. In 1612 he went to Chambery to deliver the Lenten sermon series. Turin, the glittering capital of Savoy, and Milan were on his agenda in 1613. This involved, in part, the installation of the Barnabite order in Annecy and also allowed Francis to visit the tomb of Charles Borromeo. Thus Francis and Jane communicated often by letter.

With a few exceptions, our knowledge of this mutual correspondence is one sided. It was customary in that era to keep letters, and Jane collected Francis' missives faithfully. Francis did the same, but after his death his collected papers were entrusted to her. For some unknown reason, she chose to burn all of her own letters that he had amassed and annotated. We don't know if it was out of humility, fear that they were too confidential, or concern for the order's reputation. Nevertheless, his side of the exchange provides something of a view into the nature of their bond.

> O God, my dearest daughter, how tenderly and ardently I feel the sacred bond and the good of our holy unity! I preached a sermon full of flames this morning I was so aware of it. I must tell you how much I wish for blessings for you! You cannot imagine how I was impelled at the altar to commend you to our Lord forever and ever.[8]

> . . . I protest, but I protest with my whole heart, which is more yours than mine, that I feel keenly the privation of not having seen you today. Tomorrow with God's help I will come and speak with you a good hour before the sermon and we will speak of our challenge, which my dear daughter, you will find very agreeable and worthy of our heart, which is so indivisible.[9]

The two spoke of their hearts as one, united in the love of God and each other:

> I am impatient, my dear daughter, that this heart that God has given us is uniquely and inseparably given to and linked to its God by this holy unifying love, which is stronger than death and all else. My God, my dearest daughter, let us fill our heart with courage and from now on let us perform miracles for our heart's advancement in this celestial love. And let us note that Our Lord never gives you intense inspirations for the absolute perfection of your heart unless he gives me the same will. For he wishes us to know that it is but one

> single aspiration for the same thing by the same heart and that, through unity of aspiration, the Sovereign Providence wants us to be one single soul in pursuit of the same goal for the purity of our perfection.[10]

The warmth expressed in the bishop's letters was typical for the period. Although some expressions might seem flowery or excessive to the modern ear, it was part of the art of writing letters. Honorific salutations and declarations of high regard and affection were common. Yet those that flowed between the two founders were especially warm. They reflect the extent to which Jane and Francis knew their bond was one of love, a chaste affection focused on discerning and doing God's will. This did not halt all outside comment. In fact, some detractors criticized Francis for spending so much time with women. In part this was viewed as potentially suspect behavior. But those who believed that episcopal ministry should be directed toward persons of social importance, influence, and (presumed) superior capacity, thought spending time with the opposite sex was a waste of time. But this did not deter Francis. Although he was a firm advocate for women and clear that they were capable of heroic sanctity, he was also a man of his time. Expanding on Saint Paul's dictum that God works through weakness, he held that God often operates through the lowly, the underestimated, and the "weaker" sex.[11]

Gradually the relationship between the two friends shifted even more. While Francis remained Jane's guide and confessor, he observed her rapid spiritual maturation and came to regard her as his equal. In fact, scholars have suggested that much of his knowledge about advanced states of prayer, about which he wrote so compellingly in his *Treatise on the Love of God,* was gained from his intimacy with Jane and the early daughters of the Visitation.

———•◆•———

Their little community grew quickly. Entrants came from varied walks of life but were culled primarily from the nobility or cultured middle classes. They were mostly young women such as fun loving Claude de la Roche, a childhood companion of Jacqueline Favre's; the capable Peronne-Marie de Chastel, daughter of a captain in the Duke of Savoy's army; and the mystically inclined Marie-Aimée de Blonay, who had known Francis de Sales from her earliest years. By the end of 1610 the Gallery House had attracted a dozen members.

The original three founding sisters—Jane, Charlotte, and Jacqueline—made their formal oblation on June 6, 1611. They took simple vows, not solemn, in canonical terms. Instead of taking perpetual vows, they renewed their vows each year, which better fit their form of life. Together with Francis, the sisters chose a black muslin fabric for the modest veil they would wear as a sign of their commitment. They designed a silver reliquary cross modeled on the one that Francis wore. It bore images of flames, a cross, a heart, and the letters M and A, a possible initial for Mary or a reference to *mons amor,* the mount of lovers, de Sales' name for Mount Calvary.

His theological vision and formative conversations imbued the institute with his distinctive charism. But it was Jane de Chantal, foundress and first superior, whose administrative skills and constant guiding hand ensured that its characteristic spirit would continue to be realized. The details of everyday life were gradually enshrined in a Custom Book. Additionally, Mother de Chantal was responsible for the ongoing guidance of each of the young women who entered or, as the community grew, for the training and oversight of those responsible for each Visitandine's development. In this task Jane's experience as mother of several very different, biological children came into play. Her approach to formation was instinctively and deeply maternal: she had a keen sense of developmental stages. A young girl flush with adolescent enthusiasm and energy must be led gently, her immaturity overlooked in inessential matters. She sought to inculcate this sensitivity into those sisters who would aid her in formation.

> I exhort you, my dearest daughter, to encourage them [the novices] to advance in their love of their heavenly spouse as much as you can, but do it with a spirit of gentleness, patience, and charity, which will in turn help you shoulder all their little weaknesses—their negligence, tardiness, and failings—without ever being surprised so that their perfect confidence in you might never be disturbed.[12]

A more mature sister must be challenged, again with gentle insistence, to grow in self-control and self-sacrifice, as the following letter makes clearer. Jane wrote it to a spiritually mature woman, a superior, who wished to display humility by becoming a domestic sister.

> My dearest daughter, it would be out of the question for me to flatter you or treat you too delicately since you place so much trust in me and allow me to speak freely. I think Our Lord has given you a spirit that can overcome its strong

natural inclinations, as worthy as these may seem to be. To move beyond them is the greatest sacrifice you can make to the Lord.

As for that old hankering of yours to be a domestic sister, take my word for it, our blessed father's advice, to "ask for nothing and refuse nothing" is far superior to this desire of yours or any other self-chosen practice of humility. I admit that God surely wants you to be most humble, but in the way he chooses, and not according to your fancy.[13]

Jane was similarly sensitive to the foibles and gifts of differing personalities. Her goal was always to win hearts, to capture the love and loyalty of her daughters in religion even while she led them up the steep pathways of the mountain of crucified love. In this way they would eagerly follow her lead as she taught them the arts of living Jesus. As hidden as it was in the obscurity of alpine Savoy, the Visitation was to be a living sign to the world of the divine relational mystery of love that its name implied. Always her letters to her spiritual daughters stressed the ways this spirit might be realized.

> I beg you, my dear sister, govern your community with a great expansiveness of heart; give the sisters a holy liberty of spirit and banish from your mind and theirs a servile spirit of constraint. If a sister seems to lack confidence in you, don't, for that reason, show her the least coldness, but gain her trust through love and kindness. . . . The more solicitous, open, and supportive you are with them, the more you will win their hearts. This is the best way of helping them advance toward the perfection of their vocation.[14]

CHAPTER NINE
. . . . . . . . . . . .

# Conflict and Growth

The Visitation of Holy Mary was animated by the reforming spirit that swept through the Catholic world during the early seventeenth century. The spiritual luminaries that Francis had met in 1602 at the Paris salon of Madame Barbe Acarie were now sowing fresh seeds on the French ecclesial and social landscape. After her husband's death, Barbe Acarie and several of her daughters joined the Teresan Reformed Carmel that she and Pierre de Bérulle had imported into France from Spain. Bérulle brought to fruition his dream of revitalizing the French clergy when he established the French Oratory dedicated to the spiritual nurture of the diocesan priesthood. From the fertile soil of the Oratory other branches of the French spiritual renewal sprouted. Vincent de Paul founded the Congregation of the Mission to serve the poor and invigorate faith through preaching domestic missions. With Louise de Marillac, de Paul founded the Daughters of Charity to serve the urban poor. Jean-Jacques Olier and Jean Eudes created seminaries to educate and form priestly shepherds who could bring their flocks to a fully realized faith.

Soon the Visitation and its founders began to capture the imagination of others beyond the borders of Savoy. Several pious women of the wealthy mercantile city of Lyon in southeast France were taken with the notion of founding a congregation like the Visitation nearer to home. After several failed attempts at community, they turned to Annecy for help. The Visitation was a diocesan foundation under the ecclesial oversight of the bishop. Other religious groups of the Catholic reform such as the Jesuits, were structured to answer directly to the papacy. Older monastic orders like the Benedictines had their own organization that transcended diocesan boundaries. But the Visitation was a canonically simple congregation. If it were established in Lyon, the presiding bishop, Denis de Marquemont, would be obliged to take on its oversight.

De Marquemont admired Francis but had firm ideas about what he thought an appropriate French religious group should be. He insisted on following the instructions from the Council of Trent that required enclosure for women's communities. Nor could he imagine influential French families sending their daughters with their substantial dowries to a religious congregation whose members renewed their vows yearly, not in perpetuity. In 1615, Francis visited Lyon to persuade his influential colleague to accept his vision of the Visitation with its simple yet flexible organization. Following the visit the two exchanged a lively correspondence, each arguing his position. Ultimately, Francis had to decide either to retain the foundation only as a local congregation, or to introduce changes and allow it to grow. Weighing the options, he chose the latter. The community's inner spirit would not be altered; they would still recite the Little Office of Our Lady and practice mainly interior asceticism. But they would be reconstituted as a religious order observing enclosure and formal vows. The impromptu visits to neighbors would be curtailed.

Throughout her active life, Jane had always been drawn to seclusion. So she admitted that the decision was in keeping with her own inner promptings. But it would take three years of correspondence and administrative activity before the community could be formed. Jane traveled to Lyon to begin the process of forming a new community in the spirit of the Visitation. She would part with Jacqueline Favre, who became the superior of the order's second monastery.

Francis' intuition that the wider Church was eager for such an innovation in religious life seems to have been accurate. The Annecy community soon outgrew the little Gallery House. A larger structure, designed specifically for their life with a formal church, enclosed walls, and blocks of cells, was built down the hill close to the town walls. The move was completed by 1615. The call for monasteries increased from cities all over France: Moulins, Grenoble, Bourges, Dijon, and eventually Paris itself. By the end of Jane's life, eighty-two Visitations of Holy Mary had been established. Most of their beginnings were presided over by Jane or one of the early entrants in Annecy.

While Mother de Chantal was busy in giving life and form to this new communal exercise in living Jesus, both in Annecy and throughout the continent, Francis' second literary creation was coming to public attention. His *Introduction to the Devout Life* had been a smashing success since its first edition in 1609, so much so that pirated copies came on the market. The definitive version appeared in 1610. Francis was pleased by the popularity of the slim manual that encouraged devotion among the laity.

He also desired to make available his more foundational vision of the world of intertwined human and divine hearts. He planned to pen a work on love tentatively titled *The Book of Holy Charity*. It would be an exposition on the entire spiritual life, both in theory and practice, directed toward any heart anxious to grow in love of God. It would be a magisterial treatment of the "history of the birth, growth, and diminishment of the workings, qualities, advantages, and excellence of divine love."[1] The resulting manuscript was published in 1616 as *Treatise on the Love of God,* a work of astounding erudition. Its language is typically straightforward, direct, affective, and rich with images. At root it is a story of a passionate, loving God who created humankind in the divine image and likeness and with the innate desire to return love to God. The *Treatise* sought to weave together the contemporary emerging language of abstract mysticism into the language of Scripture and theology. In this fabric, Francis threaded the warp of personal experience through the woof of the historic tradition of the Church.

The book explores the means by which love of God might be enhanced or obstructed, especially through prayer, ranging through various forms of meditation and contemplation. It also treats of discernment of the divine will in a distinctively Salesian way. Considering God's ultimate will, unknowable from a human point of view, Francis posits that there are two modalities through which that will might be partially known: the "signified" or "declared" will of God, and the "will of God's good pleasure" or God's "permissive will." A person can grasp the first of these through prayer and a well-formed conscience. Scripture, Church teaching, and wise mentors can help in making a wise decision, aligning one's personal actions in accordance with the signified will. The second, God's permissive will, is understood through the events of a person's life, especially circumstances outside human control. The task then is to align oneself graciously, trusting that God's gracious Providence is at work. Francis teaches the art of living *between* these two wills, exercising vigorous human effort when called for, and gracefully surrendering that effort when necessary.

Commentators have noticed that the central chapters of the *Treatise* on mystical prayer owe a debt to the witness of Jane and her first companions. Prayer was at the heart of the Visitation and, as Mother de Chantal would later write, most Visitandines seemed drawn gradually into a simple, wordless, contemplative gaze upon their beloved. She termed this the prayer of simple surrender. The bishop's attentive direction of the institute influenced his descriptions of deepening degrees of divine-human intimacy. Jane's own prayer experience would follow the classic kenotic pattern of Christian discipleship: dying to self in order to rise in Christ. The *Treatise* closes with the insight that "Calvary is the mount of lovers. All love which does not spring from the Savior's passion is a perilous plaything.... In our Lord's passion, love and death blend so inextricably that no heart can contain one without the other."[2]

Book II of the *Treatise* deals with this paradox of union with the Crucified One as the height of mystical encounter. Throughout her life Jane was privy not only to the delights of divine love, but to the desolations common in a deeply plumbed interior life. In a letter Francis wrote in 1612, he counsels her to accept these privations, for they signal the process of self-emptying if one is to live with the Savior's heart. The letter directly addresses the theme that the bishop would later explore in detail in this part of the *Treatise*.

> It is the height of holy resignation to be content with naked, dry, and insensible acts carried out by the superior will alone . . . you have expressed your suffering well to me and there is nothing to do to remedy it but what you are doing: affirming to our Lord, sometimes aloud and sometimes in song, that you even will to eat as the dead do, without taste, feeling, or knowledge. In the end the Savior wants us to be his so perfectly that nothing else remains for us, and to abandon ourselves entirely to the mercy of his Providence without reservation.[3]

Mother de Chantal understood, at least in faith, that the path by which she was called was a part of the landscape of love that led her closer to her divine lover. In 1614, she wrote to her director suggesting such:

> I am overwhelmed with things to do but I do believe that everything will be all right. I have a great desire to fulfill God's will. That is why I ask you again to let me know what I should do to realize this. I have impulses I cannot describe and a joy which says to my soul that this great God is leading

me and making me capable of his love even while I am aware of my soul's incapacity. Pray to him that he will give me the strength to do whatever is required.[4]

This prayer would be answered two years later in a manner Jane might not have expected.

---

It was customary for sisters to take personal time for an annual retreat away from the community in order to refresh themselves and delve deeper into the intimacy with God at the core of their vocation. Mother de Chantal had chosen the traditional theme of detachment for her prayerful consideration. Perfect love of God, while intrinsically linked to love of neighbor in the Salesian vision, also mirrors divine love imaged in the sacrifice of Christ on the Cross.

In May, Jane took time to reconsider her vows and reflect on the extent to which she had realized the unconditional surrender to her divine lover, which her heart desired. Ironically, as she entered her retreat, her friend Francis fell gravely ill. She found herself preoccupied and unable to pray. From her solitude she wrote to him and he, sensing that some crucial interior shift was taking place, gently guided her by letter. At first, her letters had been filled with sentiments of concern: she wondered if she should leave retreat. Then they changed tone as she recognized that the excessive worry about Francis was an obstacle to being attentive to God. Likening himself to a midwife encouraging the weaning of a child, her director gradually began to aid his friend in the detachment for which she had prayed.

> You must not take any kind of wet nurse, but you must leave the one who nonetheless still remains and becomes like a poor little pitiful creature completely naked before the throne of Divine Mercy, without ever asking for any act or feeling whatsoever for this creature. At the same time, you must become indifferent to everything that it pleases God to give you without considering if it is I who serve as your nurse. Otherwise, if you took a nurse to your own liking you would not be going out of yourself but you would still have your own way, which is, however, what you wish to avoid at all costs.[5]

Jane's response was to be both overjoyed and desolate. On one level she still clung to the habits of her heart. But on a deep, interior level she began to know herself as free, as unclothed as a newborn, dependent entirely on the sheltering embrace of a nurturing God. She wrote expressively to her friend and spiritual father, Francis:

> My God, my true father, how deep has the razor cut? Can I remain in this feeling long? At least our good God, if he so pleases, will hold me firm in my resolutions as I wish. Ah, how your words have given my soul strength. How it consoled and touched me when you wrote, "What blessings and consolations my soul has received to see you utterly naked before God." Oh, may Jesus grant you to continue to be consoled by this and me to have this happiness.
>
> Alas, my only father, I have been reminded today of that one time when you ordered me to denude myself. I replied, "I don't know what is left" and you said to me, "Haven't I told you my daughter, that I will strip you of everything?" Oh God, how easy it is to leave what is outside ourselves. But to leave one's skin, one's flesh, one's bones, and penetrate into

the deepest part of the marrow, which is, it seems to me, what we have done, is a great, difficult, and impossible thing to do save for the grace of God. To him alone then glory is due and may it be given forever.[6]

This extraordinary exchange of 1616 marked the beginning of a new phase in the spiritual friendship that the two shared. To all outward observations they continued as before: both busily occupied with the future of the order, Francis also with the myriad demands of his office. But interiorly something had shifted. The passion that initially fueled their relationship, which increased as they shared the labors of the new family they created, now entered profoundly into the Passion of Christ itself. Self-gift. Abandonment. Surrender to God alone. The mother superior never revealed her inner desolations nor the trajectory of her deepening surrender to the outside world. She was regarded with great esteem and displayed the gentle, cordial spirit of the Visitation to all who came her way. But more visible sorrows that could not be hidden lay in store for her during these years.

Chapter Ten
. . . . . . . . . . . . .

# Trials

Despite her entry into a vowed life, Madame de Chantal had never abandoned her children, and she remained responsible for arranging their adult futures. Francis had supported her in this. The scene that her eldest, Celse-Bénigne, had staged when his mother left Dijon indicated the boy's temperament. At fifteen, her strong-willed son had left school to live the glamorous life of a Parisian nobleman. Given to gambling and carousing, he tried his mother's patience at a distance. Francis sought to allay Jane's anxieties in his calm, protective way, and also to correspond and meet with Celse-Bénigne as a wise, steadying presence in his life.

The bishop also took a quasi-paternal interest in Françoise who, unlike her docile, older married sister, was fiery and willful. One recorded incident sheds light on her relationship with the gentle bishop and his guidance. He happened to run into her one day strolling down the streets of Annecy while her mother was away on community business. He noticed her fashionable dress replete with ribbons, and bows, and a plunging neckline. The bishop greeted the girl pleasantly, exchanged a few good-humored remarks, and then produced from the folds of his garment a few pins with which he discreetly rearranged her garment.

By 1617, neither Celse-Bénigne nor Françoise was married. As was her duty, Jane tried for the next several years to rectify this situation. Marie-Aimée was happily wed, but also a cause for grievous concern. Although the young baroness had been pregnant several times, she had miscarried and her health suffered. The girl was made even more vulnerable in May when she learned that her husband, Bernard, on campaign with the army of the Duke, had succumbed to an epidemic raging through the soldiers' camp. The nineteen-year-old girl bore the sad news bravely. But soon she discovered that she was pregnant again. Finding her own estate too lonely without her cherished Bernard, she decided to lodge with her mother in the convent in Annecy. Well before term, in the middle of a September night, Marie-Aimée went into labor and gave birth to a tiny premature boy. Jane was wakened and hurried to her side just in time to baptize the infant who died immediately. As the young mother sensed she was on the cusp of dying as well, she requested to be clothed in the Visitation habit. Bearing her grief bravely, Jane had the bishop and her other daughter, Françoise, quickly summoned. As Marie-Aimée in these last days had expressed a desire to join the community, a ceremony of profession was performed and last rites given for the young woman whose spirit Jane and Francis had once agreed was most in keeping with their own.

Marie-Aimée died in her mother's arms at midnight the next day.

Jane felt profound grief at the deaths of her daughter, son-in-law, and infant grandchild. But the work of the community she and Francis had founded demanded attention. In 1618, the Visitation of Holy Mary in Annecy received canonical approval from Rome. It was established as a formal cloistered religious order with permanent vows under the auspices of the Bishop of Geneva, Monseigneur de Sales. The bishops responsible for Visitations in other locations followed suit. For the next five years Jane, the mother superior, was constantly on the road overseeing new foundations. Her letters to the freshly installed superiors of these various houses again show her gifts as a spiritual guide. She often found herself having to gently, if firmly, remonstrate against the harshness and overzealous impulses of some of her sisters in religion, who were charged with formation of their communities.

> In the name of our divine Savior, I beg you and urge you to govern according to his spirit and that of our vocation, which is a humble, gentle spirit, supportive and considerate of all. In order to govern in this manner, my dear, you must not act according to the strength of your natural spirit, nor according to your inclinations which lean in the direction of austerity. What we are asking you, my daughter, and without further delay, please, is to be most gentle in thought, word, and action, and to treat your own body and those of your sisters in a more kindly manner than you are in the habit of doing.

> What good does it do to put bread on the table for someone who doesn't have teeth that can chew or a stomach that can digest it? So, without stalling any longer, let me emphasize once again that we do not want to hear any more talk of your gruffness and severity with the sisters and yourself.[1]

As the order grew, the establishment of each new house brought unique challenges. The Lyon monastery had accepted as an entrant one Madame de Gouffiers, a disgruntled transfer from the order of the Paraclete. Entranced by the stories circulating about the Visitation co-founders, at first she seemed like the ideal entrant. But this enthusiast, on a leave from the Lyon community in order to disaffiliate herself from the Paraclete, took it upon herself to travel to Moulins. There, without anyone's knowledge or permission, she interested the bishop and a group of pious women in setting up a Visitation. Jane and Francis learned of this unauthorized and audacious effort after the bishop of Moulins had given his approval. They sent Charlotte de Brechard to oversee the foundation and to ensure that the true spirit of the order was inculcated. But Madame de Gouffiers was offended that Jane herself did not come, so she left and was next heard of attempting a similar self-appointed foundation in Paris. Unresponsive to the founders' pleas that she settle down as a dutiful daughter of the Visitation, she lost interest in the entire enterprise and moved on.

The wealthy, young widow Madame de Tetre was another challenge for the Moulins community. After the death of her husband, she had scandalized her family with an affair and the birth of a child outside of wedlock. Her family was determined that she withdraw from society and enter a convent. While the Visitation generally did not admit women without a true vocation, her family pressed the issue and Madame de Tertre did seem at first to have a calling. But it turned out that she did not. She had a separate house erected for herself on convent grounds. (Although this was a common practice of rich patronesses in unreformed monasteries at the time, it was not done in the Visitation.) She dressed fashionably and lavishly entertained whatever visitors she wished. This went on despite reprimands from her superiors and the founders. When Charlotte de Brechard's term as superior was over and she was transferred to Nevers, Madame de Tetre threw a fit. With her vast wealth she tried to become a patroness at the Nevers Visitation so that she could have privileges there as well as at Moulins. The orders' public persona was compromised as the two affected bishops came into conflict over which diocese should receive the handsome sum that the wealthy widow's patronage supplied. After many years of this behavior, Madame de Tetre had a disconcerting dream that prompted a genuine conversion. She tore up the documents that guaranteed her special privileges as patroness of the community and entered the Visitation novitiate in order to adopt the life of a true Visitation sister. She died less than two years later.

Perhaps the most harrowing foundation Jane was called upon to execute was in Paris. Despite its glowing reputation in other regions, in the sophisticated capital of France the new order appeared to many as a provincial upstart. This snobbery masked an underlying fear that once Parisians had met Mother de Chantal, postulants would flock to her and more established orders would cease to attract entrants and their dowries. When Francis was in Paris on diplomatic business, he had gone ahead and prepared the ground for what he considered an essential foundation, getting permission from the local ordinary and scouting locations.

His co-founder was at the time busy forming a fledgling community in Bourges, the city where Jane's brother, André, was the archbishop. André was always very attached to family and he assumed that his sister would soon become the permanent superior of his town's monastery. (He thought this even though the constitutions required that superiors not be elected for more than two successive terms of three years.) When it became clear to him that after the six months she had been given to attend to the requisite business, Jane intended to move to the capital, her brother balked. André went so far as to declare that he would forbid her any transportation to leave the city. She simply replied that then she and her entourage would walk the seventy miles to Paris. Then he acquiesced and sent his splendid episcopal carriage for his sister's journey.

Although Jane and her little group arrived in Paris in splendor, they had few resources. Dowries from postulants would be required. Few postulants presented themselves and the sisters endured several years of extreme hardship. A first temporary dwelling was located between a noisy tavern and a gambling den. Most of the community fell ill due to poor sanitation. They had scant money for even a daily ration of bread. Even when they relocated to a more suitable location and began to receive postulants, a plague broke out in the capital and most of the population fled to the countryside. As the plague subsided, winter set in, but the community lacked enough fuel and blankets to keep warm at night. Nevertheless, the situation gradually improved. A better house was purchased in a residential quarter on the rue Saint Antoine, which was near the city limits. The surrounding forests in that area provided a modicum of pastoral calm.

---

Even with the burdens of leadership required by the Paris venture, Jane's own children continued to occupy her thoughts. Celse-Bénigne, as high-strung as always, got embroiled in a quarrel with another hot-headed youth and agreed to serve as second in a duel (an illegal practice under both state and Church law). He was charged but escaped capture by fleeing the city. His likeness was hung in effigy in a public square. Jane was concerned for her son, though his actions certainly complicated her efforts to establish the legitimacy of her order in the public eye of watchful Paris. Eventually she arranged a judicious marriage for her son with the de Coulanges family. By 1619, he settled down and wrote to his mother that even if she had never left the world, she could not have provided better for him than she did.

Jane's daughter, Françoise, had a temperament similar to Celse-Bénigne's, and also caused her mother to worry. With a love of luxury and a flirtatious nature, Françoise had rejected a string of suitors. Finally, much to Jane's relief, Françoise agreed to a match with the wealthy Burgundian Count Toulonjon, a man her senior who was very much in love with her. They married in 1620 with a lavish wedding (though Jane tried unsuccessfully to gently reign in some of the extravagance).

The foundress remained in Paris three years, then returned to Dijon. During this time Francis was often in the capital when he was not on the road carrying out his new responsibility as almoner for Victor-Amedée, Prince of Piedmont and heir to the Savoyard realms, who was soon to be wed to Princess Christine of France. Royal marriages were highly sensitive diplomatic liaisons as much as personal covenants, and Francis would spend enormous energy attending to the interests of his duke as the wedding approached.

During these years he also entered a pastoral relationship with Angelique Arnauld, the youthful abbess of the Cistercian convent of Port Royal. She would become known to succeeding generations as one of the figures associated with the crisis of Jansenism that came to roil the Catholic Church. Angelique's family had given her over to religious life as a child, which was customary in wealthy families with political and monetary investments in ecclesial offices. She became entranced by stories of Francis and entertained the thought that she might seek reassignment to the Visitation. The two met several times and a cordial correspondence continued the conversation. In the end, Francis, with Jane's concurrence, felt the abbess should stay and flourish where she had been planted.

Although Francis passed through Paris during these years, the work that he and Jane had to do left scant time for them to meet or speak. Periodically Jane's longing to share her inner life with her friend appeared in the letters they exchanged. Otherwise, their missives mainly concerned the business of the order. She voices her desire in a note from 1621:

> When I allow my heart to feel the incomparable joy of kneeling at your feet again as you give me your blessing, and I see this happening in my mind's eye, then I am suddenly overcome with sadness and the tears start, for I know I shall weep when, in God's mercy, I see you again. But I turn quickly away from the thought and don't allow myself to dwell on it. It is impossible for me to long for a meeting of set purpose; I leave everything that concerns me entirely to God and to you.[2]

Francis' replies reflect a practical wisdom tinged with regret. This note from 1622 followed an appeal delivered by the Paris community to Annecy and Francis that Jane remain with them as superior even though her term was up and she privately wished to return to Savoy. In it he evokes his beloved mountainous Savoy and contrasts it with the teeming urban capital of France.

> Oh if only God had arranged things so that we need never part company, how delightful that would be! But just think how this would work out in practice: our mountains would spoil Paris and would block up the Seine, and Paris would starve our valleys if it were here in our mountain land. One day, or rather, in eternity which is our goal, we shall always be present to one another; that is, if we live in this place of passage according to God's will.[3]

The bishop's poignant words were to be prophetic, for the two friends were destined to see each other face to face again only twice more.

Chapter Eleven
• • • • • • • • • • • •

# Ending and Beginning Anew

The year 1622 continued to be crammed with activity for both Mother de Chantal and Bishop de Sales. Francis presided at the annual chapter of the Feuillants, a reformed Cistercian order, attended to the Duke of Savoy and his court in Turin, and traveled on other ecclesial business to Avignon and Valance. Francis and Jane had met very briefly in October when he passed through Dijon. He asked her to visit several new foundations and to make her annual retreat before they could meet again in Lyon. Jane arrived at the Visitation in Lyon as the courts of France and Savoy converged there to celebrate King Louis' recent victories over the Huguenots in southern France. Francis was traveling with the Savoyards. Despite their busy schedules, he and Jane stole time for a meeting.

On December 11, the bishop appeared in the parlor of the monastery and found Jane seated across from him behind the cloister grill. She had brought two lists lest she forget all the issues they needed to settle. One list concerned Visitation administrative concerns. The second was personal: it had been too long since she had spoken to her longtime confidant about the depths of her inner life.

Because his time was limited, Francis stressed that they must attend first to the issues confronting their community. With some regret Jane slipped the second list into her pocket. They spoke for some time, but royal responsibilities pressed in and it became clear that a further meeting would be needed. It might not happen amid the current confusion, but Francis promised that when they met again at home in Annecy they would focus on her private concerns.

Jane left the next morning for the Grenoble monastery. Because housing in Lyon was limited due to the presence of the courts, Francis had lodged in the gardener's quarters on the Visitation grounds. From there he appeared before the assembled royalty.

On Christmas Eve, he caught a chill but continued with his schedule: he presided at Eucharist at midnight at the Visitation, celebrated the second Mass of Christmas for the court at the Dominican church, then returned to the Visitation where he preached the third Mass for the feast. When day dawned he received two postulants into the community, bid a formal farewell to the French Queen Mother, gave a conference for the sisters on his favorite motto: "ask for nothing, refuse nothing," and attended to his vast correspondence the next day.

On December 27 he collapsed at his desk and, despite the urgent ministrations of the doctors, he died on December 28.

The diagnosis was apoplexy caused by a rupture of the cerebral artery.

In Grenoble, Jane seems to have had a premonition, but she left there for Belley. Because her friends who had received the sad news wanted her to celebrate the feast of the Epiphany with serenity, they didn't tell her about Francis' death. Worried that she had not received any word from him for some time, she asked the Visitation chaplain why Francis hadn't written. The priest reluctantly handed her a note from Francis' brother Jean who had just succeeded his elder brother as bishop of Geneva.

> When Monsieur Michel put the letter . . . in my hand my heart beat wildly. I drew myself close to the presence of God and his will, greatly fearing that there was something painful to be learned in this letter. In the small space of time it took to recollect myself in God, I understood the words that I had heard in Grenoble: "He is no more," the truth of which was clarified for me by reading that blessed letter. I fell to my knees, adoring the divine Providence and embracing the holy will of God, which included my incomparable affliction, as best I could.[1]

Mother de Chantal wept gently for much of the next twenty-four hours, even as she continued to attend to the necessary affairs of the Belley Visitation. She revealed only to her intimates the true extent of the blow she had received. To her brother Andre she wrote:

> You say you want to know what my heart felt on that occasion. Ah, it seems to me that it adored God in the profound silence of its terrible anguish! Truly, I have never felt such an intense grief nor has my spirit ever received so heavy a blow. My sorrow is greater than I could ever express, and it seems

as though everything serves to increase my weariness and cause me to regret. The only thing that is left to console me is to know that it is my God that has done this, or, at least, has permitted this blow to fall. Alas! My heart is too weak to support this heavy burden; how it needs strength! Yes, my God, you put this beautiful soul into the world, now you have taken it back; may your holy name be blessed! I don't know any other song except, "May the name of the Lord be blessed."[2]

The bishop's body was returned to Annecy and lay in state in the Cathedral Saint Pierre for the innumerable mourners who came to pay respects. On January 29 his funeral Mass was celebrated. Then, while the tomb in the monastery crypt was being prepared, the coffin was carried across town. It was placed on the high altar of the Visitation church close to the choir grill, where Madame de Chantal and the sisters gathered for prayer. It remained there for several months.

One day, Jane asked permission from the presiding superior to go into the church where her friend's remains lay. She knelt down beside it, pulled out the second list from the folds of her habit, and proceeded to pour out her heart. He had, after all, promised that when they met again in Annecy they could share these private concerns of hers. In later references to this moment, Jane recalled that in some way she felt that Francis had heard her and that she was made aware of his wise counsel. That intuited counsel, born of their long friendship and leavened with her own good judgment, would continue to nurture their beloved Visitation of Holy Mary into full flower.

Chapter Twelve

# Final Years of Faithful Service

Jane's story, of course, did not end with Francis' death. For nineteen years she continued faithfully to labor on behalf of the vision of a world of human and divine hearts to which her mentor and friend had introduced to her many years before, and which was realized both in their friendship and in the community they had created. These later years were marked by the increased popularity of the Visitation charism and the successful implanting of its spirit in communities all over Europe.

This taxing work was all hers. Because the monasteries were scattered across the landscape, distant from one another and institutionally bound not by formal structures but by the filial bonds of love, it would have been easy for the Visitation's particular spirit to dissipate. But Jane provided leadership that encouraged familial rapport. In 1624, she presided over a meeting at Annecy of all the first mothers of the far-flung order. In

1635, she undertook a general tour of all the houses on French soil. She labored to create the Custom Book that described the order's customary practices and the spirit with which they should be carried out. Yearly circular letters containing news of each house were mailed. They included detailed death notices that celebrated the lives of each flower in the garden that Francis had described as the "hidden violets" of the Church.

As founding mother, Jane carried on a vast correspondence with all the superiors as well as other Visitandines who requested her advice. Always, she encouraged them to proceed in the gentle spirit that Bishop de Sales had embodied. Not all her correspondents, however, were her sisters in religion. A case in point was one Noël Brulart, Commander de Sillery, an admirer of the order who consulted Jane about an audacious dream he nurtured. He hoped to found a theological training program for lay persons. Jane's ongoing guidance as he attempted to make his dream a reality displays her deep Salesian wisdom. This involved, as she and Francis had posited, living between the "two wills of God." Not that God actually had two conflicting wills, but that human beings have access to the ultimately unknowable divine will through two general avenues: first, the ways of discernment (i.e. prayer, conscience, Church teaching, Scripture, the advice of wise mentors), and second, through the unavoidable events and circumstances of one's life. The art was to live between these two wills; to act boldly as one experienced God's signified will unfolding in plans, dreams, and opportunities, but to surrender gracefully and flexibly to the unavoidable context in which one found oneself. Jane's letters to Commander de Sillery display her gifts of spiritual guidance. At first she encouraged him to pursue his dream, but when it became clear that such a program was too far ahead of its time to gain support, she counseled him to respond without bitterness. She wrote of this paradoxical spiritual art to Brulart in 1633:

> I have such a complete and devoted concern for your true good that there is nothing at all I wouldn't endure to obtain it for you. This good is nothing less than a peaceful, quiet response to the lights and inspirations which our Lord gives you. But, you know, I am not saying this so that you will zealously search out ways to carry out your response. On the contrary, God wants you to temper your over-eagerness by calming all this ardor, reducing it to a simple assent of your will to do good quietly—and only because it is God's will. In the same way, yield lovingly to the divine will when it allows you to fail to perform some good deed or to commit some fault. Resign yourself to not being able to resign yourself as completely and utterly as you would like, or as you think our Lord would like. . . . Abandon all your desires for advancement and perfection; hand them over completely into God's hands. . . . Have only a pure, simple, peaceful longing to please God. . . . Trust him to bring about these results at the right time for his glory and your benefit.[1]

Alongside her burgeoning community and the many who sought her advice, Madame de Chantal's surviving children continued to occupy her heart and days. Celse-Bénigne was favorably married. Welcome news arrived in 1626 when his wife gave birth to an infant girl (who would become the noted French letter writer, Madame de Sevigné). Sorrow struck the following year, however, when Celse-Bénigne was killed in battle at the siege of the Isle de Ré. His young widow, Marie de Coulanges, died only a few years later. Françoise was the only one of Jane's children to outlive her. As the once rebellious girl became a mother herself, she and Jane became close. None of Françoise's children survived infancy. The letters that passed between the now grieving younger woman and her own mother are touching in the way they communicate the spiritual resilience that had sustained the older woman through her many losses.

That resilience would be tested again and again in Jane's later years. The great plague that swept through France between 1628 and 1631 claimed the lives of neighbors, friends, and some of her sisters in religion. In 1637, other diseases carried off all three of her cherished first companions at the Gallery House (Charlotte de Brechard, Jacqueline Favre, and Anne-Jacqueline Coste). In 1641 her brother André Frémyot, Archbishop of Bourges, died. Over the years he too had come to rely on his sister's judgment and spiritual counsel.

Always mindful of Francis, the absent friend whose love had sustained her in a "bond of perfection" that was stronger than death itself, Jane devoted herself to promoting his cause for canonization. In her later correspondence she consistently referred to Francis as "blessed," a holy, even saintly figure. The deposition she prepared for the tribunal that gathered to assess his cause reveals both her intimate knowledge of him as well as her deep esteem. She could attest wholeheartedly to his love of neighbor:

> I am not afraid of saying, as I fully believe, that he had this virtue to a most eminent degree and that he faithfully practiced it to the last moment of his life with the utmost perfection. In all the nineteen years that I had the happiness of knowing him well, both before and after I became a nun, I never knew him to fail to do for his neighbor all the good

> that lay within his power. He never spared himself in this service; I am quite sure of this, and have seen and experienced more of it than I can ever tell you.
>
> He loved God and man and man in God, and said that he did not want to mean anything to people, or people to mean anything to him, except in God. He was full of charity, loving souls truly and each in a different way, "for this is how God chose to make my heart," he said. "I want to love my neighbor so much, so very much. Yet I feel that I love God only, and every soul for his sake; and everything that is not God, or for God, is as nothing to me."
>
> He once wrote to me: "When shall we be really steeped in the sweet and tender love for our neighbor? When shall we really see his soul in our Savior? Alas, if we look at him in any other way, we run the risk of not loving him purely, faithfully, and each one alike. But who could help loving him in our Lord, putting up with him, and bearing his faults? Who could then find him unattractive and tiresome? For that's where our neighbor really is, right in our Divine Savior's heart, so beloved and so lovable that the lover dies for love of him."[2]

Jane's carefully composed deposition, delivered during the first canonical process, gave insight into the vision of a transformed world that he and she shared. But Jane was not the only person who desired to see Bishop de Sales held up to the universal Church as a model. His own family, important political and ecclesial figures from Savoy and France, and his daughters of the Visitation worked tirelessly to that end. Mother de Chaugy, Jane's secretary and niece by marriage, who had joined the community sometime after Francis' death, was an especial advocate.[3]

Jane's reputation grew but, unbeknownst to her admirers, the Mother foundress' inner path was troubled. For years she had struggled with questions about faith. The ever-occurring losses of those closest to her pierced her brave heart. An episode recorded in 1632 gives a glimpse into the interior experience of the widow-superior. She was with other members of the community at recreation when she fell into an abstracted reverie. It was the feast of Saint Basil. When her sisters asked her what she was reflecting on, she replied:

> My dear daughters, Saint Basil and most of the fathers and pillars of the Church were not martyred. Why do you think this was so? . . . For myself, I believe that there is a martyrdom of love in which God preserves the lives all of his servants so that they might work for his glory. This makes them martyrs and confessors at the same time. I know . . . that this is the martyrdom to which the daughters of the Visitation are called, in which God will allow them to suffer if they are fortunate enough to wish for it. . . . What happens is that divine love thrusts its sword into the most intimate and secret parts of the soul and separates us from our very selves. I know one soul whom love had severed in this way who felt it more keenly than if a tyrant with a sword had separated her body from her soul.[4]

Those gathered understood that she was speaking about herself.

In December 1641, Jane was on the road fulfilling her community obligations. She had set out from Paris, where she had a long talk with Vincent de Paul, and then made her general confession. Francis had charged him with ecclesial oversight of the Visitation monastery in the capital. Jane then visited three other foundations, but at Nevers she displayed signs of a bronchial illness. When her daughter Françoise arrived to accompany her on the journey to Moulins, Jane uttered these prescient words.

> Goodbye, once more, my very dear sisters. I don't know whether we shall meet again in this life; we must leave that to Providence. If it is not in this world, it will be in eternity. I shall often visit you and I shall be looking at you with the eyes of my spirit—not that I really know what this means, but I do know that I know all of you very well.[5]

Arriving at Moulins, she collapsed. The physicians diagnosed pneumonia and pleurisy. For several days she remained bedridden but continued to dictate necessary letters. Her last letter was a general farewell to all the convents, asking the sisters to stay loyal to the order's distinctive spirit of unity, humility, and gentleness. On December 13 she asked the sisters to read to her Saint Jerome's account of the death of his spiritual friend Saint Paula's, the record of Francis' own death written by his nephew, chapter six of the *Treatise on the Love of God*, and Saint Augustine's relation of his mother's death. She passed away peacefully between six and seven in the evening that same day.

Far away in Paris, Vincent de Paul, who had long admired Francis de Sales and who had been an intimate witness to Jane de Chantal's later life, reported a vivid dream that came to him the night Jane died. In the dream he saw a bright globe, as of fire, rise above the earth to join with a second resplendent globe. These two then rose together and were absorbed in the radiance of a greater, brilliant, fiery globe.

# Epilogue

In 1665 Francis de Sales was canonized and thus recognized as a saint of the Roman Catholic Church. Jane de Chantal was similarly honored in 1767. In 1877 Saint Francis de Sales was declared a Doctor of the Church. He is known popularly as the Doctor of Divine Love.

In 2002, on the occasion of the fourth centenary of Francis' ordination, Pope John Paul II wrote of the late bishop of Annecy. His words can be applied equally to Jane de Chantal for the two friends' hearts were, they knew, but one.

> Doctor of divine love, Francis de Sales did not rest until the faithful accepted God's love, to live fully in it, turning their hearts to God and uniting themselves with him (cf. *Traité de l'amour de Dieu: Oeuvres complètes*, IV, pp. 40ff.). This is how, under his direction, many Christians walked on the path of holiness; he showed them that all are called to live an

intense spiritual life, whatever their situation and profession, for "the Church is a garden filled with infinite flowers where there are flowers of different sizes, colors, fragrances: in brief, of different perfections. For they each have their price, their grace, and their substance, and make a most pleasing perfection of beauty in the gathering of of their rich variety" (*Traité de l'amour de Dieu: Oeuvres complètes*, IV, p. 111).

A man of great goodness and kindness, who knew how to express God's mercy and patience to those who came to speak with him, he taught an exacting but serene spirituality based on love, for loving God "is the sovereign happiness of the soul for this life and for eternity" (*Letter to Mother Marie-Jacqueline Favre*, March 10, 1612: *Oeuvres complètes*, XV, p. 180).[1]

# Prayer in Honor of Saints Jane de Chantal and Francis de Sales

Gracious and loving God,
you give us glimpses of your own divine heart
in the gentle, humble heart of your Son.
You give us glimpses as well
in the hearts of Saints Jane de Chantal and Francis de Sales,
who declared that, in you, they had but One Heart.
Teach us to *Live Jesus*,
to allow the gentle heart of the Savior
to become our own hearts
so that we might love one another
as we have been loved.
Amen.

# Reflection Questions

1. The Salesian spiritual tradition founded by Saints Francis de Sales and Jane de Chantal has been described as profoundly "optimistic" in that it assumes humanity's essential goodness and God's desire that all persons be saved. Francis does not deny the reality of sin but privileges the power of divine love. What do you understand this to mean? Does this correspond to your own sense of spirituality?

2. The vision of an interconnected world of divine and human hearts is at the core of Saints Jane and Francis' spirituality. Are you drawn toward this way of thinking about the relationship of God and human beings and the relationship of human beings to each other? Why or why not?

3. Have you thought of friendship as a genuine form of love related to all other loves? What friendships, especially spiritual friendships, if any, have brought you closer to God?

4. At the end of the *Treatise on the Love of God* Francis de Sales writes, "Calvary is the Mount of Lovers." Given what you have learned about the Salesian spiritual perspective, what do you think this means? Have you experienced this in your own faith journey?

5. Francis de Sales is said to have claimed that the best method of prayer is no method at all. Yet he also wrote about and recommended any number of approaches to prayer. Why do you think this is so? What methods or practices of prayer have you found fruitful?

6. The *Introduction to the Devout Life* encourages all those who love God to live a devout life adapted to their own circumstances. How do you do this? How might you grow in this?

# Chronology

1567—Francis de Sales is born August 21 in Thorens, Savoy, to François de Nouvelles (Monsieur de Boissy), and Françoise de Sionnaz.

1572—Jane Frances Frémyot is born January 23 in Dijon, France, to Bénigne Frémyot and Marguerite de Berbesey.

1573—Birth of Andre Frémyot and death of his and Jane's mother in Dijon.

— Francis, along with his three cousins, is sent to the school for young noblemen at La Roche-sur-Foron in Savoy.

1575—Francis continues his schooling at the *College Chappiusienne* in Annecy, Savoy.

1578–87—Along with his cousins and tutor, Francis enters the *College de Clermont* in the Latin Quarter of Paris.

In this school run by the Society of Jesus, he studies the Jesuit humanistic curriculum, the *ratio studiorum*, and is captivated by the mystical reading of the *Song of Songs*.

1586–87—Francis undergoes the first phase of the mystical "crisis" that will shape his lifelong spiritual vision.

1588–91—Francis enters the University of Padua in Italy to study civil law as well as canon law. Jesuit Antonio Possevino becomes his director.

1591—The second phase of Francis' mystical "crisis" takes place confirming his "optimistic" spiritual vision. He graduates from Padua.

1592—Jane marries Christophe, Baron de Rabutin-Chantal, at Bourbilly, France.

1593—Francis renounces his inheritance and announces his intention of becoming a priest. He receives Holy Orders and is installed as provost to the bishop of Geneva, who resides in exile in Annecy.

1594—Francis is sent as a missionary to the Chablais region to reclaim the territory for the Catholic faith. He writes *The Controversies*.

1596–1601—Birth of Jane and Christophe's children: Celse-Bénigne, Marie-Aimée, Françoise, and Charlotte at Bourbilly.

1597—Francis has a meeting with Theodore Beza, Calvin's successor, in Geneva. Forty Hours celebration at Annemasse takes place.

— Francis becomes co-adjutor of Geneva.

1599—In Rome, Francis is approved as successor to the bishop of Geneva.

1601—Jane is widowed when Christophe is killed in a hunting accident.

— Monsieur de Boissy, Francis' father, dies.

1602—Francis travels to Paris in January on diplomatic missions. He meets Catholic reform luminaries at the salon of Madame Acarie. He refuses an invitation from King Henry IV to relocate to Paris.

— Jane and her children take up residence with her father-in-law at Montelon.

— After a retreat under the direction of Jesuit Father Fourier, Francis is consecrated bishop at Thorens on December 8.

1603—Francis is sent to the regions of Belley and Gex to reestablish the Catholic faith.

1604—Francis preaches the Lenten Sermon series at Dijon, hosted by Andre Frémyot, Archbishop of Bourges. At her father's invitation, Jane comes to Dijon for the series.

March 5: Francis and Jane first encounter each other at the church of *Sainte Chapelle* in Dijon. They agree to meet again.

— May: Francis returns to Gex.

— August: Francis and Jane meet again at the Shrine of Saint Claude in the Jura Mountains. They agree to a formal spiritual direction relationship. After she returns to Montelon, they begin to correspond.

1605—May: Jane travels to Thorens, Savoy and consults with Francis.

— Francis begins pastoral visitations and the reform of his large diocese.

1606—With his friend Antoine Favre, Francis founds the Florimontane Academy in Annecy.

1607— Madame de Charmoisy ("Philothea" of *Introduction to the Devout Life*) takes Francis as spiritual director.

— May–June: Jane travels to Annecy. Francis reveals to Jane his plan for a new community.

— October: Francis' sister, Jeanne de Sales, dies while staying with Jane in France.

1608—Francis crafts a preliminary version of *Introduction to the Devout Life*.

1609—Jane visits Annecy for the third time.

— October: Jane's daughter, Marie-Aimée de Chantal, marries Francis' brother, Bernard de Sales, at Montelon, France.

1610—Madame de Boissy, Francis' mother, dies. Jane's youngest daughter, Charlotte de Chantal, dies.

— March: With her daughter Françoise and longtime friend Jeanne-Charlotte de Bréchard, Jane departs Dijon for Annecy to establish the new community. She stays several weeks at Chateau de Sales where Marie-Aimée is setting up household. Celse-Bénigne is put under the tutelage of his uncle André Frémyot.

- June 10: The Congregation of the Visitation of Holy Mary at the "Gallery House" is founded in Annecy. Jane, Jeanne-Charlotte de Bréchard, Jacqueline Favre, and Anne-Jacqueline Coste (as outsister) are the first community members.
- The final version of *Introduction to the Devout Life* is published.

1611—Francis returns to Gex twice.
- Jane and her first companions have their profession ceremony at the Gallery House in Annecy.
- Bénigne Frémyot, Jane's father, dies in Dijon.
- Jane holds the first annual chapter of the Visitation.

1612—After their period of formation, Jane and Jacqueline Favre begin visits to the poor in their neighborhood.

1613—Francis travels to Turin and Milan on diocesan business and makes a pilgrimage to the tomb of Charles Borromeo.

1615—Reciprocal visits occur between Francis and Denis de Marquemont, Bishop of Lyon, concerning establishment of the Visitation in France.
- The first French foundation of the Visitation occurs at Lyon.
- Having outgrown the Gallery House, the Annecy Visitation community moves to the "Grand Visitation," their formal, new quarters designed expressly as a house for religious located near the town walls.

1616—Francis redrafts the Constitutions of the Visitation.
- The *Treatise on the Love of God* is published.
- Jane's retreat of 1616 marks a new phase on her relationship with Francis.
- The Visitation at Moulins is founded.

1617—Bernard de Sales and Marie-Aimée de Chantal die.

1618—The Visitation becomes a formal, enclosed religious order.
- Francis sojourns in Paris to arrange the upcoming marriage of Victor-Amadée, Prince of Piedmont, and Princess Christine of France.
- The Visitation at Grenoble is founded.

1618–1641—Nearly eighty Visitation monasteries are founded in Savoy, France, Switzerland, and Italy—among them Paray-le-Monial (1626) and Troyes (1631), which would later become centers of Salesian influence.

1619—Victor-Amadée, Prince of Piedmont, marries Princess Christine of France. Francis is appointed grand almoner.
- Francis meets with Angelique Arnaud several times at Maubuisson near Paris and at Port Royal.
- The Paris Visitation is founded. Vincent de Paul is charged with oversight of the Paris monastery.

1620—Françoise de Chantal marries Count de Toulonjon.

1621—Jean-François de Sales, brother of Francis, is consecrated as bishop and made co-adjutor to his brother.

1622—Jane leaves Paris after three years and travels to monasteries in Dijon and Lyon.
- At the request of Gregory XV, Francis presides over the General Chapter of the Feuillants at Pignerol. He travels to Avignon and Valence.
- December 8: Triumphal entry of Louis XIII into Lyon where the courts of Savoy and France converge. Francis is grand almoner.
- December 11: Jane and Francis have their last meeting at Lyon.
- December 24–25: Despite an illness, Francis preaches the three Masses of Christmas.
- December 27: He holds a last conference with the Visitandines at Lyon and then collapses.
- December 28: Francis de Sales dies.

1623—January: Jane receives news of his death.
- Francis' body is transferred to Annecy and his funeral is held on January 29.
- Celse-Bénigne de Chantal marries Marie de Coulanges.

1624—The First General Chapter of the Visitation is held at Annecy.

1626—Celse-Bénigne's daughter, the future Madame de Sévigné, is born.

1627—Celse-Bénigne dies.
- Jane draws up a deposition for the process of canonization for Francis.

1632—While visiting her daughter, Françoise, Jane meets Françoise-Madeleine de Chaugy, niece of Count Toulonjon, who will become her future secretary and biographer.

1635–37—Jane undertakes a general tour of Visitation monasteries in France.

1637—Jane's first three companions in the Visitation die.

1638—Jane crosses the Alps to make a foundation at Turin.

1640—Jane's brother, André Frémyot, dies.

1641—Jane visits the Paris and Moulins monasteries.
— December 13: Jane dies at Moulins.
— In Paris, Vincent de Paul, praying for Jane's recovery, receives his vision of three globes of fire.

1665—Francis de Sales is canonized.

1767—Jane de Chantal is canonized.

1877—Francis de Sales is named a Doctor of the Church.

1909–30—The present-day Basilica of the Visitation in Annecy where the two saints are buried is constructed.

# Notes

## CHAPTER ONE

1. Most of the names in this account are rendered in their original languages. But, as is customary, names of the two main figures in this biography, François de Sales and Jeanne Françoise Frémyot de Chantal, as well as other saints who are well-known in the English-speaking world, will be addressed by the names that are more familiar to an English-speaking audience: for example, Francis de Sales and Jane Frances de Chantal.

2. A *seigneury* was a position of authority in the feudal world of Savoy. The lord or seigneur would have been the owner and administrator of extensive property deeded to him by his overlord. He would thus be an agent of and beholden to his patron. The Duke of Savoy was the patron to whom Francis' family owed allegiance.

3. Francis de Sales, *Oeuvres de Saint François de Sales*, édition complète d'apres les autographes des Religieues de la Visitation du

premier monastère d' Annecy, (1892–1964), XIX, Lettres IX, 13. Translated by author.

4. There are many biographies of Francis de Sales either written in or translated into English. Among the most recent of which I have made use in this joint story are André Ravier, *Francis de Sales: Sage and Saint*, translated by Joseph D. Bowler (San Francisco: Ignatius Press, 1988); Joseph Boenzi, SDB, *Saint Francis de Sales: Life and Spirit* (Stella Niagara, NY: De Sales Resource Center, 2013). I have also relied on my own study of the friendship between the two: Wendy M. Wright, *Bond of Perfection: Jeanne de Chantal and Francoise de Chantal*, new enhanced edition (Stella Niagara, NY: De Sales Resource Center, 2001).

## Chapter Two

1. Saint John the Almoner was a seventh-century patriarch of Alexandria remembered for his almsgiving. His legend was well-known throughout the Middle Ages and in early modern devotional literature. He became the patron of the crusader order of the Knights Hospitaller that had its origin in caring for the sick in Jerusalem during the Crusades.

2. Perhaps the best full biography of Jane de Chantal is Elisabeth Stopp, *Madame de Chantal: Portrait of a Saint*, 2nd edition (Stella Niagara, NY: De Sales Resource Center, 2002). Also see André Ravier, *Saint Jeanne de Chantal: Noble Lady, Holy Woman*, translated by Mary Emily Hamilton (San Francisco: Ignatius Press, 1989).

## Chapter Four

1. The "nobles of the sword" were France's oldest class of landed and titled nobility who owed service and loyalty to the king. The newer "nobles of the robe"—of which Jane's father was a member—were those holding official positions in government, such as president of the

regional parlement or provincial appellate court. They were not landed or titled by heredity.

2. On the Forty Hours Devotion, see Jill Fehleison, *Boundaries of Faith: Catholics and Protestants in the Diocese of Geneva* (Kirksville, MO: Truman University State Press, 2010).

## CHAPTER FIVE

1. Francis de Sales, *Oeuvres,* XII, Lettres II, 321. Translated by the author.

2. Wright, *Bond of Perfection*, 34.

3. Boenzi, *Saint Francis de Sales*, 56.

4. Wendy M. Wright, "Saint Francis de Sales (1567–1622) and the Conception of the Virgin Mary," *Marian Studies* LV (2008): 135–158.

## CHAPTER SIX

1. Stopp, *Madame de Chantal*, 64.

2. Ibid., 60.

3. Francis de Sales, *Oeuvres, III, Introduction a la Vie Devot*, 23–25. Translated by the author.

4. Wright, *Bond of Perfection*, 70.

5. Stopp, *Madame de Chantal*, 74.

6. Wright, *Bond of Perfection*, 76.

7. Ibid. 72.

8. On the world of intertwined human and divine hearts, see Wendy M. Wright, "'That Is What It Is Made For': The Image of the Heart in the Spirituality of Francis de Sales and Jane de Chantal" in *Spiritualities*

*of the Heart: Approaches to Personal Wholeness in Christian Tradition*, edited by Annice Callahan, RSCJ (Mahwah, NJ: Paulist Press, 1990), 143–158.

9. Wright, *Bond of Perfection*, 80.

10. Stopp, *Madame de Chantal*, 76.

## Chapter Seven

1. Jane de Chantal, *St. Francis de Sales: A Testimony by St. Chantal*, trans. by Elisabeth Stopp (Hyattsville, MD: Institute of Salesian Studies, 1967), 138–139.

2. Ibid., 95–96.

3. Ibid., 67–68.

4. Ibid., 82–83.

5. Wright, *Bond of Perfection*, 122.

## Chapter Eight

1. Stopp, *Madame de Chantal*, 110.

2. Francis de Sales, *Oeuvres VI, Entretiens Spirituelles*, 54–57. Translated by the author.

3. Ibid., 56–63.

4. Wright, *Bond of Perfection*, 152.

5. On Salesian spirituality as a response to the violence of the era, see Thomas A. Donlan, "The Reform of Zeal: François de Sales and Militant Catholicism During the French Wars of Religion" (Ph.D. diss., University of Arizona, 2011).

6. Wright, *Bond of Perfection*, 103–104. Also on friendship, see Terence McGoldrick, *The Sweet and Gentle Struggle; Francis de Sales on*

*the Necessity of Spiritual Friendship* (Lanham, MD: University Press of America, 1996).

7. Daniel P. Wisniewski, OSFS, "The Eternity of Friendship in the Spirituality of St. Francis de Sales" in *Encountering Anew the Familiar: Francis de Sales' Introduction to the Devout Life at 400 Years*, edited by Joseph F. Chorpenning, OSFS (Rome: International Commission on Salesian Studies, 2012), 95–110.

8. Wright, *Bond of Perfection*, 102.

9. Ibid., 149.

10. Ibid., 150.

11. On the question of gender in the early modern context, see Barbara R. Woshinsky, *Imagining Women's Conventual Spaces in France, 1600–1800: The Cloister Disclosed* (Ashgate, 2010).

12. Wendy M. Wright, "Jane de Chantal's Guidance of Women" in *Modern Christian Spirituality: Methodological and Historical Essays*, edited by Bradley C. Hanson (Atlanta: Scholars Press, 1990): 119

13. Ibid. 126.

14. Francis de Sales, Jane de Chantal, *Letters of Spiritual Direction*, translated by Peronne-Marie Thibert, VHM, selected and introduced by Wendy M. Wright and Joseph F. Power, OSFS (Mahwah, NJ: Paulist Press, 1988), 59.

## CHAPTER NINE

1. Francis de Sales, *Oeuvres, IV, Traite de l'Amour de Dieu*, 8. Translated by author.

2. Wendy M. Wright, *Francis de Sales: Introduction to the Devout Life and Treatise on the Love of God*, second edition (Stella Niagara, NY: De Sales Resource Center, 2005), 160.

3. Wright, *Bond of Perfection*, 155.

4. Ibid., 158.

5. Francis de Sales, Jane de Chantal, *Letters of Spiritual Direction*, 80–81.

6. Ibid., 81.

## Chapter Ten

1. Wright, "Jane de Chantal's Guidance," 121.

2. Stopp, *Madame de Chantal*, 179.

3. Ibid., 180.

## Chapter Eleven

1. Wright, *Bond of Perfection*, 189.

2. Ibid., 191.

## Chapter Twelve

1. Francis de Sales, Jane de Chantal, *Letters of Spiritual Direction*, 188–189.

2. Jane de Chantal, *Testimony*, 66.

3. We owe much of our knowledge of Jane and the early Visitation to the memoires and work of Mother de Chaugy.

4. Wright, *Bond of Perfection*, 154.

5. Stopp, *Madame de Chantal*, 245.

## Epilogue

1. John Paul II, "Letter on the Fourth Centenary of the Episcopal Ordination of St. Francis de Sales." Given November 23, 2002. Libreria Editrice Vaticana: https://w2.vatican.va/content/john-paul-ii/en/letters/2002/documents/hf_jp-ii_let_20021209_francesco-sales.html.

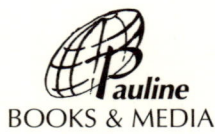
## BOOKS & MEDIA

The Daughters of St. Paul operate book and media centers at the following addresses. Visit, call, or write the one nearest you today, or find us at www.paulinestore.org.

**CALIFORNIA**
   3908 Sepulveda Blvd, Culver City, CA 90230 — 310-397-8676
   3250 Middlefield Road, Menlo Park, CA 94025 — 650-369-4230

**FLORIDA**
   145 S.W. 107th Avenue, Miami, FL 33174 — 305-559-6715

**HAWAII**
   1143 Bishop Street, Honolulu, HI 96813 — 808-521-2731

**ILLINOIS**
   172 North Michigan Avenue, Chicago, IL 60601 — 312-346-4228

**LOUISIANA**
   4403 Veterans Memorial Blvd, Metairie, LA 70006 — 504-887-7631

**MASSACHUSETTS**
   885 Providence Hwy, Dedham, MA 02026 — 781-326-5385

**MISSOURI**
   9804 Watson Road, St. Louis, MO 63126 — 314-965-3512

**NEW YORK**
   64 W. 38th Street, New York, NY 10018 — 212-754-1110

**SOUTH CAROLINA**
   243 King Street, Charleston, SC 29401 — 843-577-0175

**TEXAS**
   Currently no book center; for parish exhibits or outreach evangelization, contact: 210-569-0500, or SanAntonio@paulinemedia.com, or P.O. Box 761416, San Antonio, TX 78245

**VIRGINIA**
   1025 King Street, Alexandria, VA 22314 — 703-549-3806

**CANADA**
   3022 Dufferin Street, Toronto, ON M6B 3T5 — 416-781-9131

¡También somos su fuente para libros,
videos y música en español!